Wondrous
Transformations

Wondrous Transformations

A Maverick Physician, the Science
of Hormones, and the Birth of the
Transgender Revolution

Alison Li

The University of North Carolina Press • Chapel Hill

This book was published with the assistance of the Lilian R. Furst Fund of the University of North Carolina Press.

Designed by Lauren Michelle Smith
Set in Arno Pro and ChaletBook by codeMantra
Manufactured in the United States of America

Cover art: Harry Benjamin, courtesy of Library of Congress.

Library of Congress Cataloging-in-Publication Data
Names: Li, Alison, 1963– author.
Title: Wondrous transformations : a maverick physician, the science of hormones, and the birth of the transgender revolution / Alison Li.
Description: Chapel Hill : The University of North Carolina Press, [2023] | Includes bibliographical references and index.
Identifiers: LCCN 2023008556 | ISBN 9781469674858 (cloth) | ISBN 9781469674865 (ebook)
Subjects: LCSH: Benjamin, Harry. | Endocrinologists—Biography. | Sexologists—Biography. | Transgender people—Medical care—History—20th century. | Gender transition—Hormone therapy—History—20th century. | LCGFT: Biographies.
Classification: LCC R154.B438 L5 2023 | DDC 616.40092 [B]—dc23/eng/20230405
LC record available at https://lccn.loc.gov/2023008556

Contents

A Note on Terminology

It is immensely important to use the right language in speaking about people, but language is evolving rapidly, especially in referring to transgender individuals, so that terms that were common a few years ago are considered inappropriate today and those that we use today will no doubt soon be superseded as well. Trying to write about transgender matters in a historical context becomes particularly complex because not only the terminology but the concepts have changed. Individuals and behaviors that were once grouped together in one category are now considered separate, while other categories of people, once considered distinct, are now drawn together under one umbrella. Sexological terms of the past such as "invert," "homosexual," "transvestite," and "transsexual" are no longer in common usage and may be offensive to some readers, but because these terms are critical in describing historical concepts and categories that differ from our contemporary understanding, I have tried to use them carefully when required by the context. The terms "male" and "female" are used to refer to biology; the terms "man" and "woman" or "masculine" and "feminine" are used to refer to self-identity and social categorization.

I have used initials or pseudonyms for all of Harry Benjamin's patients unless they have publicly identified themselves or have already been identified by other scholars. Transgender individuals are identified by their chosen names and pronouns and in accordance with their public gender presentation. The use of a transgender person's pre-transition "dead" name is offensive to many, but when this name may be of historical significance (for example, in the case of those who were public figures prior to transition), I have included this information in the notes.

Preface

It seemed a reasonable proposition.

Dr. Harry Benjamin drew the estrogen solution into his syringe with a practiced hand. His patient had asked for help, and he believed that an injection of hormones would be an entirely practical and effective treatment for her suffering. The only problem was that, in 1949, virtually every other medical, legal, and social opinion in the United States was arrayed against him.

Val Barry (pseudonym) had been born with male physical characteristics but since early childhood had worn girls' clothing and taken on traditionally feminine chores around the house. Her parents supported her living as a girl, even ensuring that her school accommodated her with appropriate washroom facilities. Barry explained to the doctor that she felt herself to be a woman and that she desperately wanted to change her body to fit her sense of self. In Harry Benjamin, she found a sympathetic listener and someone who was willing to help.[1]

In 1949, Benjamin was sixty-four. He had a broad, genial face and a courtly manner that put his patients at ease. As a gerontologist, he had for decades offered hormones to help his patients ride out the turmoil of middle age and old age. In his Park Avenue office in New York and his summer office in San Francisco, he had treated an elite clientele including prominent businessmen, actresses, and opera singers. But Barry was very unlike his typical patient.

In our world today, transgender issues are a part of popular conversation and public policy, so it is perhaps difficult to grasp how dramatically different Benjamin's stance was from that of virtually any other American physician and sexologist of his time. Even his colleague Alfred Kinsey, the sex researcher, was puzzled. Most medical practitioners would have seen Barry as having a psychiatric problem and assumed their task was to help change her mind to fit her body. In contrast, Benjamin took her account of herself seriously and was willing to help her change her body to fit her mind.

Barry was not the first transgender person to seek or use medical means to change her body, but she approached Benjamin at a critical juncture in history. By 1949, significant developments in science and medicine had created a situation in which Benjamin could reasonably consider offering her the treatment she sought. Within a couple of decades, transgender identity would gain political force, a medical label, and institutionalized systems of care; Benjamin would play a pivotal role in this remarkable transformation. By the early 1960s, those who were interested in what was then called "transsexualism" were likely to find their way to his office. In 1966, he would publish the groundbreaking book *The Transsexual Phenomenon*, the first major work to define transsexualism in clinical terms and to argue for compassionate treatment of those whose internal sense of gender did not align with the sex they were assigned at birth.[2]

As a historian of science and medicine, I first encountered Dr. Harry Benjamin in connection with a very different episode: in the 1920s, Benjamin achieved some fame—and perhaps notoriety—as the physician to popular novelist Gertrude Atherton, who claimed she had been rejuvenated by his glandular treatments. Atherton went on to write the best-selling novel of 1923, a fantastical story of a woman made young again by a mysterious medical therapy; the book was turned into a hugely popular film, splashing Benjamin's name across newspapers around the country. This rejuvenation treatment was, however, considered highly questionable by many in the medical establishment.

So, I wondered, how did Benjamin, this purveyor of Jazz Age rejuvenation treatments, somehow come to be called the "Father of Transsexualism"?[3] And how did his story connect with a broader scientific development: the rise of the science of hormones, which burgeoned in the early twentieth century? Endocrinology is the study of hormones, the chemical substances that are secreted into the bloodstream by endocrine glands such as the thyroid, pancreas, adrenals, testes, and ovaries. These hormones then travel to tissues and organs in distant parts of the body where they can exert powerful effects. In the 1920s and 1930s, hormones were touted as the keys to understanding all aspects of life, from metabolism and growth to criminal behavior, sex, and aging. But more than this, endocrinology held out the possibility that scientists and physicians might actively manipulate and control these functions, conquering not only endocrine diseases such as diabetes mellitus but perhaps even aging itself—that they might reshape bodies, society, and even human destiny. In lockstep with the explosion of endocrine science came a proliferation of commercial hormone products that would soon become available for a wide range of medical purposes. For a time, hormones claimed a place in the cultural imagination similar to the one held by genes or neuroscience today. Hormones gave Benjamin and his contemporaries a striking new vision of the human body and mind as malleable.

Who was Benjamin and how did he come to possess not only his unorthodox perspective of his transgender patient but the conviction to act upon it as well? My search drew from archives in New York, Chicago, San Francisco, and Berlin and most importantly the Kinsey Institute in Bloomington, Indiana, which houses Benjamin's papers. Poring through letters and diaries, speaking with his colleagues, and immersing myself in the historical scholarship, I began to uncover the story of a complicated but thoroughly intriguing man—charming, audacious, and ambitious, generous and difficult in turns.

I started to appreciate that Benjamin's openness to unorthodox expressions of sexuality and gender was a long-standing characteristic. As a medical student in Berlin, he toured glittering drag shows with a physician and activist who was campaigning to decriminalize homosexuality. Later in the United States, he didn't hesitate to take on controversial issues such as championing the rights of sex workers. But the richest vein of material I found came in the stories of his interactions with his patients, some of whom became lifelong friends. Benjamin was above all a clinician, and for many of his trans patients he was the first medical practitioner who looked them in the eye and treated them with sympathy and respect rather than fear, disbelief, or disgust. Benjamin's 1949 meeting with Val Barry has sometimes been characterized as a watershed event—his first medical encounter with a transsexual patient and a radical break with his work in gerontology—but a closer examination of his career instead reveals a story of continuity characterized by a long fascination with the transformative potential of hormones.

One of the dangers in taking a biographical approach to history is that it can unduly emphasize the efforts of one person at the expense of contributions made by the many and can reduce to a personal struggle what is actually the story of larger social forces at work. In a biography of a physician in particular, there is a risk that patients will be portrayed as passive sufferers who are acted upon and "saved" by the doctor. There are good reasons why historians have become wary of biographical approaches to history, especially anything that might hint of a hagiographic account of a "great white male." Social historians who have instead uncovered the stories of forgotten and marginalized people have greatly enriched our understanding of the past.

Despite that, I was drawn to writing the life of this one man precisely because, in giving attention and space to a single story, we see so clearly the rich contingencies, complexities, and contradictions that form an actual life. Lives are messy and motivations mixed—and very often not clear even to their owners. And new ideas don't unfold in a systematic fashion. Benjamin's perspective on transgender identity drew from many sources of inspiration, and he arrived at it by following a meandering path formed by war, financial necessity, and chance events. It was not until he was in his sixties, as he was contemplating a quiet retirement, that he would take his first tentative steps into the field for which he is now best known.

Thanks to the growing scholarly literature in trans studies, as well as memoirs of trans people themselves, it is possible to set the story of Harry Benjamin against the broader tapestry of trans experience. Benjamin's understanding of trans identity and medicine evolved over the course of the three decades in which he worked in the field, shaped through a vigorous process of collaboration and negotiation with his patients and trans colleagues, in addition to a network of colleagues specializing in sexology, psychology, and psychiatry who were actively untangling sex and gender. He interacted with well over a thousand trans patients and strove to understand their experiences and to get to know them both inside and outside the clinical setting. But in the end, his perspective remains that of a physician. Trans lives of the past were rich and varied and cannot be reduced to a medical framework of diagnosis and treatment. It is critical to appreciate that Benjamin's viewpoint—and thus the focus of this book—captures only a very narrow slice of what it meant to be transgender in the mid-twentieth century. And even within this limited medical framework, it is important to recognize that trans people were active agents in shaping their relationship with their doctors, not just passive subjects. As the science and medicine of hormones and ideas of sex and gender evolved, many trans people avidly followed developments, shared information in their networks, and used their growing knowledge to advocate for themselves.

Benjamin enjoyed a reputation as a maverick and pioneer among his contemporaries, but this image can be misleading. Although the literary form of biography necessarily focuses our attention on the activities of one person, we must be careful not to let this focus draw us into thinking that Benjamin was the prime motive force in these complex developments. What we can say, however, is that many of the roots of today's transgender revolution threaded through the office of this genial gerontologist some seventy years ago. It is in following the strands that influenced his life and thought that we gain perspective into how one doctor came to see people in a new light and, in doing so, helped us not only rethink what it is to be male or female but also envision what it might be to move beyond these long-held categories. More broadly, his story asks us to consider an idea that has come to pervade our world: that we are all, at least in part, creatures of our hormones. The emergence of this hormonal view of life—and its associated technologies for fashioning the self—ties the story of Harry Benjamin to us all.

Chapter 1

That Which Sets in Motion

Often we are much too proud of what we think we do know, and do not realize how much there is left to be known. We may be inclined, at times, to think contemptuously of the knowledge of doctors of only a hundred years ago. How will the doctors of a hundred years hence view our present "knowledge"?
—Harry Benjamin

"Now describe," their host demanded. "How does the patient look? What are his physical and mental characteristics?"

It was a Wednesday evening in 1915, and Harry Benjamin was gathered with about a dozen fellow physicians in the offices of Joseph Fraenkel on New York's Upper East Side. Fraenkel presented the complete case history, diagnosis, and symptoms of one of his patients to the group and then invited the members to speculate. What would they expect this person to be like? How would he look? How would his personality manifest? This was an exciting experience for Benjamin, who felt grateful to have been invited to join this select group. Their leader, the dignified but wild-haired Fraenkel, struck Benjamin as a brilliant and original thinker who approached medicine with the mind of an artist.

After the participants had a chance to voice their hypotheses, Fraenkel brought the patient into the room to meet those assembled. Ah! Who had been right? Who was wrong? And why? It was a fascinating intellectual game, but more importantly it served to dramatically illustrate Fraenkel's contention that a person's entire constitution was shaped by the functioning of the endocrine glands. It was for this reason that this group gathered every Wednesday evening: to learn about the endocrine glands, or as they then referred to them, the "glands of internal secretion." And it was here, during these stimulating sessions, that Benjamin would discover the subject that would become his consuming passion: the hormones.[1]

The ruminations of these evenings fell on fertile soil. In 1915, Benjamin was ready for a new direction to his life. At thirty years old, he was modest of stature and careful of dress, with a small, neatly tended mustache. In photos of this time, you can sense a gentle warmth in his smile, but perhaps a touch of hesitation as well. Life in New York City was not easy for a newcomer. He was far from his native Berlin, though he was thankful to be in relative safety while war ravaged Europe. Like many immigrants before him, he had spent the last two years working to improve his English while scrambling to make a living with an assortment of odd jobs. Now that he had qualified for a medical license in New York, he gamely returned to the work for which he was trained: the practice of medicine.

Using twenty dollars of borrowed money, he set up a private practice in the back parlor of a boardinghouse at Lexington Avenue and Seventy-First Street. That one room served as his office, examination room, and treatment room by day and his bedroom by night. For his services, he charged two dollars for a consultation and three dollars for a house call, while his rent cost him six dollars a week.[2]

That year he was joined by his sister. Edith was five years his junior and a light soprano. She specialized in musical comedy, but when, in wartime Berlin, such entertainments were discarded in favor of patriotic plays, Edith decided to follow Harry to America. In a newspaper announcement of her arrival, she looks buxom and bejeweled, her curves draped in an ornate gown while a large feather sweeps from her hair. She picked up English quickly and, unlike her brother, soon spoke with barely a trace of a German accent. Edith spent the next few years performing throughout New York State in frothy English- and German-language productions that, according to one reviewer, featured "catchy music, pretty girls . . . stunning costumes," and a plot that required "no deep thinking." When she was between engagements, she took a room upstairs at the boardinghouse in which Harry lived. By the following year, the two siblings were able to send for their widowed mother, Bertha, who sailed on the last boat to bring Germans to the United States.[3]

Benjamin's fledgling practice was slow. He managed to make a little extra money assisting a busier practitioner, but even so, at times, even the most trifling financial obligation proved daunting. As he recalled in later years, "Six dollars a week rent is a lot if you don't have it." One evening he and Edith discovered that they did not even have enough money between them for a square meal. Just at that moment, a nurse telephoned from a nearby home for elderly men asking Benjamin to sign a death certificate. Half an hour later, they had three dollars and felt absolutely rich. "Death had been kind to us," Benjamin mused.[4]

What had sparked Harry Benjamin's interest in hormones? This had not been an obvious choice. During his days as a medical student in Germany, Benjamin had instead been deeply concerned with the treatment of tuberculosis, which was the leading health problem of his day. But by 1915, he was ready for a fresh start. In those years, medicine still had little to offer the tuberculosis sufferer besides isolation, nourishment, and the rest needed to give the patient's body a chance to fight off the infection. Benjamin had already seen much illness and death and knew very well a physician's sense of futility at the bedside. Now, immersed in the prosaic reality of general practice, he yearned to be able to do something more than simply dole out what he had learned in school and collect his fees. For him, the emerging science of hormones offered not only intellectual stimulation but also the tantalizing possibility of finding new treatments for his patients.

He had just one small but significant experience with using hormones in therapy. A few years earlier, as a new graduate, he had taken a job as assistant to a physician in the spa town of Salzungen in southern Germany. One day, his employer sent an elderly patient to him for his opinion. The woman had already been to most of the other physicians in town and had been treated for a wide array of vague symptoms. She had been left with the principal diagnosis of "idiocy." Benjamin, however, thought he recognized something that he had learned about in medical textbooks: myxedema, a condition resulting from an under-functioning thyroid gland.

Benjamin may have been thinking back to an important breakthrough some twenty years earlier in 1891, when physicians began to use extracts of thyroid tissue to treat people who suffered from myxedema. Their reasoning was that if the thyroid glands normally secreted a substance that was necessary for health, perhaps a physician could replace what was missing in the patient's defective thyroid by administering preparations made from the thyroid glands of animals. In a case history from England, a forty-six-year-old woman had become increasingly lethargic over the course of four or five years. Her speech had become slow and drawling and her memory dim, and she had lost interest in meeting people. She was strangely sensitive to cold, and her skin was so dry that it peeled off her continually as a veil of fine white powder. Most tellingly, the disease had reshaped her face: her expression was dull and languorous, her lips badly swollen, and her eyes so puffy that she found it difficult to look upward. These were classic signs of myxedema, and they foretold a bleak future of wild delusions and finally death. Inspired by recent laboratory reports, the woman's physician, George Redmayne Murray, took fresh sheep thyroid tissue, ground it up, and squeezed it through a fine handkerchief. Then, drawing the turbid pink liquid into a syringe, he injected it into the loose skin between her shoulder blades. As he repeated these injections over the course of three months, the patient improved slowly but marvelously. The swelling of her hands and lips diminished, her face became expressive, and she became able to look up again. More importantly, her thinking cleared, her memory improved, and her speech grew quick and fluent. For the first time in years, she felt able to walk in the streets without a companion. To her family and friends, as well as her physician, her recovery must have seemed the most wondrous transformation.[5]

Two decades later, Benjamin thought he recognized the same thyroid deficiency in his patient in Salzungen, even though her case seemed more pronounced and of longer duration than any he had ever encountered. He eagerly reported his theory to his employer but was met with the somewhat bemused condescension of the older man at the young doctor's "fancy diagnosis." Undaunted, Benjamin pestered a local pharmacist to acquire some thyroid tablets—which, in 1912, were relatively rare—and he prescribed them to his patient. To everyone's delight, the woman who had not spoken for years not only began to speak again but to make sense. Benjamin quickly gained a minor renown for his miraculous-seeming cure of a patient everyone else had given up on. What a satisfying sense of efficacy that must have been for Benjamin, to see a patient so clearly returned to health as a result of his direct intervention; what a sense of power he must have felt to have a patient's life so markedly improved by his ministrations. Benjamin speculated that if he had wanted to stay on in that spa town, he could have made a nice living.[6]

For endocrine enthusiasts, thyroid extracts for myxedema were just the beginning. There was growing optimism among some scientists that the endocrine glands might not only provide treatments for glandular deficiencies but also possibly hold the secrets to more fundamental questions such as the nature of sex and sexuality, personality, behavior, criminality, development, and aging. In 1905, the endocrine secretions had been given the name "hormones" by the British physiologist Ernest Starling, from the Greek ὁρμάω (ormao), which means "to excite, arouse," or "that which sets in motion." Starling set out a theoretical framework that would prove to be fruitful: he described hormones as chemical messengers that were released by the endocrine glands into the bloodstream and that acted on distant tissues and organs throughout the body. The hormone theory was in sharp contrast to the prevailing idea that the body was controlled through the nervous system, and it postulated an intriguing level of regulation that existed below conscious awareness.[7] But much remained to be known about the nature of these substances. How did tiny amounts of these hormones have such marked effects on far-flung organs and tissues? And if these hormones could so powerfully influence mental and physical characteristics, might it be possible for doctors to manipulate them to affect changes in people? Cure disease? Make people stronger, smarter, taller? Maybe even control human behavior to shape society as a whole? For Benjamin, the possibilities were thrilling.[8]

Over time, Benjamin's medical practice grew, developing a core of what he liked to call his "GPs" or "grateful patients," some of whom would continue to consult him decades later. As a private practitioner, Benjamin did not find many opportunities to use the ideas he discussed at the Wednesday night group. Despite the excitement about the possibility of using the glands in medicine, only two effective hormone treatments had been developed: thyroid extracts were fairly well established in medical practice, and, by 1901, adrenaline was isolated and commercially produced, quickly becoming a useful addition to the doctor's bag for raising blood pressure, treating asthma, and controlling bleeding and for cardiac resuscitation. There were no doubt physicians who were uncritical or perhaps overly optimistic in their use of glandular products, but there were also many very sincere and earnest practitioners and drug manufacturers who strove to make good quality glandular products and test their efficacy. Some of these treatments worked and some did not, and some of these results were carefully recorded and published in medical journals.[9] At the same time, the glandular idea was finding a foothold in the popular imagination, a fact that unscrupulous—or at least, overly enthusiastic—vendors were only too ready to exploit. At best, their products were of uncertain efficacy, since they were not yet in any standardized or regulated form. At worst, glandular extracts (usually some sort of dried tissue or other) were being flogged as cure-alls and were no better than quackery.

One day, Benjamin received a frantic telephone call from a patient, a young woman. He dashed over in a taxicab to find her five-year-old boy in bed and the woman and her husband almost in hysterics.

"He must have eaten them this morning but I only discovered it now!" the young mother cried.

Two days earlier, Benjamin had prescribed thyroid supplements for her, and she had brought home a bottle of one hundred tablets. The child had swallowed them all. Aghast, Benjamin quickly examined the young fellow. He finally allowed himself a sigh of relief when he found the boy completely fine, with a regular pulse, normal temperature, and no gastrointestinal discomfort. In fact, Benjamin reckoned the boy probably felt far better than he did himself at that moment. After a very long night, Benjamin returned to examine the boy once more; again, he was able to reassure the parents that their child was perfectly fine.

But, as Benjamin left, the young mother astutely asked him, "What kind of medicine did you prescribe for me?"

Benjamin could not remember what reply he managed to come up with. One thing was clear: he had lost that woman as a patient that day. Moreover, her pointed question fed a nagging doubt of his. He had to admit that the boy "might have just as well eaten bread crumbs." It made him wonder whether any of the successes he had achieved with hormone treatments had owed more to his having cast a psychological "spell" on his patients with his own confidence than to the virtues of the products themselves.[10]

Characteristically, though, Benjamin remained firm in his faith in hormones. He would, throughout his life, show a tenacious commitment to an idea once he had accepted it. Even if the hormone products of the time were of doubtful value, he felt sure the idea behind them was promising. And, at the very least, the Wednesday night meetings gave him a welcome intellectual respite from his days of treating aches and coughs and struggling to make rent. The other physicians made good company; Benjamin thought of them as fellow nonconformists and found their conversations lively and stimulating. Their leader, Joseph Fraenkel, was a gifted clinician and cultured intellectual who had arrived in the United States from Austria in 1892. A lover of music, literature, and art, Fraenkel moved in wealthy circles and graced many a fine table. He was a lecturer in medicine at the Cornell University Medical College and had cofounded the Neurological Institute of New York in 1909, the first hospital in the Western Hemisphere devoted to treating diseases of the nervous system. Fraenkel was Benjamin's senior by almost two decades and rangy, with sensitive features and distinguished good looks. According to one colleague, he inspired an almost godlike reverence among his patients because of his acute observations and quiet success in diagnosis and treatment. Socially, he made a compelling figure, speaking with enthusiasm, humor, and eloquence and employing a picturesque—and in Benjamin's view, rather peculiar—choice of words, in his strong Viennese accent.[11]

As Fraenkel guided his colleagues through those evenings, he shaped for them a vision of the endocrine glands that was more expansive than anything Benjamin had previously encountered. Fraenkel saw the endocrines not only as potential treatments for specific deficiency diseases but as the key to understanding the human constitution. He pictured a number of constitutional types, each of which was dominated by the function of a particular endocrine organ that shaped not only the illnesses individuals might be susceptible to but even what their temperaments and bodies were like.

To illustrate his ideas, Fraenkel offered several different types of exercises. In one, the group was introduced to a patient and told his or her clinical history. Could the participants deduce the patient's present illness and complaints? In a second exercise, the physicians were allowed to meet and examine a patient and hear his or her complaints. Now, could they reconstruct the person's past history and illnesses? And finally, in a third exercise, the group was supplied with a complete case history, past and present, as well as a current diagnosis and symptoms and were asked to deduce the patient's physical appearance and mental characteristics. They learned from Fraenkel that a malfunctioning thyroid might make some individuals irritable; a problem pituitary might make them gentle, kind, and obese; overproductive adrenals might turn them assertive and hairy; a faulty thymus, juvenile and childish; and defective gonads, secretive.[12] Fraenkel then invited the patient into the room and the participants could see for themselves whether they had been correct. These intellectual puzzles proved fascinating, but just as significant for Benjamin was the fact that he learned to think of the patient in a holistic way, that is, to look not just at a disease, a symptom, or an organ but at the entire physical and mental outlook of a person.

Constitutional ideas had currency in the United States in the 1920s and 1930s. They were, in part, a reaction against the reductionist direction that was ascendant in scientific medicine, one in which the experimental sciences such as bacteriology, physiology, and biochemistry were given priority. Constitutional medicine was an attempt to restore a more holistic vision of health and to value the clinical art and judgment of the individual physician in grasping the elusive and idiosyncratic qualities of the individual patient.[13]

Sadly for Benjamin, this stimulating time would end too soon, thanks to Fraenkel's colorful personal life. Several years earlier, Fraenkel had served as friend and physician to the composer Gustav Mahler and his wife, Alma, during Mahler's term as director of the Metropolitan Opera and the New York Philharmonic, until he returned to Europe in his final illness in 1911. Not long after the great composer's death, Fraenkel dashed to Vienna to declare his love to the charismatic Alma. He whisked her off to Corfu to court her, but Alma spurned him cruelly and went on to marry her longtime lover, the architect Walter Gropius. Fraenkel returned to New York brokenhearted but would a few years later fall in love with the opera singer Ganna Walska and marry her within ten days of meeting her. Fraenkel's marriage in 1916 would mark the end of the Wednesday night gatherings.[14]

For Benjamin, however, the rich stew of ideas that he had tasted during this brief interval was enough to change the course of his career. In time, he would realize that some of the speculative elements of their discussions failed to hold up under scrutiny, but from this start, he would grow in his conviction that the study of the endocrine glands led to therapeutic possibilities far beyond what had yet been achieved. "The seeds had been planted," he would one day say.[15]

Chapter 2

Beginnings

The oldest photograph we have of Harry Benjamin shows him at the age of twenty-four, eyes steady, chin firm, resplendent in the uniform of the Prussian Guard. He looks as if he might be about to march onto the streets of Berlin with his fellow guardsmen, rifle at the ready, boots beating a sharp tattoo. A reader coming to this book to learn about Benjamin's work in transsexualism and envisioning him as a medical maverick in the rollicking New York of the 1960s might find this image somewhat disconcerting. What we need to remember is that for Benjamin, becoming a sexologist had not really been his plan, and winding up an American was completely unintentional. It was a series of calamities, both personal and global, that brought him to that strange pass. And if he would one day become an advocate for the marginalized, it might have something to do with the fact that he had always felt himself to be something of an outsider. To understand why, we have to go back to the beginning.

Harry Benjamin was born 12 January 1885 in a Berlin that was perhaps not as different from New York as one might think.[1] In the late nineteenth century, visitors to Berlin were often moved to compare it to New York or Chicago rather than to the great capitals of Europe—and this was not usually meant as a compliment.

Berlin had been made the capital of the newly unified German nation in 1871 and over the next four decades would be utterly transformed from a swampy provincial town to one of the most populous cities in the world, third only to London and New York in size, propelled by rapid industrialization. From its asphalt paving and telephones, to electric streetlights, trams, and trains, it exemplified the modern metropolis in every way. By 1914, it had become the showcase of a dynamic new Germany, leading the world in steel production, chemical manufacture, and electrical engineering as well as being home to great cultural ferment and scientific advance. Kaiser Wilhelm II aspired to emulate, indeed surpass, the other great cities of Europe by erecting massive neoclassical structures for state and cultural institutions and laying broad boulevards meant to rival the Champs-Élysées. Some visitors found Berlin's lack of deep cultural roots, the preoccupation of its citizens with commerce and industry, and the abrasive newness of everything made the imperial capital seem rather ostentatious and crass. Rather . . . American. Others, like Mark Twain, who called Berlin the "Chicago of Europe," admired it as a beacon of progress and modernity.[2]

Harry's father, Julius Benjamin, was born 1847, the son of a merchant in Schwedt an der Oder, a town in the northeastern part of Brandenburg, close to the Polish border.[3] He and his family were among the thousands of Jews who made their way to Berlin to seek a better life. While Berlin, like virtually any place in Western society, was not free of anti-Semitism, it was there, perhaps more than in any other part of Germany, that Jews achieved a significant level of respect. As they flourished, Jews from other parts of Prussia poured in to join them, so that by the middle of the nineteenth century some 80 percent of Prussia's Jewish population lived in Berlin.[4]

The Benjamin family ran a department store, and Julius was able to acquire an education. He met and married Bertha Hoffman, the daughter of a middle-class businessman, whose family was originally from the northwestern part of Prussia, Westphalia.[5] Their first child, Harry, was born in 1885, followed by Walter in 1888 and Edith in 1890.[6] Harry had a warm home life, happier than average he thought, with a father who was a friend to him and a mother who devoted herself to her family. Their family life was marked by art, music, and a good deal of patriotism. Julius made his living as a banker, and the Benjamin household enjoyed a growing affluence. They boasted one of the first gramophones on their block.[7]

But it was also a home in which ambivalence—indeed a profound conflict—about identity seems to have been poured into its very foundation. In the Berlin of Harry's childhood, many German Jews, especially among the well-to-do, chose to convert to Christianity and marry Gentiles. Germany's Jews had the highest level of assimilation of any in Europe. Their choices were no doubt complex ones involving not only personal matters of faith and love but also the strong cultural draw of the society in which they lived and the social and economic advantages of assimilation. Harry's father, Julius, was among those who chose to convert. Harry's mother, Bertha, was Christian—like about two-thirds of Germans, a Lutheran. Harry and his siblings would be raised Lutheran, though religion did not play much of a role in their upbringing. Harry did, however, remember his mother as both anti-Semitic and anti-Catholic. In the one photograph we have of Bertha Benjamin, she stands calmly beside her son, dressed in rich black lace, her hair upswept, one hand draped on his shoulder. She and her son share the same broad face. Looking at her picture, one might sense a certain softness in her pillowy cheek, but the firm set of her lips and the long furrow inscribed between her brows belie this initial impression. The young Harry once asked his mother why, given her views, she had chosen to marry a Jew. "Papa was different," he recalled her explaining.[8]

Harry's familial tensions reflected a deeper poison at work in his society. Some Jewish families acquired great wealth and could be seen in the dress circle of the opera and driving in their finest carriages along Unter den Linden, Berlin's grandest boulevard, and in the last decades of the nineteenth century it would be precisely this wealth and success that would also bring envy and resentment and with it the disturbing rise of a new form of anti-Semitism based not on religion but on specious notions of race. Using justifications drawn from ethnography and anthropology, certain ideologues argued that Jews as a racial group could never be assimilated, no matter how many generations they had lived in Germany, no matter what their contributions to German culture.[9]

But on the whole, Harry's memories of his childhood were happy ones. At the age of five, his father took him and younger brother Walter to catch what was likely his first glimpse of America, in the form of Buffalo Bill Cody's Wild West Show. The troupe fenced in an area south of Berlin's Tiergarten—a vast urban zoo—and filled it with over 200 performers and an equal number of buffalos, horses, and mules. One can imagine Harry and Walter watching wide-eyed as the cowboys tamed bucking broncos and Annie Oakley shot glass balls tossed high in the air. At the end of the night, audience members could mill around the performers' tents, admiring the horses and gawking as the Native American performers made supper around a flickering fire. Harry would never forget that he had gotten to shake hands with Buffalo Bill himself.[10]

Harry was also thrilled to have spotted Otto von Bismarck, Germany's Iron Chancellor. Easily recognized by his signature walrus mustache, Bismarck could often be seen around the capital those days. Bismarck had achieved German unification in 1871 and continued to rule until 1890 by putting together a coalition made up of industrialists, landed aristocracy, and the military. But while the reins of political power lay in these conservative hands, the nation also fostered a thriving bourgeoisie. Harry grew up in a time and place in which the aspiring middle class could realistically hope for richer opportunities for their children. Prussia's educational system—which included free, compulsory primary education and standardized examinations and teacher education—was admired and emulated by many other nations, including the United States. After primary school, which typically ended at fourth grade, several strands of secondary schooling were available to those who could afford it, the most academic of which was the humanistic gymnasium, which was intended for university preparation. This route was open not only to those of aristocratic heritage but also to a new elite that now included the sons of businessmen, lower civil servants, and skilled workers, a group for whom it became increasingly realistic to pay a hefty tuition and temporarily forgo the earnings that a promising son might make, in anticipation of future advantage and prosperity.[11] The Benjamins were one such family. In 1891, Harry was enrolled in the preparatory school (Vorschule) of the expensive and prestigious Königliches Wilhelms-Gymnasium, which was nicknamed "Shiny Leather Shoes" for its well-shod student body. Housed in a stately neoclassical building at Bellevuestrasse 15, the school must indeed have had a beautiful view of the Tiergarten spreading lush and green to the north, while a bustling Potsdamer Platz at the other end of the street would have offered its own temptations of grand hotels and cafés, winehouses and beer palaces, theaters, dance halls, and grand modern department stores that gave Berlin's affluent a taste of cosmopolitan splendor with specialty goods imported from around the globe.

At gymnasium, Harry was introduced to a broad humanistic education founded on classical antiquity. He was not interested in student organizations and, other than playing tennis, was never keen on fencing and other sports, thus avoiding the dueling scars of some of his peers. Like other gymnasium pupils, he would not have had a uniform but may have worn a cap, the color of which differed by school and year. A strict formality was observed, with teachers and principals addressed by their titles—Herr Studienrat or Herr Oberstudiendirektor—and upperclassmen addressed by their surnames.[12]

It was during his days in gymnasium that the tension undergirding his sense of identity broke to the surface. "Papa's Jewishness was a problem," Harry would recount. His family's name was regarded as Jewish even though they were not, nor did they have many Jewish friends. At the Königliches Wilhelms-Gymnasium, where half his fellow students were the scions of aristocratic families and another large group came from the wealthiest Jewish families, he felt like an outsider as he never had before and never would again. The Christians considered him a Jew, while the Jews regarded him as a Gentile. It was an experience not merely of being marginalized as a member of a minority group but of having an internal sense of self that conflicted with what others assumed of him.[13]

He would later claim that his school experience had not caused him any pain, but the truth of its impact on his young psyche might be suggested by the fact that he developed behavior problems. Although he had previously been a good student, he began having what he called "an unruly period," getting into trouble with his teachers and cutting classes. In 1898, when he was thirteen, his father pulled him out of school. Harry finished his secondary education at the Dorotheenstadt Real-Gymnasium just north of the Brandenburg Gate, near Berlin University. Here the social climate suited him far better. Harry remembered it as an easier school but one at which he learned more. The Real-Gymnasium was a newer type of secondary institution that had, in recent years, become an alternate route to university. Unlike the humanistic gymnasium, it emphasized the modern languages and sciences rather than classical humanities; Harry took Latin—but no Greek or Hebrew—and German, French, and English, natural history, physics, chemistry, mathematics, history, geography, drawing, and religion. His school days were spent deciphering Cicero, Schiller, and Shakespeare, poring over the periodic table, and peering into microscopes and cabinets full of South American butterflies.[14]

But what path would he take? Harry's father's example might have inclined him to choose a career in business; his brother, Walter, would follow their father into selling stocks. His mother's passions, on the other hand, might have steered him toward art and music; Harry's sister, Edith, would study music. Under their mother's tutelage, Harry developed a lifelong love of music and especially of opera. While his sister favored comic musical theater, Harry found himself moved by more serious works such as Verdi's *La forza del destino* and *Aida*, with their tragic stories, resonant choruses, and dramatic musical lines. He exulted in the soaring grandeur of Wagner's *Lohengrin* and *The Flying Dutchman* and the exquisite lyricism of Mozart.[15] Opera, theater, music, and literature would become "dangerous rivals" to his studies in those days. In one of his notebooks from this era, he kept pages and pages of lyrics from operatic arias and lieder, all transcribed in his neat, flowing script.[16] The high-blown emotions of this world would resonate deeply for him and set the register of his emotional life.

The Berlin of Harry's youth was a fantastic place to indulge such passions because the city boasted close to a dozen opera houses, from the magnificent Royal Opera House to several smaller, private establishments. Many of the leading lights of the world operatic stage found their way to Berlin during this time and were treated almost like the rock stars of today—Enrico Caruso was mobbed by a crowd of 30,000—and the young, like Harry, were among the most ardent fans. Harry insinuated himself into the world of actresses and divas. Unlike other schoolboys, he developed something of a second life, traveling with the opera crowd as a youthful admirer. He successfully attached himself to the house physician of one private opera house, the Theatre den Westens, and trailed him backstage amid props, drops, and greasepaint. When Caruso made his Berlin debut, Harry eagerly watched both the dress rehearsal and opening night. Days later, when Caruso developed acute laryngitis, Harry's physician friend invited him to come peer down the famous throat.

"Want to take a look at those vocal cords?" he asked. "They are enormous."

The great Caruso graciously consented to this examination, and Harry boasted of this experience until the end of his days but would admit, "I was so excited that I did not see anything."[17]

At the age of fifteen Harry fell in love, but with a thirty-year-old actress who was engaged to a German officer. This was "always tragic," as Harry put it, never more than a "love at a distance," but as it turned out, long, unrequited passions would become a recurring theme in his life. At sixteen, Harry developed a mad crush on soprano Geraldine Farrar, America's first diva of international renown. Farrar was just nineteen years old when she dazzled Berlin in her 1901 debut at the Royal Opera House as Marguerite in Gounod's *Faust*. Celebrated for her dark, elegant beauty and acting talent as well as for her rich voice, she would remain in Berlin for three years, captivating the kaiser's court and attracting the amorous attentions of the crown prince himself. Harry could not afford to hear her sing very often but spent many days standing outside her house, hoping for a glimpse. He amassed a huge collection of her picture postcards, which he was never to relinquish. In these sepia souvenir photographs, Farrar appears as an innocent maiden with long raven tresses, a glittering queen, or a Wagnerian bride. Harry claimed to have once danced with the young Farrar, and he would cherish this memory for the rest of his life.[18]

Our first direct glimpse into Harry's inner life comes from a locked diary that he began on 6 June 1904 at the age of nineteen. This private space reads like a repository for all the mutterings of anguished adolescence and the antisocial interior dialogue that one usually knows better than to share aloud. At one o'clock the day before, the school's principal had appeared at the door of the classroom and announced in an icy tone that Harry and four others were to be held back from writing their final examination. Harry paled. This would mean an additional six months "bearing the yoke" of school. "Lord in heaven!" Harry wrote. He could not believe his ears. After he had regained some of his composure, he looked around the classroom to catch the faces of some of the other unfortunates; he thought one fellow whom he dubbed "Fat Ulle" looked as if he were trying in vain to summon up the grammatical rules of the *Dativ* and *Accusativ* cases; the angular features of another chap, "the Hedgehog," seemed to grow even sharper in contrast with Ulle's plumpness. Harry stifled a laugh, but seeing the principal looking so calm and businesslike, without a single word of consolation, he was seized with a tremendous rage. When he tried to get up, he felt dizzy. The ride home later that day was a misery, his companions showing no sign of comprehending how he felt. He would not regain his composure until later that evening. Writing in his diary, he congratulated himself on having a personality that viewed matters that could not be changed as obstacles to be overcome.[19]

In the morning, he visited the monumental Pergamon Altar on Berlin's Museum Island. He was reveling in the muscular struggles of Achilles and Telephos on the ancient frieze when he felt rudely interrupted by the arrival of a group of ladies in a cloud of perfume. Harry quipped that this proved an assault to the senses worthy of a mythological battle. He mused condescendingly that these ladies probably understood as little about the ancient story carved on the walls as Telephos's mother would have understood about modern art, and he rather thought they had come only to be able to say, no matter how bored they were, "we have seen Ancient Greek excavations that we liked very much" (or perhaps they would say "Roman," he added, patronizingly). He was determined, however, not to get into a rage. "I am certainly not an enemy of women," he claimed in his diary, but "a friend of all women's emancipation."[20]

Indeed, as a young man, he was struggling to sort out his feelings about men, women, and sexuality. When he was nineteen, his second great love, "Mimi," made her first appearance in his diary. He wrote that his love for her "grows daily, even hourly." And then when the joyful day arrived that he finally passed the exams that had plagued him for so long, he attributed his fortitude to his constant thought of her, his "Schützenliesel," whom he pictured smiling so seductively at him. His passion for Mimi would become a pulsing motif of his young manhood.[21]

He also noted in his diary that he had read Émile Zola's psychological thriller *La bête humaine*, which he found repulsive and disquieting. Its protagonist, a murderous railway man, is driven by mental illness to kill women again and again. Harry reassured himself that while he could understand such cravings on some intellectual level, "thank God" that even the slightest sensation of such a lust was "completely alien" to him, and he thus felt safe in reading such literature as it could do him no harm. It did not help that his head was already swirling with images of sexual atrocity, having spent the morning of this particular diary entry in a local courtroom, listening in on such a case. Maupassant's *Bel ami* similarly left him upset; the novel's manipulative protagonist successfully rises to power by exploiting one powerful, intelligent woman after another. "One must not believe in divine justice," Harry reckoned. "One will be disappointed in life too often."[22] While he was put strangely off kilter by these literary explorations, he ended a subsequent diary entry with a sigh of resignation. How he longed "to study literature, art history, nature . . . everything, everything," that is, to truly acquire a comprehensive education. If it were not for the fact that he would soon have to take a job to feed himself, his dearest wish would have been to become a private scholar. But that of course was impossible. One had to be sensible, he realized. "Why? Because it doesn't help to do otherwise. Who knows what shape my life will take," he mused. "And yet," he reflected, "thank God, we can't look into the future."[23]

And so, he had to turn his mind to more practical matters. What career should he pursue? In this, his choice may have been shaped not only by the expectations of his family but by the fertile environment in which he found himself. Germany at the turn of the century, and Berlin in particular, was a hothouse of scientific discovery, so it is easy to understand how an intelligent, curious, and ambitious young man might readily be caught up in the excitement. Advances in chemistry, physics, and engineering gave rise to developments that were central to the success of German industries, from robust dynamos and innovative street lighting to synthetic dyes in fabulous shades of alizarin, magenta, and violet. But it was in the study of health and the human body that science hit at the very heart of the human condition. Fantastic new developments in bacteriology, immunology, and physiology were giving scientists a greater understanding of how the body worked in health, how it succumbed in illness, and how the scientifically trained physician might alleviate suffering. The great clinician William Osler would famously say that in the German medical science of this time, "there were new discoveries being announced like corn popping in a pan."[24] Germany was at the pinnacle of medical research, education, and clinical training; it drew physicians and scientists from around the world to imbibe the bracing air of scientific medicine, engage with the most advanced ideas, and train in the most innovative techniques. The great names of German medical science—Johannes Muller, Emil Du Bois-Reymond, Robert Koch, Rudolf Virchow, Emil von Behring, Matthias Schleiden, and Theodor Schwann—would have been a source of inspiration and pride to Harry and his classmates. So, after six and a half years at the Dorotheenstadt Real-Gymnasium, Harry graduated with his *Abitur*, the university entry qualification, at the close of the Easter term of 1905. No one was prouder or happier than his papa. Harry was twenty years old, and in the school yearbook he declared his intention to study medicine.[25]

━━━━━━

Harry Benjamin began his premedical studies at the University of Berlin in 1905. As was typical for medical students in Germany, he moved from school to school to take advantage of the opportunity to learn from many teachers. After two semesters, he went north to the University of Rostock for a further four semesters of premedical training and there, passed his preliminary medical examination. On his return home, however, he faced what would be the worst half year of his life thus far: fulfilling his compulsory military service from April to October 1908. In Berlin, the discipline, militarism, and efficient bureaucracy of Prussian culture were much in evidence. Uniforms were ubiquitous and military parades with brass bands and spiked helmets a regular sight on the streets.[26] Benjamin's own upbringing had been steeped in patriotism. His parents were deeply *Kaisertreu*—loyal subjects of their emperor—and his father, Julius, was proud of his own military record in the Franco-Prussian War of 1870–71.[27] Benjamin enlisted in the famous Prussian Guard, the elite bodyguard of the kaiser, known for their discipline, fierceness, and height (the minimum requirement was five feet seven inches). Such was their reputation that, in the war that was to come, Allied soldiers would make a special point of mentioning the fact if they had fought the Prussian Guard. In the photo from this time, Benjamin looks splendid and grave, but his calm countenance belied the misery he felt inside. He found the entire experience hateful. He despised the drilling as stupid and recoiled at what he saw as the sole aim of military training, which was to transform an individual "into a mechanical robot." The only satisfaction he felt was from learning that he had a certain skill in shooting. The day he was discharged to become a free student again was the happiest he could remember.[28]

In 1909, at the age of twenty-four, Benjamin arrived at the Eberhard-Karls Universität Tübingen to begin his study of medicine. A quintessential medieval university town, Tübingen sat at the foot of the rolling Swabian Alp range in southwest Germany, and since the fifteenth century, book-laden students had picked their way along its cobblestone lanes and climbed its narrow-staired alleyways. Benjamin's classmates included students not only from the elite but also from the broad middle class. Medical school tuition was expensive and, like his gymnasium education, would have involved a significant investment on the part of his family, but a university education was increasingly possible for someone from a background such as his. And as of 1904, women were admitted into medicine, so one or two of his fellow students were female. Benjamin had ten semesters of medical study, five of the basic sciences and five of clinical subjects. Much of this would have been delivered through didactic lectures held in large halls. Courses were not organized on a graduated level or by semester, so students could choose which to go to, and they could even attend them more than once. Lecture halls could be rowdy places where students made their opinions known by stomping their feet, creating a clamor that echoed off the steeply raked rows of wooden seats.[29]

To be a student of medicine in this decade was to enter a world of exciting possibilities but also frustrating limitations. Over the previous century, medicine had developed so much that it was possible to understand disease with a striking new clarity. Physicians had a greater ability to diagnose diseases, understand their causes, and offer prognoses as to the course they would take. The microscope allowed researchers to see the germs that caused disease; illnesses that were once thought to be the result of miasmas—bad air—could now be understood to be caused by single-celled organisms. Vaccines, better nutrition, sanitation, and public health measures—honed by this new appreciation of the microorganisms that caused disease—improved the health of the general population and increased life expectancy. But when people did become ill, the most important factors in their healing were still careful nursing, rest, food, and time. Despite the conviction among medical leaders that science was the key to a physician's success, few effective therapies had actually been introduced into medical practice. Among the few tools that physicians had gained in recent decades were aspirin, morphine, and diphtheria antitoxin. These therapies would soon be joined in 1910 by Salvarsan (arsphenamine), the "magic bullet" for syphilis.

Surgery, in contrast, had made great leaps; aided by the development of anesthesia and aseptic techniques in the latter part of the nineteenth century, surgeons who had once been kept from cutting into the internal organs by the near certainty of killing their patients through shock or infection could now forge past excising external tumors and performing amputations to devise audacious new procedures. In medicine, however, age-old foes such as tuberculosis remained unvanquished. Although Robert Koch had identified the tubercle bacillus in 1882, it remained an elusive target, and in the twenty-three years since, physicians had gained no more effective agent against TB than they had before.

But to be a student of medicine *in Germany* at this time was to gain an unparalleled education, one that was respected and envied around the world. In Germany, the teaching of physicians had undergone a fundamental change in the nineteenth century. In the great hospitals of Salpêtrière in Paris or Guy's in London, or in the policlinics in Germany, medical students apprenticed at the bedside, following clinical teachers through the wards and learning to understand injury and disease as they were manifested in real patients. In the United States, many freewheeling for-profit proprietary medical schools abounded. But in Germany, medical education came to be firmly based in universities. Moreover, a doctor's training became thoroughly grounded in the experimental sciences.[30]

One experience of Benjamin's student years would haunt him. He liked to visit and chat with a pharmacist in town. One day, a fellow medical student, a long-haired artistic type, crashed down the stairs from the apartment where he lived above the pharmacy.

"What kind of potassium cyanide did you give me this morning?" the student gasped. "It did not do anything. I . . ."

The pharmacist dashed from behind the counter, his face stricken with horror. There was a sickening thump as the student collapsed, gripped in a violent convulsion. Benjamin reached for his pulse and felt the weak final flutters of the man's life.

"Some camphor, quick!" cried Benjamin. "He's dying."

The pharmacist knelt, motionless. "It's no use," he said brokenly. He explained that the student had asked him for potassium cyanide powder to kill mice, and he had suspected nothing. Benjamin attempted artificial resuscitation while a bystander ran for a doctor, but it would be in vain. The student died under Benjamin's hands. He would never learn what desperation had driven the young man to suicide. In time, he and the pharmacist pieced together some of the grisly facts: the student had taken the poison and had lain down in bed waiting to die, but because he had just eaten a large meal, his stomach was full and the cyanide failed to come into contact with the acid necessary for its activation. After lying in frustration for an hour or more, he had scrambled down the stairs to demand an explanation. Just at that moment, the poison took hold. Benjamin witnessed his agonizing end, and all his medical training had been of little use against the enormity of one man's despair.[31]

At the conclusion of his years of study were two important examinations. The first was a lengthy set of tests that might have included a task such as a dissection. Busy teachers sometimes examined several students at a time, taking answers viva voce. Students who failed could take the test again, but three failures meant certain expulsion from medical school. The second examination required the presentation of a short thesis that was generally formulaic, involving a literature review. Benjamin studied with Ernst·von Romberg, a noted authority on tuberculosis, and his thesis focused on the recent development of a diagnostic test for TB that could be conducted in the doctor's office. He received a notation of "Good" on his thesis titled "Anwendung des Antiforminverfahrens für den Tuberkelbazillennachweis" (On the application of the antiformin procedure for tubercle bacillus detection).[32]

In 1912, Benjamin graduated cum laude. He was embarrassed that his proud father made a bit too much of the fact. At first, he was unsure of his long-term plans. He was anxious to acquire practical clinical experience in many branches of medicine, so he returned to Berlin for the winter and worked at a variety of clinics at the famed Charité (Royal Charity Hospital), the teaching hospital of the University of Berlin that had been home to medical pioneers such as Rudolf Virchow, Robert Koch, and Emil von Behring. Not wanting to depend on his father's pocketbook too much longer, Benjamin then began to look for paid employment. At this point, he took his stint in the spa town of Salzungen, where he achieved success with his myxedema diagnosis. He might have toyed with the idea of settling into a comfortable practice, but not for very long; Benjamin was eager to see more of the world. He felt too many of his peers were only too ready to settle into general practice and fill their pockets. But he had already learned much about illness and death and the futility a physician could feel at the bedside. He yearned to do more.[33]

Back in Berlin, he came to the attention of Carl Ludwig Schleich, who was then one of the great figures in German medicine. Schleich, then in his early fifties, was best known as a surgeon and the inventor of local anesthesia by infiltration, but he was also a painter, poet, and philosopher and part of a cultured set who must have made heady company for Benjamin. Among them, high science was meshed with high art; explorations of the unknown through poetry and paint were integrated with a study of the natural world. In stern, orderly Berlin, Schleich and writers August Strindberg and Otto Erich Hartleben were nearly arrested when they were found trying to measure the curvature of the earth at the corner of Unter den Linden and Friedrichstrasse.[34] Schleich knew of Benjamin's thesis on tuberculosis, so he introduced him to an intense young physician named Friedrich Franz Friedmann. Friedmann had garnered a great deal of attention when he announced in November 1912 that he had developed a treatment for tuberculosis, a serum containing a strain of tuberculosis that he had extracted from turtles in the Tiergarten, Berlin's zoo. Schleich assured Benjamin that Friedmann's work was "one of the finest things I have ever seen in medicine" and urged Benjamin to take a position as Friedmann's clinical assistant. A short time later, Friedmann was ready to take his "turtle serum" and Benjamin to America.

Benjamin was full of hope. The prospect of a trip to the New World was tempting in itself, but being part of Friedmann's undertaking seemed an incredible opportunity. He felt a little uneasiness about aspects of Friedmann's personality that he had already sensed—a certain meanness and selfishness—but whatever apprehensions he had he swallowed after a heart-to-heart talk with Schleich, who assured him he was about to have a share in an "epoch-making" discovery. In February 1913, Benjamin left Berlin for Bremerhaven, where he was to board his ship for New York. Benjamin's beloved father came to see them off. As they made their farewells, Friedmann addressed Julius: "Your son," he crowed, "has drawn the big prize in the lottery."[35]

Chapter 3

Part of That Power, Not Understood

FAUST
    Who art thou, then?
MEPHISTOPHELES
    Part of that Power, not understood,
    Which always wills the Bad, and always works the Good.
—Johann Wolfgang von Goethe, *Faust*

Harry Benjamin had been at sea for seven days when the jagged outline of New York rose on the horizon, smoky gray and shot through with pinpricks of light against a darkening sky. It was an outline as shimmering as it was elusive. Aboard the palatial SS *Kronprinzessin Cecilie*, Benjamin was an ocean apart from all he knew and loved. His overcoat must have been pulled tight against the biting air. In a photograph taken that day, his keen eyes peer from beneath the brim of a tidy black bowler. He looks subdued, perhaps a little apprehensive.

An American banker, Charles Finlay, had announced he would give a prize of $1 million if Friedrich Franz Friedmann could come to New York and demonstrate that his cure worked in ninety-five out of a hundred patients, provided that the banker's son-in-law be among those cured. Drawn by this phenomenal offer, Friedmann set sail from Germany with Benjamin as his clinical assistant and a newspaper man serving as press agent. The weekend before their arrival, the *New York Times* featured a two-page spread in the Sunday supplement titled "Has Dr. Friedmann Really Found a Tuberculosis Cure?"[1] At the pier, they were met by a mob of reporters and whisked off to a posh banquet and press conference. As Benjamin pushed through the throng, jostled by newsmen and barraged by rapid-fire English, he perhaps began to grasp the magnitude of the enterprise of which he had become part. He had plunged into modern medicine at its most intense, practiced under the acid glare of publicity and burdened with a weight of expectations.[2]

Over the next days, crowds of desperate tuberculosis patients thronged the lobby of the Waldorf Astoria Hotel where Friedmann and crew were staying. A thousand souls hunched together through the frigid night in a line that snaked up Fifth Avenue, awaiting the opening of a clinic that had been announced. Pathos-filled stories appeared each day in the papers: a sad-eyed mother throwing herself in front of Friedmann's motorcar holding her sick baby aloft; a shoemaker and his family who had walked miles before dawn only to be turned away; an escapee from a tuberculosis tent hospital in Arizona who had made his way to New York, all in the vain hope of seeing the great doctor. In New York, Theodore Roosevelt chatted with Friedmann about Goethe, Schiller, and Luther and asked if he might treat one of his associates; in Washington, President Woodrow Wilson received Friedmann at the White House and had him demonstrate his treatment before a crowd of ambassadors and dignitaries. Everywhere Friedmann and his group went, they were trailed by reporters and hailed as saviors.[3]

Benjamin's first week was a blur of visitors and meetings. He also struggled to decipher many strange new sights, sounds, and customs. He was hardly unsophisticated; after all, he had been raised in Berlin and seen Paris and Vienna. Yet everything about New York astounded him, from the skyscraping towers and frenetic traffic to the fact that the "morning" papers appeared in the evening. As he later recalled, he found it all "astonishing, sometimes overwhelming, sometimes bewildering." Someone pointed out "Diamond" Jim Brady to him, drinking orange juice at the bar at the Waldorf. He had no idea who the legendary railroad magnate was and saw only a rather heavy middle-aged man with a large diamond pin in his tie and a diamond in every waistcoat button, which he deemed in rather bad taste. He wrote home about the strange white-tiled restaurant they ate in at Thirty-Fourth Street called Child's, which looked to his eyes like a combination of a kitchen and a bathroom. One could not even order a beer there! He didn't appreciate that he was at a true New York institution, one of a chain of restaurants that had emerged to provide economical and hygienic meals to urban working people in an era when the public was newly conscious of germs and food safety. Child's was distinguished by its austere decor and waitresses who gleamed like nurses in their starched white uniforms.[4]

Benjamin found the interactions with the press particularly bewildering. His schoolboy English had been helpful in conveying Friedmann's ideas to American correspondents who had made their way to the clinic in Berlin, but here in New York, his skills proved utterly inadequate, and he had to have several of the headlines explained to him. The entire notion of a press agent was new to him, and he felt himself rather a "babe in the woods" when confronted with the slick maneuvers of their press agent, Charles de Vidal Hundt. Benjamin was shocked to read an interview that he was supposed to have given because the facts quoted were as new to him as they were to the readers; Hundt had apparently written the entire article himself.

In the halls of the Waldorf, many reporters were frustrated by the lack of information. Few were admitted into Friedmann's suite, and the rest were reduced to speculating about the mysterious sequence of knocks used by bell-hops at the door or the contents of the hushed conferences among members of what they had come to call the "Turtle Cabinet." Many physicians arrived from around the country to represent the interests of their hospitals and patients, some waiting all day only to be turned away. Only a fortunate few managed to enter the inner sanctum. Finlay brought a fellow businessman who had tuberculosis. "I have enough money to rent the whole hotel," the Connecticut millionaire told Benjamin. "I'll give your doctor all I have if he can cure me." But even he was to leave disappointed.[5]

Tensions were running high behind the scenes, however. Friedmann, characterized by one reporter as a handsome, wild-eyed genius of "extreme nervousness and intensity," seemed on the verge of collapse; physicians who had seen him were very concerned for his health.[6] Benjamin was kept busy analyzing the data from the clinics at which Friedmann had tested his serum and within weeks, he became aware there was a problem. It was not clear that any improvement could be documented. Moreover, Benjamin now realized that Friedmann expected him to "clean up" the data. Benjamin's sense of integrity was affronted. While he still had faith in the serum itself, he was troubled by Friedmann's methods.[7] At one of their daily press conferences, two patients were presented to reporters as showing signs of improvement, but when reporters asked Benjamin for his opinion, he gave only a guarded statement: "I do not care to give an opinion. . . . The time is too short to determine anything of medical value, and the final results would probably contradict any statement I might make at this time. There are so many various changes in tubercular patients that one must be very careful in deciding which ones should be attributed to the treatment and which should not."[8] His response infuriated Friedmann. Further, Benjamin's finances were becoming strained as Friedmann had as of yet failed to pay him the salary and expenses he had promised.[9] Benjamin had come to America believing he was part of an epoch-making endeavor—that he was helping to wipe out the white plague—and instead, he found himself short of funds and in the employ of someone he now suspected of being a scoundrel and charlatan. After a vociferous confrontation, Benjamin left Friedmann's party.[10] In the beginning, the American medical community had been cautiously optimistic about the turtle serum. The US Public Health Service had sent representatives to meet with Friedmann, and several hospitals and physicians had cooperated with him to allow clinical trials to be performed. By May 1913, however, the evidence was mounting that the turtle serum was a failure. Despite this, Friedmann drew the interest of a commercial concern that offered to set up "Friedmann Institutes" across the country. Soon, Friedman returned to Germany with a $125,000 in cash and $1.8 million in stock in the proposed institutes, having sold the US rights to his "cure."[11]

Benjamin, on the other hand, was stranded with little English and even less money, unable even to pay for a return ticket home.[12] Years later he reflected that he and probably many other people had good reason to regret their contact with a man he called "one of the most objectionable personalities in the history of modern medicine." The Connecticut millionaire whom Benjamin had met at the Waldorf heard that Benjamin had broken with Friedmann and invited him to New Haven. Benjamin arrived to find the man lying on a couch on the porch of his palatial home, in the advanced stages of pulmonary tuberculosis. The patient pulled out a thick wad of bills from his pocket.

"Look," he announced. "Two thousand dollars. You know where it came from?"

He explained that one of Friedmann's assistants had charged him this sum for an injection, claiming to have access to the true serum. Benjamin was aghast. When the millionaire discovered that only Friedmann possessed the authentic serum, he had confronted the assistant and threatened to call the police. The culprit reluctantly repaid the money, admitting he had administered only water mixed with glycerin. Benjamin stayed on with the wealthy man for a few more days, if only to give moral support. The patient, despite eventually getting a legitimate injection at a Friedmann Institute, died less than a year later.[13] Benjamin was left with only the memory of jostling crowds, heart-rending pleas, and bitter regret.[14]

The Friedmann episode was Benjamin's first encounter with frenzied press reportage and the contentious margins of medical orthodoxy. It would not be his last. The man who would one day be touted as the "Father of Transsexualism" was already no stranger to controversy.

Through the following summer and autumn, Benjamin learned many new things: he discovered what it was to "bounce a check" and what a "hard time" meant in America. He survived by connecting with the large, thriving German-speaking community in New York and by tapping some of the medical connections he had made to get odd jobs in medical translation and abstracting.

The glamour of the stage and screen had always captivated Benjamin, even from his student days in Berlin. He now sold tickets at the German theater in New York and roomed with a young Viennese stage actor and director. The two men worked on their English and struggled to make rent but at least three times a week managed to come up with a nickel to take in a two-reel feature at the cinema. In his diary, Benjamin penned a neat list of twenty-nine films featuring Alice Joyce, the serene, dark-haired beauty known as "The Madonna of the Screen." His roommate, G. W. Pabst, would go on to make his own first film nine years later and become one of the most influential filmmakers of the Weimar Republic.[15]

Back in Berlin, Harry's father, Julius Benjamin, threatened to charge Friedmann with unprofessional conduct with the Berlin Chamber of Physicians and Surgeons.[16] Sadly, news came to Harry shortly afterward that Julius had been diagnosed with kidney cancer. Harry dared not burden his family with his own concerns, so he wrote letters home painting a rosy portrait of his life in New York, full of false hopes and invented accomplishments. In November, he was devastated to learn that his beloved father had died. His widowed mother, sister, and brother were an ocean away, and he worried greatly for their welfare.

In grief and depression, Benjamin took a position as private physician to a farmer in Rockville, Maryland, a man who was anxious to always have a doctor by his side. The job gave Benjamin time to improve his English and brush up on his medical knowledge while offering a comfortable salary of fifty dollars a month, some of which he was able to send home to Berlin, where it was now much needed. Benjamin soon realized there was nothing much wrong with the farmer, so he practiced his own brand of psychotherapy by convincing his client to set up a makeshift cinema, the first in that town. Four nights a week they rented the town hall, and Benjamin, the private physician, became a projectionist and cashier, temporarily forgetting his troubles in the entrancing shadows of the silver screen.[17]

Finally, in the spring of 1914, Benjamin secured a job running the laboratory at the Hospital for Deformities and Joint Diseases in Harlem.[18] The facilities were spacious and brand-new, and Benjamin felt happy with his work. He was able to live at the hospital and also find spare time to study for the state board examination for his medical license. One Sunday afternoon in June, Benjamin was strolling along Seventh Avenue when a headline leaped from the newsstand: "Archduke Ferdinand Murdered at Sarajevo." Suddenly, home seemed so very far away, and his responsibilities to his family and his native land loomed. Soon after, he was asked by the hospital's board to return to Germany to further investigate Friedmann's serum. The hospital had been one of the sites at which Friedmann had tested his turtle serum, and some of the patients seemed to show improvement. Despite Benjamin's disastrous experience with the discoverer, he had never lost faith in the discovery itself. He still thought there might be something in the turtle cure; it did not seem to work on all forms of tuberculosis, but he wondered if it might be effective against certain indications.[19]

On 25 July 1914, Benjamin found himself again at the Hoboken pier of the German ocean liners. In a curious twist of fate, he sailed once again on the *Kronprinzessin Cecilie*, but this time, instead of the opulent transatlantic liner that had brought him the year before, he was on a smaller steamer of the same name. Three days after leaving port, the wireless brought news that war had broken out between Austria-Hungary and Serbia. The passengers were gripped with tense excitement. Benjamin wondered how long Germany and France might remain neutral and whether he would soon be on active duty. A week later, as the ship approached the French coast, news arrived that Germany and France were now also at war. The German-owned steamer was chased by French cruisers and swerved back toward England, narrowly escaping capture. "If we had just been a half-hour earlier I could have gotten through," the captain said. "Just a half-hour earlier."[20]

In Cornwall, the harvest was in full swing and blackberries, aloes, and hazelnuts were ripening lavishly in the hedgerows. Benjamin and his shipmates arrived on the Cornish coast at Falmouth on the morning of 4 August to what they assumed would be a neutral port, only to learn that German forces crossed into neutral Belgium the same day. That night, at eleven o'clock, Britain formally declared war on Germany. The German crew and many of the passengers suddenly found themselves enemy aliens. Over the following days, curious Cornish citizens thronged the dockside to peer at the *Cecilie* and a second German ship, the SS *Prince Adelbert*, that had arrived the same morning.[21]

For ten days, the passengers and crew waited. One of Benjamin's fellow passengers was a former Austrian cavalry officer who was a fanatical patriot; he threatened suicide if he could not go back to fight the Serbs. Other passengers rather enjoyed the novelty of the situation, in those innocent days when many assumed the war would be over by Christmas. For the German crewmen, there was a sense of revelry mixed with panic. They dived into the ship's champagne and wine stocks, began to break furniture and instruments, and even talked about blowing up the ship. Benjamin and the other passengers cautiously ventured into the kitchen to make their own meals when the cooks were drunk enough not to interfere. Most were relieved when the British finally came aboard and took possession of the ship.[22]

Days later, the German crewmen were marched off the ship and paraded through streets on their way to spend the next several years as prisoners of war. Their path was lined with curious locals in straw boaters and fluttering summer whites. A cheeky band of young boys marched alongside, looking thoroughly pleased that the opening days of war had already brought so much excitement to their remote corner of England.[23] Benjamin and the other enemy aliens who had funds of their own were released with the requirement they register at a police station.[24] Not knowing a soul in Britain, Benjamin boarded a train to London.

He wrote to his mother, brother, and sister (writing in English in concession to wartime censors): "My dearest Mama! . . . I have not heard from you since almost one month and you can probably imagine how greatly alarmed I am. . . . We all have to wait and must try to not lose hope that everything will be all right in a short time." He was worried about their finances, not knowing how he might get funds to them. He begged them, "Don't pay any debts! Don't pay the rent now! Nobody can blame you in a time like that." He assured them that he now had no intention of trying to reach Germany.[25]

The days stretched into weeks. Caught in this limbo, he filled his days roaming the British capital, watching recruits drill in Hyde Park and following

Hindenburg's victories in the *Times*. He was appalled by a street vendor's cheap jingoistic pamphlet that referred to the kaiser as a shameless "Emperor and King of Sausage Annihilators, Savages and Barbarians"—a concession to idiots, he reasoned—but on the whole was very impressed by the British. When he reported to the police station to register, the officer peeled a page off his notepad and wrote out an address, saying, "If you are a German doctor, you will be interested to know that we have a German hospital in London." This small act of kindness and respect made a deep impression on Benjamin. He wrote in his diary, "Sehr anständige Behandlung auf der Polizei"—very decent treatment by the police—speculating that a German functionary in the same situation might have acted very differently, issuing stern orders and admonitions with an attitude of superiority.[26]

While he considered himself a German patriot, he had decidedly mixed feelings about being back in uniform. When he encountered fellow countrymen, he often felt at odds with them as he had little faith in an ultimate victory for Germany. After several weeks of frustration at not being allowed to continue on to Germany nor being released to return to the United States, Benjamin insisted on seeing "the man in charge" and, remarkably, was given an appointment with a high official in the Home Office. Benjamin found himself in a huge, impressive office in the presence of an elderly, aristocratic man behind an elaborate desk. After listening to Benjamin's story, the gentleman smiled pleasantly, asked a few questions, and then shook his hand and said, "Bring me your ticket to the U.S.A. and I will give you a permit to leave England." Benjamin would reflect that it seemed that the higher an official was and "the bigger the man," the more approachable he usually was and the easier to deal with. Permit in hand, Benjamin quickly made his way to Liverpool and, three days later, on 16 September, sailed for Philadelphia. From this strange interlude, he would keep the following mementos for the rest of his life: a photograph of his fellow shipmates on the *Kronprinzessin Cecilie*, the propaganda pamphlet with the caricature of the kaiser, and the sheet of notepaper on which the police officer had penciled in the address of the German hospital, a remembrance of British civility.

Twelve days later, Benjamin arrived in Philadelphia. A year and a half before, when he had first arrived in America, there had been crowds of reporters, banquets, dignitaries, and a suite at the Waldorf Astoria. Now he arrived unheralded and unnoticed, one more face in a sea of exhausted travelers. Had the *Kronprinzessin Cecilie* been a half hour earlier back in August, he might now be in some battlefield dressing station in a gown flecked with blood. Instead, the only home address he could give to the immigration official was 1919 Madison Avenue, New York City—the address of the Hospital for Deformities and Joint Diseases. He had spent his last money on the Atlantic passage, so a visit to a Philadelphia pawnshop was required to pay for the train ticket back to New York City.[27]

From the early 1800s to 1914, the United States had a vibrant German culture. Germans were easily the largest ethnic group after Anglo-Americans, and New York had the third-largest German-speaking population in the world after Berlin and Vienna, with close to a quarter of its population speaking German. From northern Wisconsin to Texas, one could find thriving communities with clubs, theaters, and hundreds of German-language newspapers. In science and medicine, there had long been strong ties between Germany and the United States. A generation before, America's elite physicians had counted a visit to Germany as a vital part of their postgraduate training and had brought home a deep appreciation for the German tradition of scientific medicine. By the 1890s, Germans making a visit to the United States saw that the spirit of research had been absorbed and transformed in the New World, and thanks to the largesse of private philanthropy, in certain first-class institutions the equipment even surpassed that in German hospitals and laboratories. A succession of leading German-speaking scientists and physicians visited the United States, including Robert Koch, Carl Ludwig, and Auguste Forel. Paul Ehrlich was given a hero's welcome during his tour in 1904, and he in turn was enchanted by the "simple hearty existence and practical sense" of the Americans he met. German visitors often felt very much at home, noting that German was still frequently spoken by hotel clerks, managers, waiters, guides, and train conductors. When Sigmund Freud arrived in 1909, he delivered five lectures in German to a packed audience.[28]

But Benjamin settled in America at precisely the moment when everything was changing. Anti-German sentiment seeped into American culture in 1914, and by the time the United States entered the war in 1917, it would even give way to vigilante violence. Street names were changed. Newspapers shut down. German-language instruction, once an integral part of public schooling, was canceled. Mendelssohn's famous strains were no longer played at weddings, and Beethoven was removed from concert listings. Even many German medical and scientific journals were banned, and all traces of a once respected and integral culture were eradicated.

Back at the hospital in October 1914, Benjamin found the atmosphere markedly changed from when he had left in July. The Irish head nurse, according to Benjamin, ruled not only the staff but the surgeon-in-chief as well. When the first payday came, she saw to it that Benjamin was no longer on the payroll, and all the German and Austrian staff found themselves discharged. Already broke, Benjamin was chagrined to realize he had worked a whole month for nothing. But unlike the previous summer, he was now no longer a "greenhorn." He had come in contact with many eminent medical people during his time with Friedrich Friedmann, and he remained on good terms with several. One procured a position for him as first assistant to the director of the Montefiore Home Country Sanatorium in Bedford Hills. The sanatorium was a Jewish charitable institution for tuberculosis, and Benjamin was pleased to work in his field again. When the job of superintendent became available a few months later, he assumed he would make a good candidate, since he had served as acting superintendent on occasion and had a good record and many recommendations. Unfortunately for him, the institution required that the person filling the post be married and Jewish, and Benjamin failed on both counts. He was, however, still keen to have the independence of a private practice. The state board exam did not prove difficult, and in 1915 he earned his license to practice in the state of New York.[29]

If, as Freud said, the death of a man's father is the most important event in his life, his most poignant loss, then for Benjamin that loss was cruelly compounded by several more that followed in its wake: the losses of home, family, country, culture, and livelihood. What Benjamin could not know then was that the misadventure with Friedmann would ultimately prove a blessing, sparing him many evils that were to come.

Chapter 4

A Glandular View of Life

In August 1921, Harry Benjamin gazed out the window of a train steaming up the Austrian Alps. The railroad was a triumph of nineteenth-century engineering that had thrust tunnels through mountains of gneiss, slate, and limestone and raised breathtaking viaducts across plunging valleys. In summer, its locomotives hauled wealthy Viennese high up the mountains to indulge in bracing sport or to take coffee on a terrace with panoramic views.

But Benjamin was not there for a vacation. In his compartment, he began a conversation with a fellow physician, explaining that the purpose of his trip to Semmering was to pay a visit to a most eminent personage. Since he had never met this man, Benjamin was a little worried he might have trouble recognizing him at the train station.

"Steinach," the local man replied. "Oh! I don't have to describe him. When you see him you'll know him. Everybody in Vienna does."

According to his amiable travel companion, Eugen Steinach was one of the most famous of the professors at the University of Vienna, feared by his students but the object of much civic pride as well. The doctor continued by regaling Benjamin with the latest Steinach joke to make the rounds in Vienna: A woman pushing a baby carriage bumps into an acquaintance. The friend is astonished. "But, I never knew you had a baby!" she says. "This isn't my baby," replies the woman. "This is my husband. He went to see Professor Steinach and the job was overdone." The joke revealed much, for it was precisely the truth behind the humor that Benjamin had come in search of: the possibility that aging might be reversed by science.

As they neared the alpine pass, Benjamin's companion tried to assure him about the prospect of meeting the esteemed professor: "He has done some great work. You'll spend some exciting time with him!"[1]

━━━━━

Exciting time indeed. Benjamin was in Europe for the first time since before the war, and one of his chief aims, beside visiting with family, was to meet Eugen Steinach, the renowned physiologist. Some months before, a Viennese colleague of Benjamin's had offered to make an introduction for him. Steinach had graciously responded by issuing an invitation to Benjamin to visit. By the time Benjamin was able to make his way to Vienna, Steinach was taking his vacation in the mountains, so he honored Benjamin with an invitation to meet with him there.

Looking back from our vantage and knowing of Benjamin's contributions to transgender medicine, it is tempting to see his meeting with Steinach as a pivotal moment in the development of his thought and career; after all, just a few years earlier, Steinach had produced stunning experimental evidence that had shaken scientific ideas about the fixity of biological sex. But this assumption would be somewhat misleading. Benjamin was foremost a practitioner and a pragmatist. He was less interested in the startling theoretical implications of Steinach's work on sex difference than in a practical application that had emerged from it, the procedure known as the Steinach operation for rejuvenation. Not only was this operation the butt of popular jokes, but it had aroused serious attention and controversy because of the claim that it could reverse the aging process. This claim, coming as it did from a respected physiology professor and backed by his thorough experimentation, was not easily dismissed as quackery.

Steinach was waiting at the station when Benjamin's train pulled in. With his impressive bearing, he was indeed unmistakable. He had sparkling dark eyes and a long gray-blond beard. At sixty, he was more than twenty years Benjamin's senior. Benjamin thought Steinach's head looked particularly imposing.

The two men left the station on foot and made their way up the mountainside through the cool of a pine forest to Steinach's hotel. During the hourlong walk, Steinach spoke quickly and animatedly about his work. The "Steinach operation," he explained, was a surgical procedure that essentially consisted of vasoligation—or tying off—of the vas deferens, the ducts that carry the spermatozoa from the testes to the urethra. At a microscopic level, you could make out two types of cells in the testes: the first functioned to make sperm, and the second, the interstitial cells, created the hormonal secretions of the testes.

Benjamin had already spent time at the library in Berlin reading Steinach's early papers in preparation for this meeting; he tried to interject that he already knew this but found he could not squeeze a word in.

Steinach plunged on at a rapid-fire pace. The interstitial tissue, he explained, could be thought of as the "puberty gland," since it began to function at the time of puberty. He stopped and hunted in his pockets for a scrap of paper. Ligating the vas deferens meant that no spermatozoa could be discharged, he explained, sketching the anatomical structures on the back of an envelope. This, he believed, created a back pressure that caused the sperm-generating cells to atrophy. This in turn allowed the interstitial cells to multiply greatly, so that they seemed to fill the entire testes. He quickly drew a view of how the testes looked under the microscope before and then a few weeks after a vasoligation. He stopped to see if Benjamin was following him. Benjamin nodded.

"Now you see the aging process has something to do with the testicular hormone production. When this production decreases, old age sets in. Maybe it isn't as simple as that, but in any event, the connection is there. The less testicular hormone the quicker the aging process. We have to revivify the aging puberty gland, and a rejuvenation of the other organs results." The results were striking. Rats who had been lethargic and underweight, almost lifeless, would just a few weeks after the operation grow glossy new coats, gain weight, become active, and regain an interest in sex.

Benjamin felt he had a thousand and one questions that day. The professor answered many of them and referred Benjamin to his new book, *Rejuvenation through Experimental Revivification of the Aging Puberty Gland*, which documented not only the remarkable experiments on rats and guinea pigs but three striking case histories as well. The first human patients to have undergone vasoligation were described as having experienced a restoration of their physical and mental abilities. Steinach cautioned Benjamin not to take the word "rejuvenation" too literally. But, he added, "if you would ever watch two rat brothers of the same age and the same litter, one treated and one untreated, you will find the justification for the word 'rejuvenation.'"[2]

As Benjamin made his way back to Vienna later that day, perhaps the scenes flashing past his train window reminded him of the last time he had been in the Alps. Fifteen years before, in August 1906, he had taken a tour alone through Austria and southern Germany. He was twenty-one and had completed two years of university. This was one of the few times in his life that Benjamin left us a true diary, written in a neat Fraktur script and locked with a tiny key. This diary gives us a peek into the mind of an unformed young man, at turns testy, superior, and annoyed by the frictions of travel in the company of strangers and at others achingly open to life.[3]

One morning, Benjamin joined a family he had met to climb the Edelboden. As the party made its way through the windless forest, two of his companions—a father and teenage son—bellowed back and forth as they spotted one organism after another. Benjamin grimaced internally. He thought their chatter might have been mildly interesting had it not been for the relentless parading of Latin scientific names. The path rose briskly over clay and craggy limestone. At times, the sun broke through the fog and glistened on the branches with a blinding abruptness. Suddenly, they emerged into an alpine meadow where a most beautiful aspect greeted them. The mountains were magnificent, partly forested, partly bare, and ranging ever higher to rocky summits. A glimpse of snow in summer delighted him, and the sight of numberless peaks stretching into the misty distance made Benjamin wax poetic of his impression of an infinite world—"der 'unendlichen Welt.'"[4]

But just where was his place to be in this infinite world? This was the question he would mull over during this solitary journey. There were glaciers, icy mountain lakes, and cavernous salt mines. A wizened proprietress at a dilapidated hut served him watered wine and bread, and Benjamin thought to himself that she could nicely serve as the witch in the story of Hansel and Gretel. There were days of drizzling rain, inedible meals, and some very fine ones as well. And for entertainment, there was a summer festival put on by volunteer firefighters and a less-than-satisfying performance of the operetta *Das Waschermädel* (The washer-girl). Benjamin deemed the music deplorable, the libretto unbelievable, and the singing coarse, but he was rather pleased that, through a stroke of good luck, he managed a clear view of the old Austrian emperor himself, Franz Josef.[5]

While to an observer, Benjamin's travels might have looked like an enviable grand tour, for the young man himself it masked an inner turmoil. The secret underpinning the entire summer was that Benjamin was struggling with an unrequited passion. At the start of his trip, he had had a meeting in Weichselboden with the woman he referred to in his diary as Mimi and her companion, whom he called Aunt Ludy. Mimi was older than he was and a musical comedy star. She was also a lesbian. Benjamin had held a deep passion for her but had as yet dared not say anything. For the rest of his alpine trip, he thought of her. The cruelly beautiful scenes he saw out his window mirrored his wounded spirit; the high mountains, though impressive, seemed stark and forbidding. In the dark, their wildness must certainly "press upon the heart," he imagined. Every place he stopped, he thought of the fact that Mimi and Ludy had traveled the same route the year before: here his beloved had praised the food; there she was filled with dread at the sudden onset of darkness. At the mountain refuge, the Schiestlhaus, the first thing he did was to locate her name in the guestbook. In his diary, he wrote of thoughts that caused his heart to bleed, and he cursed his faithful nature that had tied his heart to her.

But it was also a time to consider philosophical questions. At Mariazell, he found himself very put off by his visit to a Catholic church, and he ruminated about why he had found it so dislikable. Benjamin mused that he was not opposed to religious rites and in fact rather liked them when they were understood to be of a symbolic nature, but on this tour he found the ossuaries "ghastly" and the objects "sprinkled" by priests to be unpalatable. If he had to try to describe his worldview, he would say he regarded himself as a monist, that is, that he believed God is expressed *in* nature and is not above it. The monist philosophy was one that would have been current in his intellectual circles as a man of science, inspired by the example of leading figures such as the physicist Ernst Mach and the chemist Wilhelm Ostwald. For Benjamin, it meant that he felt confident that all phenomena could be adequately explained through the laws of chemistry and physics alone, without resort to supernatural explanations. Above all, he thought reason should predominate. Here, we see one important side to his intellectual makeup, one that would shape his ideas for his whole life: his commitment to finding natural, biological causes for the phenomena of life. But his diary reflected a lack of dogmatism as well, an openness to an unknowable future. Whether or not he would always be a monist, he wrote, he did not know. "After all, at the age of twenty-one, I am not a finished man and not yet at the height of human understanding." It may well be that he would change his mind, he admitted—though he rather doubted it.[6]

Now in 1921, he was back in Europe for the first time since he had gone to the United States in 1913. At the age of thirty-six, he looked as trim and neat as he had when he had first left. His forehead was still unlined, though it had, year by year, inched steadily upward. He had been able to afford this journey thanks to a commission he had to bring a young female patient and her mother to Europe to consult a specialist. Once the patient was safely delivered, he was free to pursue his own interests.[7]

When he had visited Vienna all those years ago, it had been the fabled, cultured center of half of Europe, at the heart of a realm comprising fifteen nations and over 50 million inhabitants speaking a dozen different languages. He remembered it as the "gayest capitol of Europe," rivaling Paris in its beauty and in its accomplishments in the art of living. It had been, moreover, the center of modernist thought and culture, a place where writers, artists, composers, philosophers, physicians, and scientists traveled in tight-knit, interconnected circles. More so than the intelligentsia in London, Paris, New York, and Berlin, intellectuals in Vienna formed friendships across disciplinary boundaries and regularly interacted at the great salons of elite women.[8]

But after the Great War, Vienna had become a capital without an empire. Two-thirds of the Austro-Hungarian Empire had been stripped away, and in its place was a new republic. The devastating effects of the war were evident in its streets and its people. Spiraling inflation had wiped out the savings of many in the middle class. Refugees poured into the city, along with former soldiers of the Imperial Army. The Viennese were plagued by high unemployment, hunger and poverty, raging tuberculosis, syphilis, and the Spanish flu. So, for Steinach and other biologists in Vienna, the work of reviving the human body was not an abstract intellectual goal but a pressing, concrete need. Rejuvenation was not just a question of personal aspiration but an urgent social imperative.[9] As medical writer Van Buren Thorne observed in the *New York Times*, rejuvenation was of serious interest to the best of European citizenry precisely because of the ruthless wastage of the Great War. The writer and impresario Frida Strindberg passionately spoke of Vienna, once a famous medical center, now in its "stirring sunset glory," and of its continuing contribution to science: "I know nothing so grandiose and at the same time so touching as this half-starved city, with its doomed little children reaching out life to the world through Eugen Steinach, simply, nobly, as though it were a matter of course."[10]

Benjamin now found Vienna "depressing and depressed," the contrast between the glories of the past and the bleak realities of the present laid bare. Still, Benjamin found traces of beauty and gaiety here and there; he felt the Viennese managed to mingle their sense of futility with some of their old love of life, though it was now touched with a certain grim humor. At the same time, there was optimism about the possibility of social and political reform. The country's first democratic government, led by the Social Democratic Party, intervened at an unprecedented level to create public housing and social welfare programs, including childcare and healthcare initiatives that dramatically reduced infant mortality and tuberculosis rates. A deep interest in science and medicine flourished as well as a continued devotion to music, art, and theater. Many intellectuals thrived in this setting, including the founder of psychoanalysis, Sigmund Freud, psychiatrist Alfred Adler, writer and playwright Arthur Schnitzler, economist and social philosopher Karl Polanyi, philosopher Ludwig Wittgenstein, and composer Arnold Schoenberg.

In August 1921, after his memorable meeting in the mountains with Steinach, Benjamin made his way to Steinach's laboratory in Vienna, at the world-famous Biologische Versuchsanstalt (Institute for Experimental Biology), where Steinach had arranged for colleagues to show Benjamin around. This facility must have seemed a palace of scientific wonders to Benjamin's eyes.

Steinach's laboratory was housed in the shadow of a Ferris wheel in the Prater, Vienna's vast public park, in a building that was known colloquially as the "Vivarium" for the golden inscription above the main entrance. Built for the Vienna World Exposition of 1873, the structure had originally served as a public aquarium; in time, creatures such as crocodiles, monkeys, and various amphibians and marsupials had been added. In 1902, the building—which had by then become run-down—was purchased by zoologist Hans Leo Przibram and botanists Leopold von Portheim and Wilhelm Figdor, who turned it into a privately owned biological research institute. The three founders were part of a thriving Jewish haute bourgeoisie that valued culture and intellectual endeavors and were willing to invest their own money toward these ends. In contrast to the laboratories at the University of Vienna, which were underfunded and tied to traditional, static approaches to natural history, the Vivarium exemplified a modern, dynamic, and experimental approach to biology. Instead of collecting shelves of preserved specimens, the founders and their associates created a state-of-the-art facility where they learned to breed and house a vast array of living plants and animals. Their belief was that the fearsome complexity of life could ultimately be distilled into the language of mathematics and that biological phenomena could be properly understood only through the collaborative efforts of researchers in botany, zoology, chemistry, and physics. Moreover, Steinach, biologist Paul Kammerer, and their associates were committed to exploring the fluidity of the developmental process and the role of hormones in its control.[11]

In 1914, the founders had donated the institute, along with a generous endow-
ment to support its work, to the Imperial Academy of Science in Austria, making
it the largest ever private financial gift to science in the country. The institute
had survived the Great War, but since then, money for research had become
scarce. By the time of Benjamin's visit in 1921, the work of the fabled institution
was suffering. Benjamin was met by Kammerer, Steinach's laboratory neighbor
who was working alone in spacious halls that were now almost deserted. Benjamin liked him at once. Kammerer, just five years older than he, struck Benjamin as a person of both great kindness and intellect. He had large, expressive
eyes beneath tousled gray hair, though Benjamin—who was always particular
about his dress—mused that the biologist's rumpled lab coat could have used
some rejuvenation itself. Those impressions faded into insignificance, though,
as Kammerer flashed a pleasant smile and offered to take Benjamin on a tour.[12]

Most other institutes of experimental biology kept only a small number of
model organisms for their studies. At the Vivarium, however, there were almost
300 different species, from protozoa, sea squirts, fish, snakes, and geckos, to 7
species of birds and 23 of mammals. It was Kammerer's passion and vast experience in the keeping of animals that made the Vivarium truly stand out. Even as
a university student, he had kept a menagerie in his parents' apartment of over
200 species gathered from around the world. His special ability to breed these
creatures and to keep them alive over many years gave the Vivarium researchers
an unparalleled ability to trace shifts in physical form over time and to probe the
mechanisms of inheritance. His experiments required such painstaking, long-
term animal care that replicating his work was challenging for other researchers.

Kammerer made a special stop at the cages holding Steinach's rejuvenated
rats. Benjamin was startled by the striking difference between the control animals and the test subjects. Surely they couldn't really be the same age? Might
there be some mistake? No, Kammerer explained; the animals had been reared
in the Vivarium and were all carefully registered and closely observed throughout their lives. There could be no mistake.

"They really are rejuvenated," he assured him.

Steinach's young assistant, Berthold Wiesner, showed Benjamin the microscopic sections of normal testicles and those from animals that had been vasoligated. The slides from the vasoligated animals clearly showed a marked increase
in interstitial cells. Wiesner called Steinach's procedure "a royal thought."

Kammerer then took Benjamin to see the animals representing Steinach's
earlier research—what Steinach had referred to the previous day as his "old

stuff"—published eight to nine years earlier. In these studies, Steinach had transplanted ovaries into castrated, immature male rats and found that they had become "feminized": they developed breasts and nipples and even began to show maternal behaviors, such as suckling their young and allowing themselves to be pursued by males. They were also perceived as female by other male rats who attempted to mate with them. Steinach had also carried out the reverse procedure, transplanting testes into ovariectomized, immature female rats; he found that they developed male characteristics and behaviors. What was particularly significant was that the cross-sex characteristics included not only physical changes but behavioral ones. Moreover, the glands seemed to be antagonistic to each other: when the ovaries were transplanted into the castrated male, they not only produced female characteristics but suppressed male characteristics, such as the growth of the penis. Benjamin had read the papers detailing these experiments and was very impressed to see these feminized and masculinized rats and guinea pigs for himself.[13]

Steinach's work emerged from a fundamental insight that radically challenged prevailing notions of the difference between the sexes. In the late nineteenth century, investigators such as the distinguished French physiologist Charles-Édouard Brown-Séquard had begun to question the assumption that the qualities of masculinity and femininity resided in the gonads, the organs of reproduction. He postulated that these qualities came not from the testes or ovaries per se but from an "internal secretion" that these gonads produced. In 1889, Brown-Séquard reported that he had treated himself with injections of an extract he had created from the testicles of guinea pigs and dogs, which resulted in his renewed vigor and mental clarity. Gynecologists of the time saw that his idea of internal secretions could also be applied to female sex organs and the treatment of women's reproductive disorders. Brown-Séquard's work led to a growing interest in "organotherapy," that is, in using extracts of animal tissues and organs as a medical treatment.[14]

Steinach and his fellow Viennese Julius Tandler—working independently of each other—developed these ideas further. A prevalent line of thought in the study of sex difference was that the characteristics of adult men and women were dictated by the attributes of their gametes, their sperm or their eggs. Men, like sperm, were quick, active, and competitive, while women, like their eggs, were passive and nurturing. Steinach and Tandler instead promoted an idea drawn from the work of anatomists that showed the gonads actually contained two glands, the distinct cells of which could be detected under a microscope. One of these glands served the function of reproduction—producing the eggs or sperm—but a separate gland controlled sexual characteristics. One important implication of this was that sexuality of women, like that of men, was controlled not by their reproductive activities but rather by the hormones produced in a separate gland; among other things, it meant that they, like men, could have a sex drive.[15]

It is easy to imagine Benjamin wandering through these halls, entranced. He was far from New York's Upper East Side, but the speculations about glands, sexuality, and aging that had played in his head since those Wednesday night meetings in Joseph Fraenkel's office must have seemed to take on a fleshy reality in the Vivarium.

Steinach's research on aging was not derived from some misguided search for a fountain of youth. Rather, it was the logical outcome of a well-respected and broadly conceived research program that stood on firm scientific grounds. But applying the findings of animal experiments to humans was not straightforward, especially when they involved complex phenomena with a strong subjective component. How does a scientist exclude the effect of human psychology and the all-too-human ability to fool ourselves and others? Steinach, a cool-eyed experimentalist, realized that if he were to prove his theory on humans, he would have to find a way to rule out the power of suggestion. In 1918, he had collaborated with his longtime associate the urologist Robert Lichtenstern to try to find out whether aging men could be rejuvenated as easily as laboratory rats. Lichtenstern, who was impressed by Steinach's experimental results, agreed to tie off the vas deferens of three men he was operating on for other health concerns but without letting his patients know they were receiving the "Steinach operation." Then, he watched and waited. One by one, the patients reported improvements. One, a forty-four-year-old coachman, had come to Lichtenstern displaying signs of premature senility with dulling skin, graying hair, and loss of weight and appetite. He had found himself unable to work for long hours. After the operation, there was initially no change. But slowly, gradually, the patient improved. His appetite increased and he gained weight. Soon, he reported that he could easily pick up loads of 220 pounds. A year and a half later, he looked youthful and vital again and had such a luxuriant growth of beard that he needed to shave twice a day. When these results were reported to the medical community, they caused a sensation. Many surgeons soon came to study with Steinach and his associates. The Steinach operation spread quickly; by 1923, the *New York Times* would report that every major American and European city had several surgeons offering the operation.[16]

After Benjamin's visit to the Vivarium, he went to the Allgemeine Kranken-haus (Vienna General Hospital) to meet Dr. Erwin Horner, the assistant professor of surgery, one of Steinach's collaborators. Benjamin found him modest, competent, and kind. Horner allowed Benjamin to watch him operate, and then he procured cadavers from the Anatomical Institute so that Benjamin could practice vasoligation several times under his supervision. Benjamin learned to locate one of the two vas deferens by feeling for a hard strand in the scrotum and then to incise the skin and carefully lay the muscular strand free from the surrounding tissue, taking care not to injure the blood vessels and nerves. Finally, he completed the procedure by tying the duct with a length of silk thread.

Benjamin found a warm personal welcome from Kammerer, who invited him to his home on a Saturday for a frugal meal prepared by his sister-in-law.[17] This would be the start of a heartfelt friendship. Benjamin also met with the brilliant young Berlin physician Peter Schmidt, who was one of Steinach's most eager followers and who also became a good friend. Toward the end of his stay, Benjamin paid a visit to the laboratory of the world-famous radiologist Professor Guido Holzknecht. A researcher in the early days of X-ray science, Holzknecht would become a martyr to his work, dying of radiation poisoning ten years later. When Benjamin met him, Holzknecht had just had another finger amputated, burned in the course of his experiments; Benjamin would always remember his poor injured hands. Holzknecht told Benjamin that he had been very impressed by Steinach's results in the rejuvenation of men and that he believed that women too might be rejuvenated, but with one important difference: instead of a surgical procedure, the ovaries were treated with X-rays. He said he had noted similar rejuvenating effects in the women he had treated in this way. On his final afternoon, Benjamin was introduced to Steinach's "Case Number One," the first "rejuvenate" he had ever met. The patient was a strapping middle-aged male who, full of enthusiasm, told Benjamin that the operation had made him a man again.[18]

Just before Benjamin left Vienna, Steinach returned from Semmerling.

"Before you go I have to acquaint you with something that is more import-ant than all the dead and living rats—young, old, or rejuvenated," the professor announced.

"What is that?" Benjamin asked.

"You'll see," Steinach smiled.

That night, Steinach took Benjamin to the Griechenbeisl, the oldest restaurant in Vienna, in a picturesque medieval building bounded by narrow, cobblestone lanes. Founded in the fifteenth century and tucked into the oldest part of the city, the restaurant proved to be everything the professor had promised, from the sawdust on the floor to its excellent *Kalbsbraten* (roast veal) and beer.

Though he was much in awe of Steinach, Benjamin would come to be a devoted acolyte. The two men would correspond for decades. For years to come, Benjamin would make an annual summer visit to the Vivarium, and no visit was complete without a dinner where the good food and good conversation reminded him of what really mattered.[19]

During his stay, Benjamin would have been surrounded by the shattering, disruptive strains of modernism. In the dissonant music of Arnold Schoenberg, the spare, functional architecture of Otto Wagner, or the philosophy of the Vienna Circle, he might have seen the orderly worldview of his childhood crumble. In Freud's Vienna, however, perhaps the most haunting note would have been from the great interpreter of dreams himself, who suggested that even our innermost selves are hidden from us. Steinach and his associates were beginning to articulate just how motivations and drives were carried in the fluids of the glands, challenging the notion of people as captains of their own destinies. And in his experiments on the sex organs, Steinach was beginning to break down one of the most fundamental pair of categories by which humans arrange themselves: male and female. Benjamin's visit to Vienna would mark a sharp turn in his career trajectory. Whatever skepticism he might have felt about the more dramatic claims of the rejuvenation enthusiasts, from that point, he would be a follower of Eugen Steinach.

Chapter 5

A Science of Sex

Before he returned to New York, there was one more important visit that Harry Benjamin needed to pay. In the autumn of 1921, he made his way to a large, gracious villa overlooking the Tiergarten in Berlin, home to the Institut für Sexualwissenschaft (Institute for Sexual Science). The institute, established in 1919 by physician and sexologist Magnus Hirschfeld, was the first in the world dedicated to the scientific study of sex. For a brief glorious time, it drew poets and politicians, experts and ordinary seekers from around the globe, anyone who was interested in trying to understand sexuality in its many variations. Here, Benjamin would learn how Eugen Steinach's experimental work on the relation of hormones to biological sex could find practical expression.

Same-sex attraction and sexual behavior has existed through history and across cultures, but in Western society, the notion that people who felt such attractions and engaged in these acts were a particular *type* of person developed only in the nineteenth century. In Germany, the term "homosexual" was coined to describe such individuals, and Berlin became a focal point for the emergence of the idea of an innate homosexual identity and the struggle for homosexual rights. Beginning with the activism of the lawyer Karl Heinrich Ulrichs in 1867, the movement for homosexual rights took root in Germany, thanks to progressive forces that were fostered by German idealism and Romanticism. It was in this context that the first homosexual magazine, *Der Eigene* (The self-owning), was founded in 1896. The following year, Hirschfeld cofounded the Scientific-Humanitarian

Committee, the world's first homosexual rights organization, which was guided by the motto "Justice through science." Hirschfeld worked tirelessly for the repeal of Paragraph 175 of the German penal code, which criminalized sodomy. On a practical and legal level, the benign approach of Berlin police commissioner Leopold von Meerscheidt-Hüllessem also helped a homosexual subculture to flourish. The criminal code prohibited specific acts but not same-sex socialization or the places in which this happened. Beginning in 1885 with his creation of a Department of Pederasty, Meerscheidt-Hüllessem gave up prosecution of the city's same-sex bars and dance halls. He was on a first-name basis with many of those who frequented these bars, and he and his associates offered counseling to men who found themselves victims of blackmail. His example was continued into the early years of the twentieth century by subsequent police officials—Hans von Tresckow, Heinrich Kopp, and Bernhard Strewe—who headed the department with the same open-minded attitude and who had good relations with Hirschfeld.[1]

By the time of his visit, Benjamin had been a friend of Hirschfeld's for a decade and a half, a result of his early curiosity about sexual matters. Sex was never discussed in Benjamin's family except that his father had handed him an article warning about the dangers of masturbation, which included blindness and insanity. Benjamin later recollected to a colleague that he had not understood the article at all, but the message must have had some impact because he claimed, "I never masturbated."[2] In his student days, Benjamin began to open to the gritty realities beyond the walls of his bourgeois home and elite private school. Berlin was home to a vibrant night life. In the cabarets of the working class, the risqué and reprobate flourished. While tourists were told that the ladies might enjoy the cafés on Friedrichstrasse near their grand hotels, the gentlemen were advised to leave their wives behind when they toured the nightclubs of the industrial areas, where the more scandalous acts could be found. There was no red-light district or officially sanctioned brothels, but prostitution burgeoned. In Berlin, the sex workers typically employed a characteristic walk combined with a distinct look to signal to prospective clients as they strolled past cafés and restaurants.

Berlin was also home to great artistic ferment. Benjamin found himself deeply affected by theater, which forged his understanding of sexuality in a profound way. He was especially struck by the work of legendary director Max Reinhardt, who transformed directing into an art form. Reinhardt's 1903 production of Maxim Gorki's *Nachtasyl* (The lower depths) opened Benjamin's eyes to the harsh existence of people the likes of whom had never been seen onstage before; it featured derelicts and drifters, a prostitute, a thief, a card sharp, and a self-styled aristocrat whose lives collide one night in a foul lodging house. The story was bleak, un-redemptive, and morally ambiguous. Benjamin would particularly remember the 1906 premiere of Reinhardt's production of Frank Wedekind's *Spring Awakening,* which shocked its audience for its frank depiction of child abuse, rape, masturbation, homosexuality, suicide, and abortion among its teenage protagonists. The play was a forthright critique of the sexually oppressive culture of the nineteenth century and a plea for sex education, arguing that hypocrisy and oppressiveness could only result in sexuality becoming distorted in horrific ways. This message would have resonated with Benjamin. He had known a young man of nineteen—"splendid," he called him—who had been just about to enter the University of Berlin when he contracted syphilis as a result of his first sexual encounter. The young man had been raised by puritanical parents and had no understanding of sex except for what he had been able to glean from the other boys. He felt so guilty that he concealed his worsening symptoms until the spirochetes had wormed their way throughout his system. When he died six months later, his father clung to the belief that this death was a just punishment by the Almighty.[3]

A turning point in the formation of Benjamin's views came with the 1906 publication *The Sexual Question* by the Swiss neurologist and psychiatrist Auguste Forel. The book treated questions such as premarital sex, homosexuality, prostitution, and venereal disease in an unusually forthright manner, and Benjamin found its views refreshingly objective and commonsense. Forel emphasized that sexuality was beautiful, not shameful. When Forel came to Berlin, Benjamin eagerly attended his lecture even though the subject matter was the life of the ant, since myrmecology was another focus of Forel's research. At the close of the talk, Benjamin approached Forel and introduced himself. The Swiss expert generously spent ten minutes speaking with him, but Benjamin was rather disappointed that Forel, an avowed teetotaler, spent more time urging him to abstain from alcohol than discussing questions of sexuality.[4]

Benjamin's curiosity would lead him to Hirschfeld in about 1906 or 1907. As Benjamin later explained, a "girl friend" of his had introduced him to Heinrich Kopp, then the *Kriminalkommissar* (chief inspector) of the Berlin police who was in charge of investigating sexual offenses. Kopp in turn introduced Benjamin to Hirschfeld. Benjamin admired Hirschfeld's tremendous courage in his

efforts at reform.[5] Berlin was then the home to a great flourishing of gay and
gender-diverse culture, so much so that homosexuality was known elsewhere
as "the German disease." There was, however, still a great deal of secrecy and
hypocrisy surrounding the issue of homosexuality. Homosexual activity was
well known and secretly tolerated among the Prussian officer class, but in 1906
this code of silence was breached when a radical newspaper broke a story accus-
ing a close friend of the kaiser, Prince of Eulenburg, of a homosexual liaison with
another favored courtier, Count von Moltke, leading to a series of scandalous
and highly publicized civil trials and courts-martial in which Hirschfeld played
a prominent role as an expert witness.[6]

Hirschfeld testified in the hope of promoting his theory that homosexuality
was a natural variation rather than a disease or a sin. Unfortunately, the trial
instead led to an ugly backlash against homosexuals and against Hirschfeld.
Hirschfeld's identity as a Jew was also used against him in critiques marked by a
vicious anti-Semitism. Hirschfeld's courage in continuing this struggle was not
diminished even after he was beaten so badly by a group of thugs in 1920 that it
was widely reported that he died.

Hirschfeld was a pioneer in trying to understand homosexuality on a scientific basis, describing it in medical terms rather than as a moral issue. His goal in
doing this was emancipatory. He regularly took academics and foreign writers
through Berlin's nightlife in the hopes of educating them and persuading them
to his view that homosexuals were not a threat to society. Hirschfeld himself was
homosexual, though not openly so. The police chief inspector Kopp, though not
homosexual, was, according to Benjamin, a serious student of sex issues and
sympathetic to the plight of homosexuals. Hirschfeld and Kopp took the young
Benjamin with them on their rounds of the city's blooming gay subculture,
including the famous nightclub the Eldorado with its glittering drag show, where
Hirschfeld was greeted as "Tante Magnesia."[7]

What had drawn Benjamin to Hirschfeld? In one sense it is obvious that Benjamin was a curious and adventurous young man, consorting with artists and
bohemians in a setting of great intellectual and cultural ferment. On an emotional level, perhaps his own experience at school of being accepted neither
as a Jew nor as a Christian gave him a particular sympathy for those who lived
on the margins of society. We might also wonder whether he was discover-
ing something of his own sexual yearnings that might have inclined him to be

sympathetic to those whose sexuality expressed itself in unorthodox ways. His familiarity with homosexuality seems to have been limited. When he had been about fourteen or fifteen, another boy had approached him in the study room; he had initially failed to understand what the other boy intended, but when he realized that the boy was making sexual overtures, he grew annoyed because they had been good friends until then. He described to an interviewer, years later, that there was another incident in which a homosexual had "desperately tried to seduce" him after dinner in a café, but we know nothing more about this episode. Rather, I suspect that Benjamin's romantic obsession with Mimi might have played a significant role in shaping his interest. Judging from his diaries, this fixation consumed much of his imagination and energies through his early twenties. Perhaps Mimi was even the "girl friend" that Benjamin described as having facilitated the introduction to Kopp and Hirschfeld. Could Benjamin's early intellectual interest in sexual variance have been stoked by his fervent wish to understand Mimi's sexuality as a lesbian and his vain hope that she might somehow be able to return his feelings for her?[8]

As a premedical student in Rostock, he had spent the winter in the wind-swept Baltic seaport unburdening his heart in his diary, saying everything he did not have the courage to say to Mimi in life. He waited in agony for her replies to his letters and, after his grueling preliminary exams were over, rushed home to Berlin to see her, only to experience the familiar cycle of "heavenly exultation" plunging into "deathly distress"—the exultation only seldom and even then not genuine; the distress day in, day out. When he was newly returned to civilian life after his military service, he took a blow when Mimi told him not to come to see her anymore. The following day, he walked around in such a daze that he failed to properly salute his superior officer. Still on reserve, he was put under *Mittelarrest* for three long days of detention, alone with his wretched thoughts. In his diary, he thought back to the meeting he had with Mimi in Weichsel-boden: "You must think me so weak and effeminate," he said to the Mimi of his imagination. But, he reasoned, isn't it always the case that every man has something of the feminine in him, and every woman some masculine?[9] He was, however, most disappointed in himself and his lack of courage. He learned from a newspaper that Mimi had left town, and he followed her to Paris and Frankfurt. There, he finally managed a confession of his feelings in the presence of Ludy. Ludy, he thought, understood a little, though she felt perhaps only the pity that a husband who loves his wife—and knows she loves him—might feel when a friend confesses to have fallen in love with her. That confrontation was followed by a terrible night on a train, followed by more weeks of wild fantasies, "castles in the air," sentimentality straining against cautious reason, and all of it "built on an infinite longing."[10]

As his medical studies had drawn to a close, Benjamin plucked up his courage to reveal his feelings to Mimi and propose marriage.[11] Combing through his diaries from three years before, he felt a grim satisfaction in finding evidence that his feelings for her had not changed, not even an atom. When after many months he was able to see her in person again, his mind became overwhelmed and his words jumbled, knowing that so much depended on the outcome. She unexpectedly argued back. He found himself unable to mount a defense. In frustration, she told him to write out his feelings. More letters followed and more anxious waiting. He worried to himself that she had misunderstood him and that she assumed a man would want her only for her body. In his diary he protested that his love was not merely physical. Of course, he had a great respect for healthy sensuality—"it is the world-conserving principle," he said, and he would not be a normal man if there were not an element of this in his love for her—but sexual desire was only in the background to a love from the heart that was so intense he sometimes felt frightened by it. He offered her the best and the noblest of which he was capable. But at long last a reply came from Mimi and with it clarity. She completely understood him, and she rejected him, unambiguously. For Benjamin, all hope was shattered. He was left with only a dull sensation and the remembrance of their last farewell at the station, her half-turned face glimpsed through the window as the train pulled away, her harsh nod, and finally her indifference. Now, all that was left for him was to endure and to anesthetize his pain through work. He counted her the great love of his life, and he never saw her again.[12]

From the late nineteenth century, people who felt same-sex attraction or engaged in same-sex acts began to be described by various terms including "urnings," "inverts," and "homosexuals." The characterization of homosexuals included not only same-sex attraction but gendered qualities of physiognomy and behavior. Different schools of thought arose about the nature and character of homosexuals. One line of reasoning, based on German youth movements, described male homosexuality and homosocial activities as the outgrowth of male-centered culture and characterized men who preferred sex with other men as highly masculine. An alternate school of thought held that same-sex attraction was linked to cross-gender physical and psychological characteristics—that is, that male homosexuals were more feminine than other men, while lesbians were more mannish than other women. Ulrichs had characterized the homosexual male as "a female soul in a male body." Hirschfeld ascribed to this second school of thought and, moreover, believed it to be supported by recent scientific research. Beginning in 1897, on his first petition to the Reichstag, he argued that studies of embryonic development suggested that homosexuality was the result of a congenital error and as such was an involuntary condition and therefore not a legal or moral issue. Homosexuality did not fall under the category of a disease, though, according to this reasoning, it might still be likened to a developmental anomaly such as a cleft palate.[13]

Extending Ulrich's concept of homosexuality as a blending of male and female, Hirschfeld developed a doctrine of sexual intermediaries in which gendered identity and sexual attraction exist along a spectrum. In his clinical studies, he documented not only differences in sexual desire but what he felt were subtle morphological characteristics of homosexual males that distinguished them from heterosexual men. For example, he asserted that among his homosexual subjects, many had wider hips, less facial and body hair, smaller hands, and rounder contours than the average man. He proposed that each individual contains a blend of male and female physical and psychological characteristics and argued that there were potentially an infinite number of possible intermediate types. This was a theory that was eagerly taken up by activists for homosexual emancipation and, because of its scientific tone, circulated quickly among medical professionals as well, though it was not always accepted.[14]

Individuals who cross-dressed had been categorized as homosexuals. But in Hirschfeld's tours of the Berlin bars and clubs, he had come to know many people who challenged these conceptions and forced him to rethink this way of classifying people. His growing perspective that cross-dressers were not necessarily homosexual came as the result of years of sometimes angry exchanges with cross-dressers. In 1910, Hirschfeld disrupted the traditional categorization by introducing the term "transvestite" to describe men who dressed as women or women who dressed as men, arguing that how a person experienced or expressed themselves as men or women was a phenomenon that was distinct from whether they were sexually attracted to the same or other sex. These ideas were set out in his book *Die Transvestiten* (The transvestites).[15]

From 1912, Hirschfeld had begun to speculate about the chemical nature of sexual behavior and gender. Just before the Great War, he traveled to visit

Steinach in Vienna and was able to view the masculinized and feminized rats and guinea pigs at the Vivarium, just as Benjamin would do some years later. Hirschfeld recognized that Steinach's laboratory results had direct implications for his own attempts to disentangle sexual phenomena among humans. Steinach in turn learned from Hirschfeld's clinical experiences and believed that his findings on cross-sex transplantation could be applied to human phenomena. In addition to transplanting testes into castrated females and ovaries into castrated males, Steinach conducted experiments in which he transplanted both testes and ovaries into the same animals. In most cases, one or other of the grafts failed, but in a small number of animals, both glands survived, creating striking experimental hermaphrodites. Steinach suggested that homosexuality and hermaphroditism were caused by the production of both male and female secretions in the gonads. His conclusions were reinforced by Hirschfeld's clinical work suggesting that male homosexuals not only desired men sexually but also had subtle physical features that he felt showed they were "feminized" in their bodies as well.[16]

Hirschfeld's 1914 work *Die Homosexualität des Mannes und des Weibes* (*The Homosexuality of Man and Woman*) was hailed by pioneering British sexologist Havelock Ellis as the largest and "most precise, detailed, and comprehensive" work on the subject. Hirschfeld made numerous distinctions—between same-sex practices that were "situational" and those that were "constitutional," between individuals who might wish to wear the clothes of the other sex and others who, given their character, might be considered to actually belong to the other sex—and he postulated that some individuals, such as the author George Sand, might be considered to have no fixed gender at all.[17]

Defining sex and sexuality in terms of hormones brought the possibility of fluidity rather than fixity and of infinite gradation rather than an absolute male/female binary. But defining homosexuality as a biological variation was a double-edged sword. While Hirschfeld believed that finding scientific proof that homosexuality was based in biology was the best route to securing freedom from persecution for homosexuals, an alternate conclusion was also possible. If homosexuality was the result of varying concentrations of glandular secretions, could and should homosexuality be "treated" by medical manipulation of these secretions?

Steinach strongly believed that science could and should be used to treat homosexuality. He extrapolated from his early work to speculate about whether homosexuality could be "corrected" using a glandular transplant. Could the testes of a homosexual man be removed and replaced with the glands of a "normal" man? Steinach engaged his colleague the urologist Robert Lichtenstern to do this operation on a young homosexual man who had to have his testes removed because of tuberculosis. In 1918, they reported that the man developed heterosexual desires and had gone on to marry a woman less than a year later. Steinach and Lichtenstern rejected the possibility that these changes could have happened through the power of suggestion, arguing that the patient also showed physical signs of a more masculinized body. Given the scarcity of human testicles for such transplants, few of these operations were done, but there was a brief interest in these types of grafting operations. While there were some reports of initial successes, ultimately this endeavor would prove a complete failure. Medical scientists and physicians disputed whether Steinach could really have observed changes he claimed to see at the cellular level. More importantly, any behavioral changes observed in the transplant recipients soon dissipated. By the mid-1920s, the results were clearly so poor that surgeons who had attempted these procedures gave them up entirely. Hirschfeld's beliefs and practices in these matters were at times inconsistent. He tended to believe that homosexuality should not be treated, though in some cases, when his patients wanted very much to be "cured," he did refer them to Steinach. Initially he had thought that the experimental results seemed remarkable, but he argued that even if "curing" homosexuality were scientifically possible, it was not justifiable. By 1930, Hirschfeld reported that he was unable to find a single successful case of a lasting effect in the scientific literature.[18] Whatever its nature, homosexuality appeared to be tenacious.

After the war, in the newly liberal atmosphere of Weimar Germany, Hirschfeld gained support for his efforts from the social democratic government. In 1919, he achieved a longtime dream of establishing the Institute for Sexual Science, which was the first of its kind in the world. Through the 1920s, the institute was a magnet for visitors from around the world, drawing top researchers and collaborators as well as members of the public who wanted to learn about sexuality. Guided tours of the library and museum became a popular Berlin tourist attraction. At the institute, research, clinical services, public education, public policy, and advocacy were brought together. The facility housed over forty staffers in many fields of medical research as well as clinical services such as marriage counseling, treatment of venereal disease, and birth control. These activities allowed Hirschfeld to make a systematic collection of empirical data about sexuality in its many variations. The library and archive came to hold an unprecedented trove of information comprising thousands of questionnaires. The institute also had a mission to bring an understanding of sexuality to the broader public, which it did through a series of public lectures, film programs, and the publication of journals and pamphlets. It additionally provided academic-level programs for students, physicians, lawyers, teachers, nurses, and police officers. Investigations were made into biology, psychology, psychiatry, ethnography, and anthropology.[19]

The social atmosphere of the institute was joyful, transgressive, and at times startling, even to those who considered themselves avant-garde. The furnishings were described by visiting writer Christopher Isherwood as "classic, pillared, garlanded, their marble massive, their curtains solemnly sculpted, their engravings grave."[20] A photograph from the period shows Hirschfeld with his bushy mustache in a lighthearted moment, collapsed in a heap with a dozen or so denizens of the institute, variously arrayed in attire for a costume ball. They lounge, draped over one another for a moment of calm repose. At lunch, researchers paused their work and gathered with patients and visitors for convivial meals. But more than this, the institute brought together the scientific study of sex with advocacy for the rights of sexual minorities. It frequently served as a refuge from violence for sexually variant and gender-diverse individuals and offered legal advice and asylum for those accused of sex crimes.[21] The close cooperation of police and reformers during this period can be seen in the fact that Hirschfeld was able to create "transvestite passes" that served as identification to prevent the arrest of cross-dressing individuals on the grounds of public nuisance or impersonation. The institute had a large number of female domestic workers, many of whom were transgender individuals who would have had difficulty finding employment elsewhere. Some were patients who worked temporarily to pay for their treatment or rent.[22]

In 1921, Benjamin would become another in the long line of visitors to the institute. Having been introduced to Berlin's queer subculture by Hirschfeld long ago, Benjamin must have felt fairly comfortable in the presence of the transgender members of the institute's community. We do not know very much about his impressions of what he saw except that this visit reignited for him an interest in sexology, which had lain dormant for several years. He was warmly received and introduced to several of Hirschfeld's associates, including psychiatrist Arthur Kronfeld, physician Felix Abraham, and dermatologist and urologist Bernhard Schapiro. During his time in New York, Benjamin had not been able to find much literature on sex, and only the growing interest in psychoanalysis had kept the scientific study of sexuality alive for him. This was a time when Freud's books could still not be sold openly in the United States. Benjamin's visit would become the first of many that he would make to Hirschfeld and the institute through the next decade. He spent many hours at Hirschfeld's lectures, and more than once he would take part in the official tours of the institute and its museum. Benjamin greatly admired Hirschfeld's courageous efforts at reform, his popular publications of pamphlets and books, and his willingness to appear in court to testify for homosexuals. He regarded him as "the outstanding sexologist of his day." But Benjamin, always a careful dresser, found that Hirschfeld's sloppy clothing and bushy walrus mustache as well as his stinginess somewhat detracted from his appeal.[23]

Just before he left for home, Benjamin took part in a stimulating and significant conference. Hirschfeld believed that there were two requirements for homosexual emancipation: the first was the recognition of homosexuality as a biological variation, and the second was the integration of the homosexual movement with other sex reform movements, such as those for birth control, abortion rights, and marriage reform. For this reason, he organized the First International Congress for Sexual Reform on the Basis of Sexual Science, which was held 15–20 September 1921 in the heart of Berlin at the Langenbeck-Virchow-Haus, the newly opened home of the Berlin Medical Association and German Surgical Society. This meeting gave Benjamin an exciting opportunity to meet many other researchers, clinicians, and reformers in sexology. Talks included "Love in the Light of Experimental Biology," "Marriage Reform," "Origin of the Story of the Stork," and "Ceremonies among Primeval Tribes." Hirschfeld addressed the congress, expressing his hope that this event marked just the beginning of intensive research into love and sexual life. Scientists, he argued, must not be swayed by theologians or moralists but follow the implications of their research. Should that research show a belief in the sinfulness of love or sexual relations to be wrong, then scientists must demand a change in these views. His motto, he declared, was "Truth above everything." There were, he argued, no greater contrasts than war and love, one the negation of life, the other its affirmation. "Love is potentialized life," he concluded. "Life without love is merely existence."[24]

New research findings on hormones would likely have found their way into the official presentations as well as into the animated conversations in the hallways and receptions over those six days. Benjamin would no doubt have engaged with ideas about hormones in connection with homosexuality and transvestism during his time with Hirschfeld in Berlin. But for Benjamin, sexology was still just a side interest. For him, the chief appeal of glandular science was its promise in fighting aging. His main concern as a practitioner was making a living, and by the fall of 1921 he had determined that the best way he might do this was through offering the Steinach operation. On his homeward journey, he began to draft a speech with which he intended to introduce Steinach's ideas to an American audience.

Chapter 6

A Black Cloud Lifting

In the autumn of 1921, Harry Benjamin returned to New York afire with enthusiasm to promote Eugen Steinach's ideas. On 16 November, he delivered his first public paper on the topic to an audience of physicians at the New York Academy of Medicine at 17 West Forty-Third Street. In a talk titled "Preliminary Communication regarding Steinach's Method of Rejuvenation," Benjamin described several of the clinical cases he had observed in Vienna. He suggested the results were very promising, though he warned against too much excitement and unrealistic hopes.[1] The next day he wrote to Steinach with pride, "Yesterday was the big evening when your discovery was made public to the American medical world for the first time, and I consider myself fortunate indeed that the privilege of fulfilling this role was given to me."[2]

He was delighted. The evening had been a surprising success. The reception to his talk had been cordial and without the hostility that Steinach and his associate Peter Schmidt had encountered. In the early 1920s, glandular rejuvenation was very much in the air. The Russian-born French surgeon Serge Voronoff was then tantalizing Europe and America with his monkey gland rejuvenation treatments. In 1920, Voronoff made a sensation by transplanting slices of testicles from chimpanzees and baboons into the scrota of aging men. Though later dismissed as a quack, his work was regarded with considerable interest by the medical community and the public at large, albeit with some skepticism. His work would attain such widespread fame that it would inspire a new cocktail—the "Monkey Gland" made of gin, orange juice, raspberry juice, and absinthe—and even the sale of popular ashtrays depicting monkeys covering their loins. A few years earlier, Benjamin had expressed interest in Voronoff's work to colleague Dr. Max Herz, a Viennese heart specialist who was visiting New York. Herz had steered him away from Voronoff's work to the scientific studies of Steinach that he regarded as more serious, declaring, "There is no comparison." It had been Herz who facilitated Benjamin's introduction to Steinach.[3]

In the months before Benjamin's lecture, the Steinach operation had also been very much in the news, though not in a way that Steinach would have preferred. In Britain, a wealthy septuagenarian had returned to London after seven weeks in Vienna, enthusiastically touting the rejuvenating effects of the Steinach operation. Delighted with the results and inundated with letters from other men, he announced that he had rented Royal Albert Hall in order to give a lecture titled "How I Was Made Twenty Years Younger by Method of Professor Steinach." In a sorry twist of fate, he was found dead just twelve hours before the lecture. A frenzy in the news ensued.

By February 1922, New York was hearing even more about the Steinach treatment because a famous Austrian orthopedic surgeon, Dr. Adolf Lorenz, was visiting when he announced that he too had undergone the operation. He argued that the success of the treatment was amply demonstrated by the fact that he had been able to resume his celebrated work in treating crippled children. Reporters who jumped on Lorenz's story found their way to Benjamin, who disclosed that he had already treated some cases. The results had been encouraging, he said. One college professor who had been troubled by poor hearing could now hear an alarm clock tick. Another patient who had felt his memory slipping now found it had been restored and was enjoying renewed physical and mental vitality. Benjamin wanted to make it clear that the Steinach operation had nothing at all to do with monkey glands, transplants, or introducing any foreign substance. Instead, the patient's own glandular activity was revived. He speculated, "I believe that Steinach's work will be ranked next to the greatest discovery in medical science, discoveries such as the Roentgen rays (X-rays) and vaccination for smallpox."[4]

Benjamin reported enthusiastically to Steinach that the newspapers were full of Steinach's name and that the ball had really started rolling. His mail had grown so much in volume that he had had to hire a secretary to keep up with the correspondence. He assured Steinach, "I am not hiding your light under a bushel, Herr Professor." He did, however, think it wise to remain conservative, given the general animosity of the medical profession. The patients who were now arriving at his door came not through referrals from other physicians but from the lay public, thanks to his having given interviews in the popular press. Benjamin was particularly anxious to learn more from Steinach about the new treatment for women using X-rays. He told Steinach that he was convinced this procedure could be of huge importance from a financial standpoint. Two days later, Valentine's Day, Benjamin appeared prominently in a news article announcing, "Youth of Women Renewed as Well as Man's through the Steinach Operation."[5]

It had come years before, late one long sleepless night, the vision of a strikingly beautiful woman, standing alone. As author Gertrude Atherton tossed in her bed, an image had flashed in her mind of a woman rising in the front rows of a theater, turning her back to the stage and gazing at the house through her opera glasses. Atherton was well-traveled, so she knew this simple gesture was common in Europe—in fact, she had made it herself. In America, though, it would be considered shockingly forward. The woman of her imagination was poised, aloof, mysterious. Atherton felt haunted, unable to guess who this woman was or what her secret might be. For five years, this figment of her writerly imagination would remain in the theater, surveying the crowd, her story tightly furled.[6]

In February 1922, Gertrude Atherton was sixty-four years old. She gazed imperiously at the world from beneath an extravagant sweep of pompadour and bore herself with a trademark erectness. Her profile was worthy of a cameo. In the Gilded Age, she had been considered a firebrand who had flouted social convention in her personal life as well as in her writing. At this point in her life, she would have had good reason to feel satisfied with her accomplishments. Her most recent novel, *The Sisters-in-Law*, had climbed to the 1921 bestseller list alongside Edith Wharton's *The Age of Innocence* and Sinclair Lewis's *Main Street*. In Europe, where her books were found in the paperbound Tauchnitz editions, hers were the most popular of any American novels in the 1920s. She was the author of some thirty-six books written over thirty years. Most were novels, epic stories of her native California or vivid historical fictions set in distant lands. They were considered daring, even scandalous, dealing frankly as they did with sexual desire, alcoholism, and adultery. She wrote boldly about history, politics, women's suffrage, and war, and her heroines were adventurous women who defied the social roles imposed on them.

She herself had long ago strained against the roles of wife, mother, and respectable widow that had circumscribed her early life. Atherton had fled her family and San Francisco to lead a peripatetic existence taking her to New York, Munich, Paris, and London. As a reporter for the *New York Times* and for the women's magazine the *Delineator* during the war, she had borne witness to the scatter of flags marking the graves on the battlefield of the Marne and to hospital wards teeming with maimed and dying men. She had felt the shattering boom from the great guns of the Somme. A tenacious researcher, she had ventured to Cuba in the 1890s, when such a trip was all but unthinkable for a woman alone. When writing a novel about a mining baron, she had descended 1,800 feet into a Montana copper mine. When inventing the character of an accused murderess, she had convinced officials at Sing Sing prison to strap her into the electric chair. "Interesting," she commented, but the restraints had hurt, and "it was not pleasant . . . to reflect that I was sitting in the chair in which several dead men had been."[7]

But in recent years, a gnawing dissatisfaction had settled on her. In early 1922, she had returned to New York pursuing a hunch that a new book awaited her there. She chose a hotel that was home to many Old New York families who had given up their houses, a fact that appealed to Atherton's patrician sensibilities. From her window overlooking Madison Square, she would have been able to hear the roar of lions when the Ringling Brothers and Barnum & Bailey circus was playing and to watch the triple line of sporting fans wind along Twenty-Sixth Street to Fourth Avenue when there was a prize fight at the Gardens.

For many artists, musicians, and writers, Manhattan in 1922 offered an intoxicating whirl of artistic ferment and frenetic social engagements. Carl Van Vechten, the novelist, music critic, and consummate bon vivant, remembered the decade as the "splendid drunken Twenties." A twenty-five-year-old F. Scott Fitzgerald and his wife, Zelda, would be arriving in the autumn of 1922 to begin their own round of gin-infused literary teas; their experiences would later bubble up in fictional form in the tale of Jay Gatsby. The year would be a landmark one in literary modernism, opening with the publication of James Joyce's *Ulysses* and closing with T. S. Eliot's unprecedented poetry in *The Waste Land*. Obscure, fragmentary, and challenging, these works evoked the despair and disruption of the modern age. Fitzgerald would describe it as the symbolic height of the Jazz Age and would set *The Great Gatsby* in this pivotal year.[8]

A decade before, Gertrude Atherton had been in New York hosting salons, bringing together men of letters, society doyens, and leading politicians. But now, these parties no longer held any appeal for her. She felt that as a hostess she did nothing but "stand about listening to scrappy conversation," worrying whether she had forgotten to introduce guests to the celebrities they had come to meet and "wishing they would all go home." Some days, she joined the writers, playwrights, actors, and critics who lunched at the Round Table at the Algonquin Hotel, but separated in age by three or four decades from the members of this witty, wisecracking crowd, she never felt truly at ease. By now, her early reputation as a daring social critic had largely been forgotten. In literary circles, she was regarded as a bit of a hack. For her part, Atherton deplored the arrival of the flapper, with her bobbed hair, high-flying hemlines, flippancy, and hedonism. She disdained the fascination with small towns and mean lives in the work of Sinclair Lewis and John Dos Passos, what she called the "deification of the common and the vulgar." She found in them nothing to inspire or elevate. Worse yet was her despondency over her own work. Although *The Sisters-in-Law* was a bestseller and well received by critics, she herself regarded it as uneven and shallow. Her recent nine-month stint in Hollywood as part of Samuel Goldwyn's "Eminent Authors" project had been a crushing disappointment. And for the past year, she had found herself in a slump. She could not concentrate, could not create. Desolate, she feared she might never be able to write again.[9] Perhaps it is telling that among her papers is a bill from a New York attorney's office charging for services in the drawing of her will in February 1922.[10]

That winter was devastating across the Eastern Seaboard. New Yorkers woke to find that rain, sleet, wind, and freakish summer storm conditions had combined with frigid temperatures to sheathe the pavements in a brittle crust. Rumbles shook the air and jagged streaks lit the icy open spaces of Central Park.[11] In bed one morning, Atherton was reading the newspaper when an article caught her attention. It described the remarkable "reactivation" of glands by Austrian physiologist Eugen Steinach and explained that Steinach's disciple, Dr. Harry Benjamin, was carrying out reactivation work right in New York. With burgeoning excitement, she read that women all over Europe had been rushing to Steinach's clinic in Vienna; Russian princesses were said to have sold their jewels, hoping to regain the energy they would need to support themselves "after the jewels had given out." This phrase—"after the jewels had given out"—ran through her like a jolt of electricity. In a flash, she knew she had her story. She looked up Benjamin's number in the telephone book and called him at once.

He offered her an appointment that morning. Less than two hours later, she left her hotel to make her way to his office at 237 Central Park West.[12]

Cars careened through New York streets and jammed its squares, governed only by the most rudimentary of traffic regulations. Traffic lights were only emerging from an experimental stage. Seven splendid twenty-three-foot-high ornamental bronze signal towers were being erected that year along Fifth Avenue, featuring electronically synchronized clocks and 350-pound bells that tolled the hours. At the top of each sat a policeman in a small room, flipping levers to open and close colored glass windows in red, yellow, and green. Elevated trains thundered above the streets on their ironwork trestles. Subway trains hurtled below. Electrical wires swayed overhead and snaked into apartment houses and stately homes alike, powering irons, washing machines, refrigerators, dishwashers, toasters, waffle irons, mixers, percolators—just about every manner of convenience for the modern housewife.[13] Invisible waves—radio signals—were propagating through the air. Commercial broadcasting began to explode that year so that all sorts of new and marvelous sounds—from the clarion highs of the operatic diva to the stentorian lows of the news announcer, from bedtime stories, lectures, sermons, and popular concerts to baseball scores and the price of farm products—all crackled into the 1.5 million radio sets already in American households. What an age of wonders this was. High-speed elevators carried businessmen and stenographers sixty stories into the sky; burgeoning networks of trains, telegraphs, and telephones linked the nation with unprecedented speed. And everywhere New Yorkers looked, their eyes were beguiled by commercial allurements: signs painted on sides of buildings, posters on trolleys, sprawling ads in the daily paper, and billboards that mushroomed throughout the countryside. They featured face creams that promised to erase the years, modish hats guaranteeing their wearers would be at the height of fashion, and electrical devices that offered to soothe aches and pains. Advertising was becoming a sophisticated art of manipulating desire and creating needs that consumers had not realized they had. The phrases "mass market" and "brand name" would make their first appearances later this year.[14]

So what about the reactivation of glands? The glands of internal secretion had been much in vogue of late. Newspapers and magazines featured stories touting the miraculous powers of the glands—the pituitary, the thyroid, the adrenals, and especially the sex glands. Shady commercial concerns were already flogging a wide range of glandular solutions to life's problems. Dwindling sex life? Feeling weak and run down? Handbills, brochures, and newspaper advertisements offered ready help in the form of "Youth Gland Tonic," "Glandex," "Glandogen," "Glandol," and the irresistibly named gland preparation known as the "Exhilarator of Life."[15] And why not? Medical science was already responsible for wonderful gains that could be recognized by any informed person. New York City boasted a death rate that was the lowest it had ever been, and the striking drop in infant mortality meant that an estimated 22,000 children were alive who would have died under the conditions of just one generation before.[16] True, much of this could be attributed to improved nutrition and good old-fashioned sanitation, but advances in laboratory-based public health measures were of particular interest to health officials. On the very same night Benjamin had introduced Steinach's work to America, a visionary founder of the American Public Health Association was giving a keynote speech at the Hotel Astor, making the dramatic claim that public health and medicine had done so much to overcome infectious disease over the previous half century that human beings should expect a longer life—not immortality exactly, but perhaps a "life that suggests immortality." The speaker, still robust and optimistic at the age of ninety-eight, declared, "We have too long been content with the false code of the Mosaic law that limits life to three-score years and ten, with a possibility of reaching four-score years." Instead, he believed biology held the promise that human life should reach to one hundred years.[17]

───

Atherton arrived at Benjamin's office punctual to the minute. Across the street, at Central Park, the trees pressed icy fingers against the winter sky. If Atherton felt a shiver of anxiety as she mounted the steps, she was soon put completely at ease by the courtly Benjamin, who welcomed her warmly. She noted that his voice was inflected by the tones of his native Berlin, and she decided she liked him at once. He inspired an immediate confidence. Benjamin, for his part, found himself faced with a rather formidable figure. He recognized her as an accomplished writer. He later wrote to Steinach describing her as one of the most famous authors in the country, an American "Marlitt" he said, comparing her to the best-selling nineteenth-century German romance novelist.

Benjamin ushered her into his office, and she soon found herself telling him all about her idea to write a novel based on the Steinach therapy. Benjamin was only too happy to explain the science of reactivation to her. The principle behind the treatment for women was fairly simple: X-rays were directed onto the patient's ovaries, using the beam's destructive power to eradicate the ovaries' reproductive function. This, Steinach believed, would leave the ovaries free to concentrate their remaining energies on producing their internal secretion—their hormone—which would course through the body, restoring the patient's vigor, suppleness, and womanly vitality. As their conversation continued, Atherton began to speak of her own weariness and despondency. Benjamin listened attentively. Years later when she wrote about this visit in her autobiography, she would claim that her intention in going to the office that day had been to conduct research for her new book. Perhaps that is even what she told herself. But when she revealed her personal struggle, when she spoke of her yearlong bout of "mental sterility," Benjamin naturally asked why she didn't consider taking the Steinach treatment herself. It was true, he argued, that the therapy had a 20 percent failure rate, but even if it should not work for her, at least it would not hurt. Atherton made up her mind on the spot. As she explained it, "I was always ready for anything new."[18]

Once her decision was made, Benjamin's first task was to give his patient a thorough physical examination to ensure her suitability for the therapy. He never risked treating anyone with defective organs, he explained. In short order, he declared that she had the arteries of a sixteen-year-old. She was delighted. According to his diagnosis, all that was wrong with her was that her pituitary and thyroid were depleted and that she needed a fresh release of hormones into her bloodstream.

A day or two later, she returned for her first treatment, a brief X-ray irradiation that Benjamin arranged for her with a radiologist, Dr. Thomas Scholz. After that, Benjamin met her in the laboratory three times a week for more sessions. In all there were about eight treatments, which Atherton found painless and rather boring.[19]

For weeks afterward, Atherton felt only torpor. She was lethargic and slow-witted, so much so that she could barely read a mystery story, let alone sustain a conversation. All she could do was sleep for sixteen hours a day. She began to worry that she had been ruined for life, but when she telephoned Benjamin about her concerns, he laughed, assuring her that it was all working according to plan. More weeks passed and still nothing happened. Then one day, everything changed in a flash.

"I had the abrupt sensation of a black cloud lifting from my brain," Atherton recalled.[20] All was clarity and dazzling light. She flung herself at her desk and began to write.

She wrote for hours without letup. The words poured out of her. Like a geyser that had been capped, the story that had been trapped in her mind gushed forth and spilled onto the page. Now Atherton found she could march the mystery woman of her imagination out of the theater in triumph, fully confident in the knowledge of who the character was and what was going to happen to her. In May, three months after her final treatment, she returned to Benjamin's office. She announced with delight that she was writing a new novel, and what was more, she was doing so with the concentration and ability to work that she had had thirty years before. Her memory had also improved, and she was willing to swear that these good effects were due to the Steinach treatment. Benjamin examined her and noted her blood pressure was lower and that she had a generally improved appearance. But while he was pleased for Atherton, he privately acknowledged that most of the changes that so thrilled her were wholly subjective. He wrote to Steinach with this excellent news but added cautiously, "Although Mrs. Atherton is very sober and not at all a hysterical lady, I cannot rule out a psychological influence."[21]

But Atherton had all the confirmation she needed. She told a friend, "I haven't felt so thoroughly well-equipped for writing for years."[22] Atherton found she could write at a speed she had never commanded before, and she completed in five months what ordinarily would have taken her seven. The manuscript, written first by hand and then twice by typewriter, came in at 110,000 words. When the time came to send her book out into the world, Atherton, having grown disenchanted with her previous publisher, decided to approach the dashing Horace Liveright instead. Liveright was at the helm of what his biographer called "the most magnificent yet messy publishing house" of the twentieth century.[23] The founder of the Modern Library and the Boni and Liveright houses, Liveright had been after Atherton for a book for some time. She rather liked his daring, especially his willingness to upend the staid publishing industry by marketing books aggressively, treating them like any other product. No doubt, his personal qualities helped as well. He was tall and bone-thin, graced with angular good looks and a devastating charm. Aptly perhaps, his name was pronounced "Live-Right." He braved censorship battles in order to publish authors who were obscure, obscene, and revolutionary. It was he who would bring out Eliot's *The Waste Land* as well as the first American edition of Freud, at a time when American booksellers kept Freud's books under the counter. And he did all this while hosting lavish Jazz Age parties. At his office in a brownstone in the heart of the speakeasy district on West Forty-Eighth Street and Sixth Avenue, far from the older established publishing houses, visitors were as likely to meet theatrical agents and chorus girls as literary types, since Liveright was also a dramatist and stage producer. Known for serving the best bootleg liquor in town, he also treated his authors generously, establishing the later standard practice of offering advances on royalties to almost any writer of talent. He took a flying chance on the urgent new voices of modernism, publishing everyone from Ezra Pound, Eugene O'Neill, Theodore Dreiser, Sherwood Anderson, and William Faulkner to e. e. cummings, Djuna Barnes, Dorothy Parker, Lewis Mumford, and Hart Crane. Hemingway's first book, *In Our Time* appeared under his imprint.

Atherton's novel suited Liveright perfectly.[24] It was current, racy, bold, and highly controversial.[25] In the story, a stunning but mysterious woman suddenly appears in New York society. She is Madame Zattiany from Hungary, and she is soon ardently pursued by the young Lee Clavering, a critic and playwright. But Clavering fights an unsettling sense that the lady is not who she appears to be. As their courtship progresses, they spend an evening at the opera. That night, even long-dimmed sensibilities are reawakened in the crowd by the stirring performance of the great diva Geraldine Farrar, who lying almost supine in the arms of her seducer sings with such "voluptuous abandon" that she creates what seems the most explicit scene of any in operatic art. From their box, Clavering spies Madame Zattiany gazing over the auditorium "with a look of hungry yearning."

"Why do you look like that? Have you ever been here before?" he asks her abruptly.

She turns with a smile. "What a question! . . . But opera, both the silliest and the most exalting of the arts, is the Youth of Life, its perpetual and final expression," she says cryptically.

But in time, as their love grows, she can keep her secret no longer. She reveals the shocking truth: she is actually Mary Ogden, a great beauty celebrated by New York society a generation ago who has now been rejuvenated by a famous Viennese doctor. At the age of fifty-eight, Mary had been faded and worn, but now through a miracle of medical science, she has come to possess the devastating combination of maturity and wisdom fused with youthful beauty and vigor.[26]

Once Atherton delivered her manuscript to Liveright, she still had one nagging problem: she could not find the right title. Nothing seemed to work. One evening, she happened to be dining in the sparkling company of Carl Van Vechten and Avery Hopwood. Van Vechten, a critic and writer, was at the center of New York's avant-garde artistic and social scene. He would later become a key white supporter of the Harlem Renaissance. Hopwood was one of the foremost playwrights of the Jazz Age and would become a millionaire with a string of popular and often risqué farces featuring flappers, jazz, and bathtub gin; he could boast the remarkable distinction of having four plays running simultaneously on Broadway. Van Vechten asked Atherton whether she had been able to find a title. Gloomily, she shook her head. Suddenly, some lines came to her from a play by William Butler Yeats: "The years like great black oxen tread the world …" These words had made a deep impression when she had first read them years before in Munich.[27]

"Great Black Oxen?" she wondered aloud.

This suggestion met with instant and wholehearted assent.

"A wonderful title," declared her companions. But "Black Oxen," they insisted. "Leave off the great."

The next day, the fresh title was dispatched to Liveright, who accepted it with equal enthusiasm.[28] When *Black Oxen* reached bookstores in early 1923, it was roundly denounced as a threat to public morality and even banned from the public library in Rochester, New York, as being "unfit for young minds." It was also a roaring success. Atherton's decision to publish with Liveright would prove to be a rejuvenation in itself for her career. *Black Oxen* was not only one of Atherton's most accomplished works but one of the most commercially successful. For Liveright, acquiring Atherton had been a coup. She was a "grand dame" amid his roster of innovative new writers. He could have reasonably expected any book of hers to receive a cordial reception and generate a modest profit, even if readers had grown rather weary of her historical novels. But instead, she had delivered this deliciously spicy and contemporary work. *Black Oxen* would be Liveright's first fiction bestseller. Sales seem to have in no way been hampered by controversy and very likely were much helped. The first edition, at two dollars a copy, rose to the top of the 1923 bestseller list, along with Emily Post's *Etiquette*, besting Sinclair Lewis's *Babbitt*.[29]

Van Vechten, perhaps predictably given his acquaintance with Atherton, published a rave review in *The Nation* calling *Black Oxen* Atherton's most brilliant book to date, comparing her favorably to Edith Wharton as a writer of "natural temperament and genius" born with a facility for telling stories. He mused, "The exceedingly novel pivot on which the actions turn … will certainly be the cause of Mrs. Atherton's receiving letters of query from every dowdy frump who has passed fifty."[30] Van Vechten's joke was prescient. Atherton had never been shy of publicity or even a touch of scandal in promoting herself and her work, and she fully understood it to be part of the modern author's respon-sibilities. But now with Liveright and his staff working actively to flog the novel, by October, sales had topped 100,000.[31] Benjamin shipped a copy of the book to Steinach and reported to Atherton that the professor was "tickled to death" by it. For her part, Atherton regarded the glandular therapy she had received as a true scientific marvel and felt certain that her revitalized abilities were due entirely to the Steinach treatment. In Benjamin's copy of *Black Oxen*, she inscribed, "I am the mother and you the father of this book."[32]

The silver screen flickers to life. A herd of black cattle tramples down a slope, thundering, unstoppable. The words of Yeats flash across the screen: "The years like great black oxen tread the world and God the Herdsman goads them on behind." The scene changes to show an elegant New York audience enjoying the opening night performance of a new play. As the curtains close and the house lights come up for intermission, a slender woman in white rises to her feet. Standing in the front rows of the plush auditorium, she turns to face the crowd, then coolly surveys it with her opera glasses. Titters of astonishment erupt from the spectators at this act of daring. Among those watching her is the jaded critic and playwright Lee Clavering. His blasé demeanor melts, and he is transfixed by this vision. His companion, the upper-crust octogenarian Charles Dinwiddie, quips, "Evidently a European—I can't image an American woman doing that!" But as the woman slowly lowers her binoculars, Dinwiddie catches a glimpse of her face. He is rendered speechless. Running from the hall, he gasps, "Give me a drink, Lee: I've just seen a ghost!" He explains to his young friend that the woman is the very image of Mary Ogden, his old flame who had since become the Countess Zattiany. Mary had been a brilliant beauty who had conquered Old New York society some thirty years before, but the last time he had seen her, she had been an elderly widow, shriveled and spent. Later that evening as the audience departs, the question on everyone's mind is not "What do you think of the play?" but "Who is she?" Who was this stranger who looked every inch the modern woman in her Parisian gown and Marcel waves yet had such a remote, timeless quality to her? Clavering knows this alluring creature cannot possibly be the same Mary Ogden that Dinwiddie remembers. Or can she? "I don't care who she is or what she is," he declares. "I intend to meet her and know her."

This melodramatic scene opens the 1924 silent film *Black Oxen*.[33] Billed as a "subtle science fiction," the movie offered an enticing blend of mystery, romance, and fantasy. Corrine Griffith—then considered one of the greatest beauties of the silver screen—starred as the enigmatic countess. A nineteen-year-old Clara Bow had a breakout role as Janet Oglethorpe, the quintessential flapper who, in contrast to Zattiany, is foolish and pleasure-loving. Bow would go on to become the "It Girl" of the 1920s, personifying the spirit of her roaring decade. The film was a box office smash, and in its aftermath many a middle-aged woman was sent clamoring to discover whether the story of Zattiany's miraculous rejuvenation was science fiction or fact.

By January 1924, a photoplay edition of *Black Oxen* was brought out for seventy-five cents and the novel was serialized in 200 publications across the country. Atherton received over $40,000 in royalties in the first year—about half a million dollars in today's terms. And as Van Vechten had correctly predicted, she received a torrent of mail, over 800 letters, most from women hoping to recover their youth and vigor.[34] Headlines accompanying the release of the film trumpeted "Women Here Made Younger, Like Heroine in 'Black Oxen,' by Rejuvenation Treatment," and news articles reported that "Dr. Harry Benjamin, of 237 Central Park West," was the only physician in New York offering this therapy. The blurring of fact and fiction was of course not at all accidental. Publicity posters blithely merged the two. "Science Solves Secret of Eternal Youth in 'Black Oxen,'" one movie advertisement declared while pointing out its "All Star Cast." "Dr. Harry Benjamin, famous New York surgeon, and collaborator of Dr. Eugen Steinach, noted Viennese scientist and inventor of the Steinach glandular and X-ray method of restoring youth and beauty, treats scores of successful cases in America," the ad continued. "Wrinkled old age now said to be a thing of the past—sparkle, vivacity and pep restored to women and men." Below the movie stills showing a dewy Corrine Griffith gazing into the eyes of her adoring costar Conway Tearle is a photo of Benjamin looking serious and sage. The ad blared, "A picture that tells women the secret of youth and beauty, not a myth, but true."[35]

In the publicity blitz that followed, Atherton skillfully toyed with reporters. "Is Mrs. Atherton Rejuvenated Like Heroine of Book?" one article asked. "What accounts for the marvelously youthful appearance of Mrs. Gertrude Atherton . . . ?" wondered another. Although nearing sixty-seven, "Mrs. Atherton has not a single line about her clear blue eyes, [and] her double chin has practically vanished," observed the reporter slyly, displaying as evidence a pair of images, the first a photo showing the author looking a dowdy matron in 1911, and beside it a portrait of her "clear-eyed, unwrinkled," and glamorous in the present day. In the accompanying interview, Atherton told all about her dream, the woman in white standing alone at the front of the theater, Dr. Lorenz, Dr. Benjamin, the Russian princesses selling their jewels, and the birth of an idea for a novel. But about her own experience, she remained silent. When the reporter asked whether she knew of anyone who had taken the X-ray treatment, she coyly answered that she knew of two women, one in her forties and one in her fifties, both of whom had experienced clear improvements. The reporter pushed. "If the time ever came when you felt your own powers declining would you take this treatment?" She replied earnestly, if disingenuously, "In a shot!"[36]

When reporters asked Benjamin whether he had given rejuvenation treatment to Atherton, he refused to answer. In a medical presentation, however, he described the case study of a sixty-four-year-old educator who had for several years suffered an increasing lack of mental activity, concentration, and imagination. This patient had begun Steinach therapy in February 1922. Six weeks later, the patient—who was described as "very intelligent" and "not hysterical at all"—felt her brain clear, began to sleep better, and regained the ability for sustained work. The report declared, "New ideas had come to her 'like a flash,'" a choice of words that make it clear to us that this is a veiled account of Atherton's experience.

But of course, the truth behind the glamour was more complex. Benjamin realized the term "rejuvenation" was controversial as well as inaccurate. The Steinach treatment did not extend life, nor did it make people look dramatically younger. The treatment instead offered what he called additional years of "usefulness." Benjamin tried to introduce the less-loaded term "reactivation" into popular usage to reflect more modest and realistic objectives. It never really caught on. Benjamin wanted to dissuade women from considering Steinach therapy a quick ticket to beauty and youth. He revealed that he had had to turn down a number of actresses who had thought of his laboratory as "a new sort of beauty parlour," though by 1924, he claimed to have treated some seventy New York women, including some well known in society, in the arts, and on the stage. "Women are taking the treatment in increasing numbers," a news article stated, "as word of it is being whispered around from mouth to mouth." Benjamin warned that reactivation took time. In some cases, a woman might feel "a quickening of the stream of life" after only one treatment, but in general, the results did not manifest themselves for months, and the older a patient was, the more difficult it became. He considered the ideal age for beginning the therapy to be forty-five. The Steinach treatment was not magic: wrinkles did not disappear, nor did gray hair turn black, "though where new hair grows in . . . it is often the original color." But when it worked, it could be encouraging: "The body functions better and the flesh grows firmer. There is vitality, springiness, some of the joy of living that passes with the years." Patients regained a fitness for work. Women who had been physically tired and emotionally depressed found they had renewed energy, enthusiasm, and mental alertness and "ten years of added usefulness." He warned, "The Steinach treatment does not have the sensational rejuvenating effects claimed for it in some quarters." But in 80 percent of cases, it did increase personal efficiency. Echoing the words he offered to Atherton when she had first arrived at his office, he explained that every patient was promised two things: that she would not be hurt by the treatment, and that she had nothing to lose.[37] Nothing, a skeptic might add, but her money.

In the novel *Black Oxen*, Prince Hohenhauer, Mary Zattiany's former lover, visits her and asks a disquieting question: To what purpose would she direct her marvelously rejuvenated body and mind? She owes her rejuvenation to Austria, he tells her. Instead of squandering her energies in the arms of a young man, she could become a powerful player in Vienna, hosting a grand salon of the finest minds and using her powers to restore a great nation and a great people. Atherton's novel and the movie that stemmed from it, while marketed as fantasy and romance, also served as penetrating social criticism. If we could have youth again, to what purpose would we turn those added years of energy, beauty, and "usefulness"? Atherton was scathing in her portrayal of those who were actually young. The teenage flapper Janet Oglethorpe is vain and empty-headed, wasting herself in drinking, partying, and frivolous pursuits. In an era in which older voices were left unheard, Atherton provided an urgent critique, examining the Roaring Twenties' cult of youth and finding it wanting.

Benjamin and Atherton found to their surprise that the majority of the women presenting themselves for treatment were not seeking beauty and romance but were businesswomen and professionals, nurses, shop owners, and schoolteachers who were concerned that they were losing their ability to work. In fact, as one article speculated, it was even more important for these women who were "losing a grip on their work" to regain their vitality and strength than it was for married women of leisure.[38] Benjamin was cautious to keep his clinical assessment separate from his patients' subjective accounts of their experiences. He carefully recorded measurable results such as blood pressure, pulse, and weight. He explained, "considering the mentality of patients undergoing a so-called rejuvenation treatment," it was advisable to disregard what the patients said if there were no objective changes to corroborate them.[39] In male reactivation patients, sexual desire and potency were principal concerns. But in the reactivation of women, neither Atherton nor Benjamin discussed the effects on his patients' sexual health. In general, Benjamin found references to sexual matters more circumscribed in American medical circles than in European ones because of what he thought of as a more puritanical mindset. He speculated that in the United States, business interests often suppressed or took the place of sexual matters. He knew that even his male patients were reticent to discuss sexual issues, and he worried that he was missing out on data concerning improvements in libido or sexual potency. He warned that even a direct denial of this had to be accepted with a grain of salt.[40]

Atherton's heroine, the Countess Zattiany, is momentarily tempted by the pleasures of youthful love but ultimately turns away from them. At the conclusion of the novel, she refuses the offer of marriage from her young lover and returns to Vienna to take up her full power and responsibilities as a mature woman, dedicating her renewed vitality to greater social and political good. The parallel tales of Atherton's rejuvenation and that of her fictional heroine invite us to imagine what it was like to grow old in an era besotted with youth, to have one's shapely form grow flabby, to become gray and invisible, when all around it might have seemed that so many others were downing cocktails, dancing in fountains, and having a ripping good time. What was it like to feel one's mental acuity dull and the ability to work ebb away in an age that prized progress, speed, productivity, and efficiency? Then, as the Roaring Twenties plummeted into the Great Depression, how much more urgent would one's need for reactivation seem?

And, in the early twentieth century, what was it like to begin to experience one's self as a glandular being? To understand one's very flesh and most intimate yearnings to be shaped by the activities of invisible secretions? To consider the possibility that a glandular treatment might not simply heal disease but reshape one's body, desires, sensations, and mental outlook? Life presents us all with a series of metamorphoses, from infancy to childhood, puberty to prime of life, menopause, decline, and finally death. What was it like to be among the first generation to consider the possibility that we might have some control over our glandular natures? To realize that, through the manipulation of hormones, our bodies and mentalities might be malleable, perhaps stunningly so?[41]

One question that did not faze Atherton at all was whether or not it was morally justifiable to undertake rejuvenation therapy. In the novel, her heroine,

Mary, confronts her girlhood companions. She arrives slender, stylish, and smooth-skinned to stand amid a circle of stout matrons bedecked in feathers and furs and encrusted with jewels. They are almost uniformly scandalized and envious yet horrified that Mary has tampered with nature and worked against God. Mary is unruffled. Atherton too brushed off such critics: if science had made this possibility available, a woman was simply foolish not to take advantage of it, she declared.

The hundreds of letters that poured into Atherton's mail give us a poignant glimpse into the lives of regular people struggling to carry on with the burdens of their lives. One Chicago woman in her fifties wrote, "I have recently lost my husband and find it will be necessary for me to enter some line of business— but I cannot do so in my present 'let-down' state." She added, "I have read so much on the subject of the glands (all of them) as factors in our well being and I am convinced if I could have the treatments you took I would be restored to a point where life would be worth the living in."[42] Atherton answered as many of the letters as she could, feeling she had started something and that she "had no right to disappoint these eager, sometimes desperate, women." She referred these petitioners to Benjamin in New York and later to other physicians in other parts of the country as the Steinach therapy spread. "Poor Dr. Benjamin!" she remembered; "I nearly ruined him. Women besieged him, imploring him to give the treatment free of charge or at a minimum price. It was the first time they had seen a ray of light in a future menaced with utter fatigue and the clutching of younger hands at the jobs that were wearing them out."[43] Their letters open a rare window into the lives of ordinary people: how they began to conceive of themselves as glandular beings—as organisms shaped by a wild internal sea of chemicals—and how they hoped to find some relief for their cares in the marvels of science.[44]

Atherton's reactivation experience was bookended by two notable events at New York's Metropolitan Opera: the debut of Moravian soprano Maria Jeritza on 19 November 1921 and the farewell performance of American opera star Geraldine Farrar five months later, on 22 April 1922. For Benjamin, these two performances had particular resonance.

Jeritza, incandescent and riveting, had already gained the nickname "The Moravian Thunderbolt" for her spectacular rise to fame in Vienna. Debuting in the role of Marie/Marietta in *Die Tote Stadt* (The dead city), a role created for her by composer Erich Korngold, she enthralled audiences and critics with her youthful athletic figure, radiant personality, and halo of golden curls. One reviewer said, "She seems to emit [dramatic instinct] like sparks from an electric battery."[45] The performance also marked the first return of the German language to the Met since early 1917. Benjamin wrote enthusiastically to Steinach that New York was "all about Vienna right now" thanks to the publicity surrounding Lorenz's rejuvenation and the sensational success of Jeritza at the Met. "It has not been like this since Caruso's time," Benjamin explained.[46] Jeritza, flamboyant, vital, and in full command of all the power that youth and beauty afforded her, began a sensational career trajectory, one in which she was to become a lifelong friend and client of Benjamin's.[47]

At the other end of a stellar career was Farrar, Benjamin's boyhood crush. Farrar, the first true American prima donna, drew the fanatical devotion of hordes of young women who called themselves "Gerry-Flappers." Farrar was just forty years old, but her punishing schedule—some 671 performances in sixteen years at the Met—had already caused vocal injuries. Onstage, she held nothing back—"at every performance, I cut myself open with a knife and give myself to the audience," she told Carl Van Vechten—so she made the decision to retire while still at the height of her powers. We do not know for sure whether Benjamin was in the audience that day, but it is difficult to imagine he would have wanted to miss one of the most tumultuous farewells ever seen at the Met, with disconsolate fans standing three deep behind the railing, banners strung across the orchestra proclaiming "Hurrah, Farrar, Farrar, Hurrah," and the diva "almost swamped by a Niagara of flowers" as she took bow after bow, bearing a tiara and scepter handed over the footlights by her adoring public. After the curtain calls, Farrar was swept into an open-topped automobile, where she sat like a carnival queen as fans pulled her car down Broadway and "ecstatic débutantes and 'sub-debs' perched on fire escapes with bouquets and strings of ribbon, ready to shower their idol."[48]

A comet-like arrival and a rose-strewn departure: together they made manifest in operatic art the evanescence of youth, talent, and beauty, like a seventeenth-century Dutch *vanitas* painting of luscious pears that bear on their brown-flecked skin the promise of the rot to come, or a memento mori etched in voice, the golden notes of which dissipate into the Manhattan soundscape of honking horns. For Benjamin, reactivation was not a matter of extending life but of buying a few more years of vigor, creativity, and usefulness. In the background, the steady beat of days thrummed on. In her debut, Jeritza sang the heartrending aria "Glück, das mir verblieb," known as "Marietta's lied":

> How true, a sad song
> The song of true love
> that must die.[49]

It is an evocation of the tragic yet utterly quotidian truth that all life and love will end. All is fleeting. And so the question that Atherton's Prince Hohenhauer asks Mary Zattiany hovered over Benjamin's rejuvenation practice: If science truly offers a few more years of beauty, youth, and energy, to what end should one turn this marvelous gift?

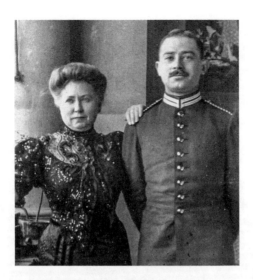

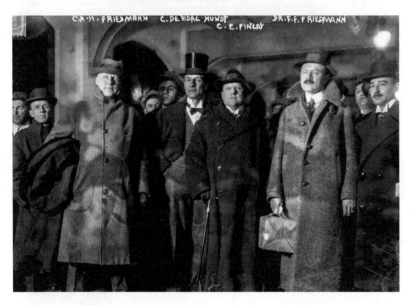

Top: Harry Benjamin in the uniform of the Prussian Guard with his mother, Bertha Benjamin, in Berlin, 1909. © UB der HU zu Berlin, Haeberle-Hirschfeld-Archiv: Harry Benjamin.

Bottom, left to right: Dr. Arthur Friedmann, brother of Friedrich Franz Friedmann; Charles de Vidal Hundt, press agent; Charles Finlay, banker; Dr. Friedrich Franz Friedmann, developer of the turtle treatment for tuberculosis; and Dr. Harry Benjamin facing reporters upon their arrival in New York, February 1913. Friedmann is carrying a package that presumably contains his serum. Bain News Service photograph collection, Library of Congress.

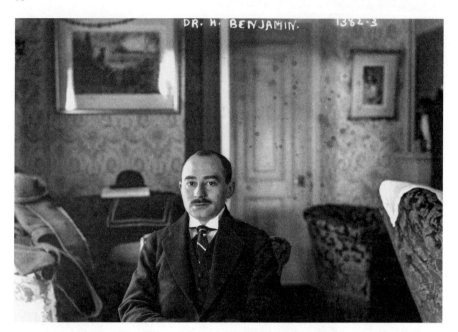

Top: Harry Benjamin, on his arrival in New York with the Friedmann party, February 1913. Bain News Service photograph collection, Library of Congress.

Right: Eugen Steinach, signed by Steinach to Dr. Benjamin and Gretchen in old friendship. From the Collections of the Kinsey Institute, Indiana University. All rights reserved.

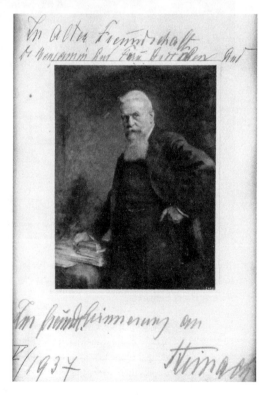

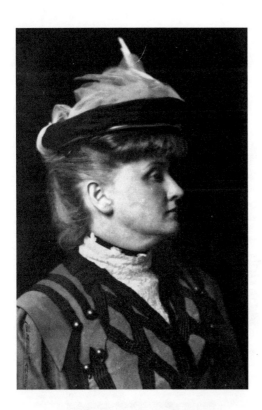

Gertrude Franklin Horn
Atherton displaying her
famous profile, c. 1904.
Library of Congress.

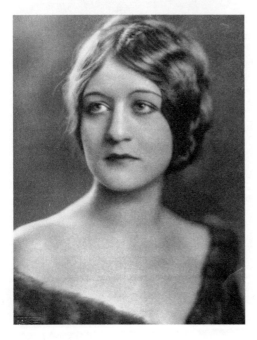

Greta Benjamin. From the
Collections of the Kinsey
Institute, Indiana University.
All rights reserved.

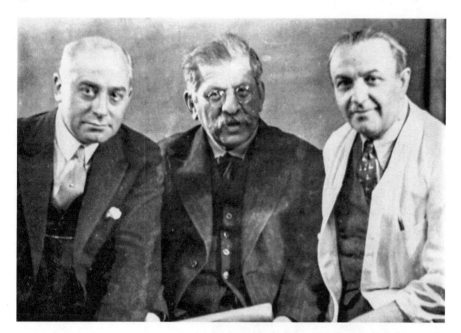

Top: Harry Benjamin, Magnus Hirschfeld, and Max Thorek meeting for the last time in Chicago, 1930. © UB der HU zu Berlin, Haeberle-Hirschfeld-Archiv: Harry Benjamin.

Right: Portrait of Benjamin taken in Vienna (probably 1937) by photographer Georg Fayer. Signed by Benjamin to Erwin Haeberle. © UB der HU zu Berlin, Haeberle-Hirschfeld-Archiv: Harry Benjamin.

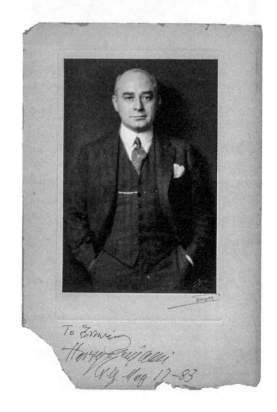

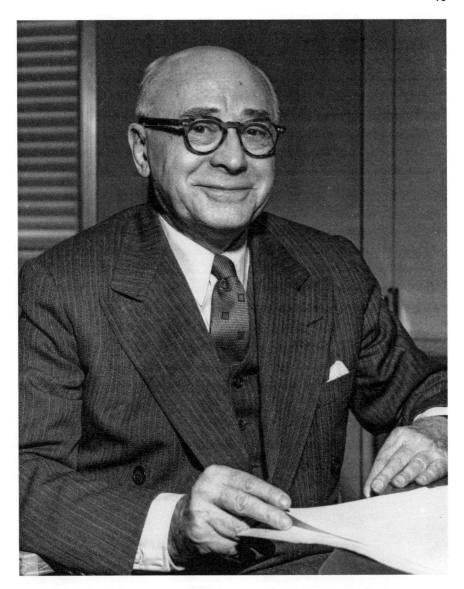

Harry Benjamin visiting the Institute for Sex Research. Photographer William Dellenback. From the Collections of the Kinsey Institute, Indiana University.

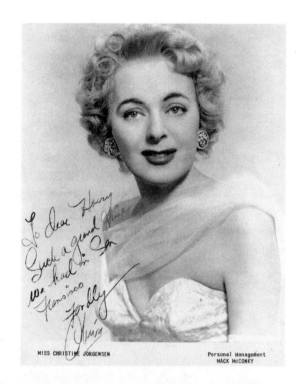

Right: Christine Jorgensen, signed "To dear Harry, Such a grand time we had in San Francisco, Fondly, Chris." From the Collections of the Kinsey Institute, Indiana University. All rights reserved.

Bottom: Harry Benjamin in his later years at the desk of his medical practice in New York. © UB der HU zu Berlin, Haeberle-Hirschfeld-Archiv: Harry Benjamin.

MISS CHRISTINE JORGENSEN

Personal Management
MACK McCONKY

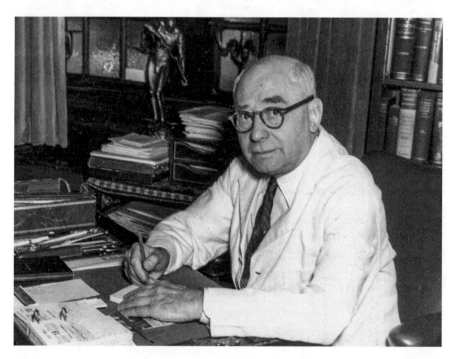

Chapter 7

In the Border Fields

The publicity surrounding *Black Oxen* drew attention to Harry Benjamin's work, and through the next decade something of the glamour of its fictional heroine, Mary Zattiany, suffused his life. It came, however, with the taint of the illicit. Glandular rejuvenation was considered unseemly, distasteful even, and generally understood as a veiled reference to the attempt to restore the flagging sexual function of older men. Benjamin tried to promote the term "reactivation" rather than "rejuvenation," which came freighted with such unrealistic expectations, but in popular discourse the rejuvenation label stuck. When observers assumed that Gertrude Atherton's novel *Black Oxen* had helped boost his practice in any significant way, however, Benjamin protested: "The only thing that did increase, at times enormously, was my correspondence." In general, he always suggested that people who wrote to him should consult their own family physician, though he came to wonder whether this, while ethical, might actually have failed to serve the patients well. He suspected that their doctors were of little help, knowing only what they had read about monkey glands in the papers. He thought these patients might simply have been left puzzled and ashamed for having asked. Perhaps they might have tried the physician's routine prescription for iron tablets or a gland tonic only to end up resigned to getting old, "to working and playing a little less, and dozing a little more."[1]

Steinach therapy was only one of the better-known glandular therapies for rejuvenation. While Eugen Steinach and Serge Voronoff, the Russian-born French monkey-gland surgeon, drew the justification for their work from elite, European scientific traditions, the American heartland produced a populist alternative as well. John Brinkley, a Kansas physician known as the goat-gland doctor, offered a folksy brand of rejuvenation and spread his message through the down-home medium of radio.[2] The reality of reactivation therapy was of course far more complicated than the popular accounts suggested. Within a year or so, Gertrude Atherton began to feel her energy lag once more. She continued to seek new and better ways of reenergizing herself. A year after the success of *Black Oxen*, she underwent a transplantation of sheep-ovary tissue with Dr. H. Lyons Hunt. She was angry when it failed to deliver the dramatic results the Steinach treatment had. She returned to Benjamin, and when he passed along Steinach's suggestion that she be given high-frequency stimulation of the pituitary, she was happy to try. Atherton remained Benjamin's patient and patron for the rest of her life, and he in turn was a loyal and attentive friend.[3]

Indeed, the power of the glands to transform bodies and minds became very much part of the popular imagination. Louis Berman's best-selling and influential book *The Glands Regulating Personality* (1921) went on to four editions and was widely spoken about. Berman, a New York physician and endocrine researcher, found his way into the conversations of Ezra Pound, James Joyce, Ernest Hemingway, T. S. Eliot, and Carl Van Vechten. In his book, Berman described the intriguing notion that personality types were linked to hormonal status. He was interested in the relation between hormones and human behavior and became convinced that glands held the greatest opportunity to promote human health and welfare. In the late 1920s, Berman began a three-year study of 250 prisoners at Sing Sing, concluding that "endocrine defects" occurred among criminals two to three times as often as in the general population and that certain crimes were associated with particular hormone disturbances. His view would develop into a utopian vision of a world that could be made more perfect through the use of hormones. His ideas were eyed with skepticism by professional colleagues, but he had a wide circle of fans.[4]

Horace Liveright, ever eager to build on the success of *Black Oxen*, tried to interest Gertrude Atherton in producing a sequel. He suggested she might draw from Berman's ideas to write a novel on the subject of those people who, like ostriches, avoid looking life in the face. He had had conversations with his doctor about this personality type and concluded it was related to adrenal insufficiency. In his bantering correspondence with Atherton, he quipped that she should pay some of his doctor's bills because her "frigid notes" to him had so increased his adrenal secretions "that I'm sure some day you'll be responsible for the fat fees that Dr. Benjamin will charge for putting me to rights."[5]

In popular fiction of the day, the glands served as signifier of the marvels of cutting-edge science as well as its temptations and dangers.[6] Arthur Conan Doyle's 1923 Sherlock Holmes story, "The Adventure of the Creeping Man," featured a professor whose behavior becomes increasingly monkey-like because he has taken a drug derived from langurs to rejuvenate himself before his upcoming marriage to a younger woman. In a 1933 short story, Dorothy Sayers's gentleman detective Lord Peter Wimsey learns of a lady in a remote Basque village with a white, puffy face, vacant eyes, drooling mouth, clammy skin, and a "dry fringe of rusty hair clinging to a half-bald scalp." She is said to suffer from "imbecility." Just a short time before, she had arrived in the village as a winsome young beauty, but now locals fear she has been bewitched. Lord Peter astutely determines that her physician-husband is the culprit; jealous of her attentions to another man, the husband has withheld the thyroxin wafers required to treat her thyroid deficiency.[7] In Sayers's 1928 novel, *The Unpleasantness at the Bellona Club*, Lord Peter meets a family who is keen on glands. The mother of the family tells him, "So very wonderful about glands, isn't it? Dr. Voronoff, you know, and those marvelous old sheep. Such a hope for all of us." The glands offer hope even for criminals, she declares: "And just to think that we have been quite wrong about them all these thousands of years. Flogging and bread-and-water, you know, and Holy Communion, when what they really needed was a little bit of rabbit-gland or something to make them just as good as gold. . . . And all those poor freaks in sideshows, too—dwarfs and giants, you know—all pineal or pituitary, and they come right again." The murderer in this novel is revealed to be an impecunious physician who shrewdly recognizes hormones to be the science of the future but has been overly eager to get his hands on an inheritance to fund his new gland clinic.[8]

In the summer of 1924, a brutal slaying brought murder, mayhem, and the influence of the glands to the front pages in real life. Nathan Leopold and Richard Loeb, two teenagers, deliberately planned the kidnapping and murder of a fourteen-year-old boy and, when captured, confessed to the crime. Their families hired Clarence Darrow to try to save the teens from the death penalty. Darrow would a year later make news in the famous Scopes trial in Tennessee, defending a teacher sued by the state for teaching evolution. Science played a key role in the Leopold-Loeb case as well. Endocrinologists brought in by Darrow produced an 80,000-word report detailing how, in their assessment, the killers were afflicted by defective hormones: Loeb, they concluded, suffered from multigland syndrome, while Leopold had a calcified pineal gland. Gertrude Atherton wrote to Benjamin asking his views on the matter, and he replied, "I feel quite certain those boys in Chicago suffer endocrine unbalance, affecting their psyche to such an extent that normal moral inhibition is entirely absent. It is hardly possible to definitely establish what gland is originally at fault, but I have the strongest suspicion that it is the sex gland which secretes a 'perverted' hormone in this case." Benjamin further speculated, "Sexual perversion to my mind plays a much greater part in the Chicago tragedy than the newspapers could possibly report."[9] The judge determined that while the scientific report added to the field of criminology, it did not affect his final judgment in the case; he was persuaded not to impose the death penalty because of the murderers' young age but sentenced them to prison for life.

Benjamin remained single throughout his twenties and thirties, but his social life was full and his sexual life prodigious. From his first days in New York, he found his way back to the world of opera singers, actresses, and chorus girls, some of whom he had known in Berlin. Often they would gather at a café on Sixth Avenue, not far from the Metropolitan Opera. He considered himself something of a ladies' man and for many years had a romance with a Bostonian woman, "a real WASP," he described her, though she was uninterested in marriage.[10]

During his first return visit to Berlin in 1921, he had met a fair young beauty with gray-blue eyes who was a stenographer at a lawyer's office. Greta Gülzow was only eighteen at the time. Over the next year, Benjamin corresponded with Gülzow, whom he called Gretchen. He was eighteen years her senior and must have seemed a dashing figure to her as well, perhaps, as a ticket out of Germany. She wrote to him by hand or secretly stayed after hours at the office to use the typewriter. Her letters were spirited, funny, and affectionate. He signed his letters "Dein Hase"—your rabbit—and called her "Urm." She enthused, "I already stand with both feet in the new world, and climb over skyscrapers to get to Central Park. I would stumble a hundred times because I cannot get to you fast enough."[11]

Her eagerness is no surprise. Life in Gretchen's Berlin had become a hyperinflationary nightmare. Thrifty, hard-working folk saw their life savings dissipating so quickly it must have felt they could barely catch their breath. Prices rose daily. Factory workers waited for their pay—sometimes tossed from a five-ton truck piled high with bank notes—then dashed to the stores to buy whatever they still could. Everything that could be bartered, pinched, or sold, was. Government presses worked through the night to print money to meet the crippling reparations required by the Treaty of Versailles, causing the value of the German mark to fall at a dizzying rate. In 1919, after the peace, it took 48 marks to buy one US dollar. By early 1922, the same dollar cost 320 marks. Gretchen told Harry that resoling a pair of shoes now cost her 600 marks and a tram ride 12 marks. "If it goes on like this," she wrote, "we'll have to put all our money in a backpack to go shopping."[12]

She begged him to give some reassurance to her parents of his intentions and his promise to look after her. Nothing could make her happier than to come to him and to find a way out of this mess—"aus diesem Schlamassel"—before she starved. She joked that her grandmother, who sat with her as she read his note, warned her that she was head over heels and that she had better come to her senses. She teased that she rather liked sending and receiving kisses through the mail as she avoided getting crushed and messing her hairstyle. But it seems Gretchen and Harry also shared a keen awareness that her social status was lower than his. Harry would later say of her that she had "no background at all" and that as a child of war, she had what he deemed a "defective education." She flirted with him, saying that she knew "Gretchen" was his favorite name but reminded him of the social rank connected with that name, a reference to Faust's Gretchen who is from a humble background. She told Harry that she was glad he didn't mind that she didn't know French; she explained that she had often tried to better herself but something had always gotten in the way.[13]

Between June and December, the cost of living in Germany leapt fifteen-fold. By late 1922, Harry and Gretchen were working out travel documents for her. He wired her US dollars. She wrote asking for more to purchase a suitcase and pay for travel to Hamburg to board her ship. She worried that she also needed the fifty dollars that new arrivals were required to possess upon landing, though she joked that if they didn't allow her off the ship, she would create such a "Berlin-style" ruckus that they would be glad to see her go.[14] By the end of 1922, the German currency had plunged to 7,400 marks per US dollar. The following year, it would go into free fall, through a million, then a billion, to a stunning 4 trillion marks per US dollar by November 1923.

In early 1923, Gretchen sailed from Hamburg and arrived in New York on 2 February, four days before her twentieth birthday. On 23 December 1925, at the age of forty, Harry married Gretchen. He would later admit that he had not been in love with her but had merely felt responsible for her. Together, though, they built a life of increasing glamour and comfort. From 1925, they had a duplex apartment on the Upper West Side in the Astor Apartments at 239 West Seventy-Fifth Street, complete with servants, a chauffeur, and a sweep of marble staircase. Newspapers from 1927 showed Gretchen looking coquettish in a stylish suit and a flapper's headband. They described her (oddly) as a German film star and reported that she was arrived from Berlin to help her husband in his work.[15] Benjamin was becoming a well-known expert on aging and reactivation therapy who was often quoted in newspaper columns. He grew accustomed to getting his suits custom-made and his haberdashery from Sulka, long favored by the carriage trade. He became a connoisseur of wines and fine foods. During this period, they had a great many friends and entertained every Saturday and Sunday, while Harry enjoyed a weekly poker game as well.[16] A social column from the early 1930s touted the "salon atmosphere and European environment" of a gathering at their home, which on that occasion included a scientist, a botanist, and a psychologist, as well as a novelist, an editor, and a playwright. Gretchen was described as "a celebrated Berlin beauty" who was much in demand both in New York and Europe as a sitter for noted artists.[17]

When in Europe, Benjamin always paid visits to famous practitioners, some of whom he consulted professionally. He was psychoanalyzed by Arthur Kronfeld in Berlin (his diary notes several appointments with Kronfeld in 1928) and by Alfred Adler in Vienna. He held Adler in great affection and gratitude for his kindness and met with him many times in Vienna and in New York. To Adler, he confided that the young woman patient whom he had escorted from New York to Berlin in 1921 had fallen desperately in love with him.[18]

Benjamin wanted to meet Sigmund Freud, and Steinach, although critical of psychoanalysis, was on good terms with Freud. He agreed to help arrange for a meeting sometime around 1928. The hour Benjamin spent with Freud would prove unforgettable. Benjamin waited in the consulting room at Berggasse 19, meditating on the collection of small symbolic figures on Freud's desk. The room was lined with heavy Persian rugs and cabinets of funereal antiquities. The famous couch had, since Freud's 1923 surgery for oral cancer, been moved to another wall so that Freud could hear his patients with his left ear, having lost his hearing in his right. Suddenly, Freud appeared from behind a hidden door. He welcomed Benjamin with polite reserve and took his seat. They proceeded to discuss a number of subjects, and the conversation eventually turned to the relationship of the body to the mind. Benjamin blurted out a wisecrack that suddenly came to him, that the disharmony of the emotions might be caused by the *dishormony* of the endocrines. Freud gave a rare short laugh. He said he agreed with Benjamin. Then he asked if Benjamin had been analyzed himself. When Benjamin replied that a brief attempt had been made by Kronfeld, Freud burst out, "But that man has a very bad character." Freud said that he admired Steinach's work very much and divulged that he had himself undergone the Steinach operation in an attempt to stem the progress of his oral cancer. He reported that he was very satisfied with the result, feeling his health and vitality had improved and the malignancy in his jaw had been favorably affected.[19]

At length, Benjamin revealed a difficult truth about his own life. He had married a beautiful woman to whom he was sexually attracted but now found he was suffering from a form of impotence, particularly with her. Decades later, Gretchen would tell a friend in sorrow that Harry had invited his mother to move in with them during their first year of marriage and that from that time on, the door to their bedroom had always remained open. Freud suddenly proposed that Benjamin was a latent homosexual. This made Benjamin furious. He had always regarded himself as something of a ladies' man. As they parted, Freud asked Benjamin not to disclose the information about his Steinach operation until after his death, and Benjamin kept that promise. Years later, Benjamin would reflect that Freud had actually been much more biologically oriented than his psychoanalytical followers; he felt that, in a way, Freud had not been "Freudian" and that the man himself would have been shocked to see what became of his doctrine in America. As well, according to Ethel Spector Person, who interviewed Benjamin decades later, Freud's unwelcome speculation about his sexuality led Benjamin to have an uneasy relationship with psychoanalysis; he would thereafter deplore it as unscientific.[20]

Was there any validity to Freud's insight that Benjamin was a latent homosexual? Could there have been anything about Benjamin's own sexuality that might explain his sympathy with sexual minorities? These questions are difficult for a historian to answer without descending to gossip. The written record gives us little guidance. We know Benjamin spoke of his many romantic attachments and sexual liaisons with women, though this in itself does not decisively answer whether he was thoroughly and enthusiastically heterosexual or whether—protesting too much—he was consciously or unconsciously hiding homosexual yearnings. Charles Ihlenfeld, a longtime colleague and friend, himself gay, is convinced there is no evidence that Benjamin was homosexual.[21] Also revealing is the testimony of Benjamin's colleague the sexologist Richard Green and

Benjamin's patient Aleshia Brevard that Benjamin had a hair fetish.[22] Brevard recalls that "he had a fetish for very thin girls with very long hair."[23] We can get a small sense of his predilections in a letter in which Benjamin asked the sex researcher Alfred Kinsey if he had yet received a catalog of "long haired ladies" from a photographer who specialized in glamourous images of women with extremely long hair; Benjamin opined of the photographer, "I think he will get away with it until somebody discovers that he may be violating the eleventh commandment: 'Thou shall not commit enjoyment.'"[24] I find this insight into Benjamin's sexual tastes intriguing. It gives us a glimpse into the secret turns— and perhaps torments—of Benjamin's own sexuality. It clicks into place like a piece in the puzzle that is Harry Benjamin, linking a fraught inner life marked by distant unattainable love interests, a fascination with the glamour of stage and film, and a troubled marital bed with a public face characterized by compassion for those marginalized for their hidden longings. But ultimately, what erotic secrets Benjamin kept, we can still only guess.

Gretchen sometimes assisted in Harry's office when he needed extra help, and some of his male patients, not knowing she was the doctor's wife, made racy comments along the lines of "testing" the effectiveness of the rejuvenation therapy on the pretty receptionist. Indeed, an aura of glamour, sex, and money framed Benjamin's practice. In public statements, he emphasized that he wanted to discourage women from considering reactivation therapy as a sort of beauty parlor treatment, but in reality, the distinction between the two was not always so clear. The beauty industry soon learned to cultivate the authority of the white lab coat and the mystique of glandular science. Elizabeth Arden's flagship salon on Fifth Avenue was a veritable temple to beauty that blended pampering, elegant bottles, and discreet services with an air of science. In a leading magazine, Arden described her meeting with Steinach to consult in the making of her hormone beauty creams. In the 1930s, she developed a "Vienna Youth Mask," a beauty treatment in which the patient's face was covered with a papier-mâché mask lined with tin foil and then subjected to diathermy, a controlled heating induced by electric currents. This echoed the use of diathermy in Steinach therapy. (Since 1923, the Steinach treatment for women had evolved from X-rays to diathermy.) Arden's rival Dorothy Gray already had a successful chain of salons and lines of creams and lotions when a newspaper story reported that she too had made a trip to Vienna to investigate Steinach's work in 1923. Reflecting on the remarkable rejuvenations she saw at a sanatorium, she mused that in her beauty business, she could make women only look younger, but here, she had seen something that could make them actually feel younger. One reporter speculated that a whole "new class" was being added to human society, that of women who had been made to look and feel younger but remained "wise with the sophistication of their years."[25]

Despite Benjamin's protests to the contrary, he was closer to the beauty parlor than he might have let on. In 1929, Gretchen successfully won a US patent for a metallic face mask to be used as an electrotherapeutic device. The device, the patent claimed, would exert a certain amount of pressure "to smooth out wrinkles" and "sagging skin." Benjamin reported this development to Steinach cautiously, knowing his mentor was likely to be appalled. He rationalized that "I look at this as a gimmick that might provide an additional income."[26]

Indeed, the budding scientific field of endocrinology itself faced challenges to its legitimacy. In the early 1920s, despite the success of thyroid hormone and adrenaline, the association of hormones with sex and monkey glands cloaked the field in such disrepute that it seemed to some that entering the field might be tantamount to career suicide for a young physician or researcher. In 1921, renowned neurosurgeon Harvey Cushing made a scathing attack against glandular enthusiasms in his presidential address to the Association for the Study of Internal Secretions, warning, "We find ourselves embarked on the fogbound and poorly charted sea of endocrinology. . . . In the enthusiasm 'to embark glandward ho!' . . . many of us have lost our bearings in the therapeutic haze eagerly fostered by the many pharmaceutical establishments."[27]

But a year later, this situation was to change. While Benjamin was busy fighting aging, another group of researchers were dealing with a disease whose sufferers would never have to deal with that problem; they would not live long enough to do so. People who were diagnosed with diabetes mellitus in childhood could usually expect to be dead within a year, perhaps two if they were extraordinarily disciplined with their diet. Their bodies failed to metabolize carbohydrates and other nutrients, leaving excess sugar to collect in their blood and poison their bodies, while at the same time they slowly wasted away. Decades earlier, researchers had shown that diabetes was linked to the function of the pancreas, a flat, pear-shaped gland tucked just behind the stomach. From May 1921 to early 1922, researchers at the University of Toronto—Frederick Banting,

Charles Best, John James Rickard Macleod, and James Bertram Collip—isolated a hormone from the pancreas that had the ability to restore the function that was missing in the bodies of people with diabetes. They named it insulin. In the weeks that followed, the medical world watched in awe as patients who only a short time before had faced a sure and imminent death were raised Lazarus-like from their sickbeds and as skeletal children were restored to abundant life. Before 1922, childhood diabetes had been a death sentence, and after 1922, it no longer was. It was as stark and simple as that.[28] At the very same moment that the fiction of *Black Oxen* poured out of Gertrude Atherton, real-life transformations were being made by the discoverers of insulin. This advance proved to be a watershed in hormone science. Many new practitioners and researchers were drawn to the field by insulin's success, and endocrine research expanded rapidly through the 1920s and 1930s.

Benjamin's relationship with Eugen Steinach was always one of a deferential disciple. Steinach could be touchy, arrogant, belligerent, and even somewhat paranoid, but he could also be the most wonderful host and teacher. During one visit in May 1923, Steinach flew into a rage about something. Benjamin wrote in his diary that the great man could be easily insulted and would not be hurried. He reminded himself, "I have—before everything else—to preserve his friendship and goodwill."[29] That same year, the German film company UFA made a feature-length documentary called *Der Steinach-Film*, which presented Steinach's research. Two versions of the film were made, one for a scientific audience and another for a popular audience. UFA—the studio later responsible for Fritz Lang's *Metropolis* in 1927 and Marlene Dietrich's first sound film, *The Blue Angel*, in 1930—premiered *Der Steinach-Film* in Berlin on 8 January at the prestigious UFA-Palast Am Zoo, Germany's largest cinema. Benjamin contracted with UFA to bring the documentary to the United States and to show it to select audiences. He was able to present it to the German Medical Society at the New York Academy of Medicine in October but found to his frustration that no US distributor was willing to take it out to wider audiences.[30] Over the years, Benjamin also tried to convince Steinach to come to the United States for a lecture tour, but the plans never worked out. Steinach grew testy with his devoted disciple, concerned that Benjamin was sensationalizing his serious science. He insisted that he would come to America only if he were formally invited by an institution.

Paul Kammerer, on the other hand, was grateful for the connection. While many people found Kammerer's erratic and highly emotional personality off-putting, Benjamin had come to regard him as one of his dearest and most admired friends. In time, Kammerer would share with Benjamin painful, personal details of his life, including his recurring bouts of depression and gonorrhea.[31]

Kammerer and Steinach had a lengthy collaboration exploring the possibility that the endocrine system might be key to understanding heredity and evolution. Specifically, they believed that sex hormones were the means by which adaptations made by one organism in response to its environment might become entrenched and then inherited by its offspring. These ideas formed an alternative to the evolutionary ideas that later became dominant that stressed blind chance in the creation of new characteristics. Kammerer often good-naturedly criticized Steinach's temperamental disposition but always said with real conviction, "Steinach is a great genius; he has ideas as original as Darwin's and as Freud's. Some day the world will recognize it."[32]

The love of music might have been one important point of connection for Benjamin and Kammerer. Kammerer was not only a talented animal breeder and experimentalist but also a committed popular science writer, public speaker, musician, and composer who socialized with Alban Berg and Gustav Mahler. Kammerer was devoted to Mahler and, like Joseph Fraenkel, developed a passion for Alma Mahler after Gustav's death. Alma spurned Kammerer's advances but accepted his offer of employment and for a time worked as an assistant in his laboratory at the Vivarium, feeding mealworms to praying mantises.[33]

Benjamin was alarmed that the financial crisis in Austria had crippled Kammerer's research. In September 1922, Benjamin attempted to raise funds for him through a scheme by which he mailed out copies of Kammerer's book on rejuvenation to the membership of the German Medical Society and asked them to send one dollar in payment.[34] As Kammerer's professional, personal, and financial life became increasingly troubled, he decided to leave the Vivarium in 1923 to try to make a living in public lecturing. He confessed to Benjamin that he had attempted suicide twice and was now so desperate that he was prepared to "crawl to America as a servant (e.g. as your lab 'assistant') or dishwasher."[35] Benjamin encouraged Kammerer that he might be able to find teaching in the United States, perhaps in one of the universities in the west. He also met with Horace Liveright to persuade him to publish Kammerer's book in the United States. Liveright was only too eager to capitalize on the success of *Black Oxen* and published Kammerer's *Rejuvenation and the Prolongation of Human Efficiency* in late 1923, with an introduction by Benjamin. Benjamin arranged a six-month book tour complete with lively promotional material playing up the connection of Kammerer to Steinach.

Benjamin argued in the introduction to Kammerer's book that it was critically important that expectations for rejuvenation be kept in check. He felt the sensationalist portrayal of rejuvenation on the stage, in literature, and in the daily papers meant that disappointment was sure to follow unless readers girded themselves with a true knowledge of the very real limitations, as well as the possibilities, of the treatment. Kammerer dedicated his book to Benjamin "as a token of sincere friendship and appreciation of his distinguished services in introducing and applying the Steinach Method of Rejuvenation in the United States."[36]

One significant intellectual commitment that Benjamin and Kammerer shared was monism. At the time, monism was a rapidly growing movement in Germany, Austria, and Switzerland. Although the work of German biologist Ernst Haeckel would have been the chief influence on German monism,[37] it is likely that Benjamin's understanding of monist ideas derived at least in part from the writings of Auguste Forel. The underlying principle of scientific monism was the unity of the human and natural world. In contrast with, for example, Descartes's dualistic view of mind and body, or with religious worldviews, monism held that everything could ultimately be explained in terms of physics and chemistry. As a neurologist, Forel was committed to explaining consciousness and the workings of the human mind in terms of physiochemical reactions. This was a view that Benjamin would remain committed to throughout his life.

Monism was also associated with broader ethical and social views, including a commitment to world peace, international cooperation, and the formation of a healthy society through eugenics. While some members of the movement would later promote race hygiene and views that would lead to fascism, other monists such as Magnus Hirschfeld preached sexual reform and tolerance. For Kammerer, a committed socialist, monism encapsulated his social and scientific ideals; his cooperative, egalitarian vision of humanity was linked to the idea of a productive version of eugenics. Today, it is difficult for us to think of eugenics as anything but a science gone horribly wrong, but it is important to remember that in the early decades of the twentieth century, eugenics was viewed as the epitome of scientific progress by intellectuals around the world and on both progressive and conservative ends of the political spectrum. For Kammerer, productive eugenics held the key to the betterment of humanity. Bolstered by his experiments on salamanders and toads, he argued that an organism might make adaptive changes in response to its environment and that these changes could at times be inherited by offspring. In contrast to the selectionist brand of eugenics that then prevailed, which advocated either negative approaches, such as forced sterilization of the "unfit," or positive approaches, such as encouraging the fertility of those considered "fit," productive eugenics held out the possibility of not only selecting from among characteristics that preexisted in nature but generating new, better traits. Disillusioned by the horrors of the Great War, Kammerer wanted to challenge humanity to take charge of its own future, arguing that better nutrition, education, and environment, as well as the use of hormones, transplants, and radiation, could ultimately improve the hereditable qualities of the human race. In place of a harsh view of nature "red in tooth and claw," Kammerer drew from his vast knowledge of zoology to show examples of mutual aid and symbiosis in nature, and he argued that humanity could deliberately reshape itself to incorporate traits promoting cooperation and the greater common good. In *Rejuvenation*, Kammerer described the endocrine system as a model of cooperation and egalitarian teamwork, in marked contrast to the nervous system, which operated hierarchically. For him, hormones were not just about sex drives, aging, or making people tall, short, fat, or thin; they were instead components of a harmonious polyglandular system that were key to the body's internal coordination.[38]

Kammerer's research generated much excitement and controversy. Dubbed "Darwin's successor" by the *New York Times*, Kammerer was met by leading scientists upon his arrival in the United States.[39] Boni and Liveright also published his next book, *The Inheritance of Acquired Characteristics*, in 1924. Kammerer's experimental evidence was compelling to many, but his case was complicated by the fact that other researchers found it difficult to reproduce his experiments, most no doubt lacking Kammerer's unusual gift for breeding and training amphibians and reptiles. His collections had dwindled from neglect during the war, and after 1921, during the years he spent on lecture tour in Britain and the United States, they grew smaller still. In a famous set of experiments done in 1909, he had found evidence of a hereditable characteristic that had been induced by a change of environment. (A land-breeding species of "midwife toads" was made to breed in water, and Kammerer claimed to find that the males developed calluses on their paws—nuptial pads—as they grasped the females during mating. He found that these pads were inherited for several generations.) In August 1926, an American researcher visited the Vivarium and examined the single remaining specimen from this experiment and announced that it appeared someone had injected India ink into its nuptial pads. The publication of his damning paper in the scientific journal *Nature* caused an international scandal, with its implication that Kammerer had faked his data.

Even today, almost a century later, observers continue to argue about whether Kammerer was a fraud or simply overly enthusiastic in his assessment of his data and whether the ink had been injected by a well-meaning assistant or perhaps even as a deliberate act of sabotage. Whatever the case, on 24 September, Kammerer took a revolver into the hills near Vienna and shot himself in the head. Many people took his suicide as evidence of his guilt. Benjamin was crushed. He had always found Kammerer a brilliant and genial associate and felt his tragic end as a true shock. Gertrude Atherton extended her sympathy to Benjamin, who she knew would be devastated: "Poor man," she wrote, "he had the temperament of an artist, not of the scientist, and was unable to take the blows of fate philosophically."[40] For some people, an association with Kammerer might now have seemed something of an embarrassment, so it seems significant that Benjamin would continue to identify Kammerer as his dear friend even years later. Perhaps as significant is the fact that Benjamin's approach to endocrinology would continue to be shaped by the polyglandular vision of cooperation and interdependence that Kammerer had shared.

One of the chief objections of medical authorities to the glandular therapies of the era was that organ extracts were sometimes used rather indiscriminately, often in inventive combinations linked only tenuously to demonstrable clinical effects. In the 1920s, the Harrower Laboratory in Glendale, California, was one of the most prolific manufacturers of organotherapeutic formulas, including "pluriglandular products" that brought several different organ extracts together into one convenient product. Harrower offered everything from "Antero-Pituitary" tablets for "Defective Children, Mongolism, [and] Epilepsy" to "Thyro-Pancreas compounded with Ovary" for "Functional Hypertension in Women."[41] Medical scientists urged a more rigorous approach, which consisted of first demonstrating that the removal or destruction of a particular endocrine organ created a characteristic syndrome, then that administering an extract of the organ relieved that syndrome, and finally that the activity of that extract could be measured by a chemical or physiological test.[42] It became increasingly apparent to those in the field that the road forward for endocrinology lay in the hands of biochemists. Through biochemistry, individual hormones could be isolated and purified and their activity could be ascertained through physiological tests. They could also then be mass-produced and made available for therapeutic use. By the early 1920s, a number of laboratories around the world were engaged in endocrine research, particularly in the area of the sex hormones, and the field gained a sense of heated competition as several different groups converged on key problems. One researcher likened this period to an endocrinological gold rush.[43] In St. Louis, Missouri, in 1923, Edgar Allen and Edward Doisy isolated a hormone from the ovary that could induce sexual maturation in immature female animals. Further research was hampered, however, by the limited quantities of the raw materials. This changed when, in 1926, other researchers discovered that placentas were another rich source of this female sex hormone. Still others discovered that urine, and even more so the urine of pregnancy, was also an excellent source. By 1929, the female sex hormone was purified in crystalline form by Doisy, Sidney Thayer, and Clement Veler in St. Louis as well as by Adolf Butenandt in Göttingen. Ernst Laqueur and his team in Amsterdam also obtained a similar material in 1930.[44]

The American Medical Association (AMA) had for decades been securing the boundaries of orthodox medicine by battling what it considered alternative medicine, fads, and quack remedies. The association established a propaganda department (later called the Bureau of Investigation) to gather and disseminate information on health fraud and quackery and to advise physicians. After 1923, the AMA also published the popular journal *Hygeia* to give health information to lay people as well. Benjamin and his glandular therapies fell under suspicion with organized medicine; the Bureau of Investigation assembled a small file on him, including press clippings as well as articles that he had sent to them. In the documentation, bureau director Arthur Cramp noted that Benjamin had appeared on the program of an organization called the American Association for Medico-Physical Research, which he deemed belonged to that "'twilight zone' of professionalism . . . whose membership consists of quacks, near-quacks and faddists." From 1926 on, the AMA's journal editor, Morris Fishbein, suggested that the bureau reply to physicians' inquiries about Benjamin's offerings with this statement: "The Benjamin treatment is in no way established, and the preponderance of evidence is that it is scientifically unsound."[45]

Fishbein held a powerful position in organized medicine, helming the AMA's journal from 1924 to 1949 with a crusading fervor to stamp out quackery. He was a prolific writer and a witty and energetic speaker, giving up to 300 speeches a year and appearing frequently on the radio as the representative of American medicine.[46] In 1925, he published the first of a series of humorous popular books that debunked medical fads. It was titled *The Medical Follies* and bore the lengthy subtitle *An Analysis of the Foibles of Some Healing Cults: Including Osteopathy, Homeopathy, Chiropractic, and the Electronic Reactions of Abrams, with Essays on the Antivivisectionists, Health Legislation, Physical Culture, Birth Control, and Rejuvenation.* Horace Liveright, who had made such a success with Atherton's *Black Oxen* and Kammerer's *Rejuvenation* two years before was now only too happy to stir up controversy by publishing their arch-critic, Fishbein. In his book, Fishbein argued that much of the evidence in support of the Steinach operation might merely be the result of nutritional or environmental influences or even the deposition of fat that normally occurred when the gonads were damaged. "To the uncritical reader," he argued, these reports of rejuvenation "carry conviction that the goal for which Faust traded his immortal soul, and for which Ponce de Leon sought unsuccessfully, has been found." But when one more carefully analyzed the data and separated what was proven from the unproven, what was physiological from the psychological, it became clear that it did not add up to proof of the extension of the human lifespan, he declared. Where Fishbein saw true hope for prolonging life was in the conquest of infectious disease. "One by one great infectious diseases and plagues have been brought under control," he explained. Hygiene, nutrition, and clean water and milk supplies had already reduced the incidence of tuberculosis, typhoid, yellow fever, and malaria. "Everyone knows from his own casual observations that a great many more people are living to a ripe old age nowadays than did formerly."[47] Fishbein believed progress lay with the rigor of the laboratory scientist.

Three years earlier, in August 1922, Fishbein had introduced novelist Sinclair Lewis to the bacteriologist and writer Paul de Kruif. Lewis, whom De Kruif remembered as "a lank, towsly, red-haired figure," had just completed the manuscript of his novel *Babbit* and was hunting about for a heroic protagonist for his next book. Lewis in turn recalled De Kruif as "a huge young man who might, except for his super-intelligent face, have been a prize fighter." De Kruif had been an assistant professor at the University of Michigan and a researcher at the Rockefeller Institute. The conversation of the three men ended up lasting all night, and at two in the morning they were still shouting philosophy at each other. Lewis realized that the heroic figure he was looking for might be a bacteriologist, and that in De Kruif he had found a perfect technical advisor who could teach him not only about microbes but about the ethos of scientists as well. Their collaboration, which included months of research traveling from leper asylums to Barbados cane fields, led to the publication of Lewis's *Arrowsmith* in 1925, which tells the story of a country physician who makes his way to become a researcher in the premier scientific institute of the day but then, in the pursuit of personal integrity, renounces those trappings of success to retreat to the woods to conduct pure research uninterrupted. The figure of Martin Arrowsmith, a noble research scientist and courageous warrior against infectious disease, was the first of its kind in American fiction, and the book marked the emergence of the scientist as a new cultural hero. Expectations that had once been pinned on priests were now increasingly transferred to the practitioners and institutions of scientific medicine. *Arrowsmith* would go on to win the Pulitzer Prize in 1926.[48]

Benjamin, however, was relegated to the company of "quacks, near-quacks and faddists." In Fishbein's 1926 *New Medical Follies*, he named Benjamin the "prime exponent of the Steinachian miracle."[49] Moreover, Fishbein mocked the reasoning of the Steinach procedure's adherents. He described them replying with a "cynical shrug of the shoulders" when confronted with conflicting evidence from the laboratory. These practitioners, he jested, could point with pride only to their case records and letters of testimony, a form of reasoning that Fishbein dismissed: "Here is as simple a gesture as might be made by a moron, but hardly the sort of thing one expects from a scientist." Benjamin was incensed. His motives were questioned and his mentality likened to that of a "moron." He wrote Fishbein, saying, "You have attacked me personally with weapons that cannot possibly be called clean," namely misquotations and willful misrepresentation.[50]

Benjamin was neither an uncritical believer nor a callous fraud. From his perspective, he was depending on the research of a highly respected experimental scientist. In his own practice, he tried to document his results as well as he could. In a 1925 article for a medical journal, he reported a survey of 114 cases he had treated, 77 percent of which he found to have had a successful result, using both objective and subjective measures.[51] The weakness in these claims was the lack of scientific controls. What he did not show was a comparison with patients who had *not* received such treatment. Given the well-known psychological factors that might be involved, this seemed to his critics a distinct failure. In presenting a collection of case studies, Benjamin was not out of step with his contemporaries—the notion of randomized, controlled clinical experimentation was only in its infancy—but the rigorous norms of laboratory science were progressively coming to shape scientific medicine. Primarily a practitioner rather than a researcher, Benjamin presented data in a manner that seemed increasingly less convincing as the years went by. It would not be until the 1940s, though, that today's gold standard of the double-blind clinical trial would be introduced, a trial in which neither the patient nor the health professionals know whether an experimental treatment or a placebo is being given.[52]

In his confrontations with Friedrich Franz Friedmann, it is clear that Benjamin was capable of viewing clinical results with a critical eye. In his private statements to Steinach about Atherton's reactivation, it is also clear he was conscious of the need to rule out psychological factors that might affect his patient's outcome. And in his publications, he distinctly argued that reactivation was about adding vitality to midlife, not about extending the life span. He said, "The Steinach Operation is no cureall, no wonder treatment, that will revolutionize medicine, but it has definite value in balancing endocrine disturbances, relieving symptoms of old age and prolonging efficiency—no more and no less." It pained him to realize that his work attracted such pronounced opposition from medical circles as well as from laypeople, and he attributed this not only to misconceptions and the exaggerated claims of "medical pirates" but also the popular association of reactivation to sex. He railed against Fishbein's reactionary stance and his equating of Steinach's painstaking experimental work to the unwarranted assertions of the most flagrant of charlatans. He believed that, while a practitioner should be wary, it was equally important to always keep an open mind. No progress could come without it. Benjamin ended a 1927 article by expressing his confidence that those who had managed to maintain "sufficient mental flexibility" would be happy to welcome new ideas. Quoting Goethe's *Faust*, he concluded:

A mind, once formed is never suited after;
One yet in growth will ever grateful be.[53]

For the next three years, Benjamin stewed about what he felt was a grave injury to his reputation. He made numerous visits to Liveright's office threatening a lawsuit and fired off letters to Fishbein and many officials at the AMA. From their private correspondence, it is clear that Liveright and Fishbein did not take him seriously, dismissing him as hotheaded and without any basis for a libel suit.[54] Moreover, Fishbein and his colleagues regarded Benjamin as an outsider and a shameless self-promoter and felt confident that if it came down to a legal fight, they would have no trouble collecting a thick stack of depositions from "all the leading physicians of New York City" opposing Benjamin's views.[55] Despite Liveright's efforts to calm him down, Benjamin was not put off. In March 1929, he formally brought a $250,000 suit against Horace Liveright Inc. and Morris Fishbein for libel.[56]

Fishbein's lawyer warned Fishbein, "The case is a dangerous one."[57] Benjamin had come to believe Fishbein's writing "hostile, malevolent and unfair" and his methods of attack underhanded.[58] He tried to publish letters to the editor in various medical journals in his own defense but found the vehicles of organized medicine largely closed to him. Sympathetic colleagues stepped in to mediate, including Chicago surgeon Max Thorek, who had himself studied testes transplantation and vasoligation.[59] Thorek visited Fishbein at his office in 1929 and hesitantly brought up the subject of Benjamin's suit, thinking it might be a delicate subject. He was surprised to find that Fishbein simply smiled and said, "Dr. Benjamin must be misinformed about me. I bear no malice toward him. I don't see wherein he found justification to enter suit against me." He added that he had never voluntarily hurt Benjamin, nor had he intended to embarrass him. When Thorek suggested that Benjamin had felt hurt that Fishbein had not replied to his letters, Fishbein replied, "Why should I? Dr. Benjamin has written to almost every officer in the American Medical Association." Thorek was shocked and wrote to Benjamin saying that, if he had indeed done this, he had made a grave mistake. Fishbein was not only very powerful but respected and well liked, while "there are a lot of fellows that do not like you," he told Benjamin. He warned Benjamin that if he were to continue his libel suit and lose, the whole of organized medicine in New York might "take a crack at" him and make life "damned unpleasant." He advised, "I know that you will get huffed and hot under the ears but I am your friend and wish you well for you are a learned man and I know you do not belong to a class that can afford to antagonize the organized profession." Even if he felt in his heart that he had been treated unfairly, Thorek advised him to show that he was "above petty things." He pleaded, "Be on the right side of the fence, Harry, even if you are hurt and in time you will be recognized and it will all work out to your advantage."[60] Benjamin, however, was not assuaged. His legal action would be painfully protracted, dragging out well into the next decade.

———

The fact was, however, that laboratory scientists were beginning to challenge Steinach's claims. In the early 1920s, zoologist Carl Moore and his team at the University of Chicago carried out a series of rigorous tests of the hypotheses behind the Steinach operation. They found that, while at times the degeneration of the reproductive portion of the testes did indeed lead to an increase in the interstitial cells, this did not actually result in an increase in the production of male hormone. In further experiments in five different species of laboratory mammals, they found no evidence that testes transplantation or the ligation of the vas deferens produced an increase in the male sex hormone.[61]

Whether or when Benjamin ever lost faith in the efficacy of the Steinach operation is not clear. He would continue to perform operations and speak about it in lectures well into the 1940s. Perhaps most significantly, he believed in it sufficiently to have had the operation himself. Its appeal lay in the fact that, unlike injecting foreign hormones derived from animals, the operation was thought to stimulate the patient's own glands into renewing their production of hormones. What is clear, however, is that as reliable hormone products became commercially available, Benjamin did not hesitate to integrate them into his practice. In the 1920s, he began to use commercial female hormones in concert with the Steinach treatment of diathermy for his women patients. By the end of the decade, he was even ready to jump into the hormone gold rush himself.

In 1928, Benjamin began a new venture with Benjamin Harrow, a physiological chemist and science writer at City College of New York.[62] Harrow had come from his native England to study and then teach first at Columbia University and, after 1928, at City College. Harrow frequently wrote newspaper articles and book reviews on topics such as vitamins, nutrition, and the glands. In his popular book of 1922, *Glands in Health and Disease*, Harrow was critical of the overblown claims made by enthusiasts, describing them as facts mixed with fancy, and warning, "imagination, not sufficiently tempered by self-criticism, is apt to enlarge a molehill into a mountain." He acknowledged that, thus far, achievements in the study of the glands could only be said to be modest when they were judged by careful scientific standards, but the possibilities, he argued, were "limitless."[63]

During his time at Columbia, Harrow had gotten to know the esteemed Polish chemist Casimir Funk. Funk was already well known for his research on factors in food that were essential for life; in 1912, he had been among the first to formulate the concept of vitamins and had coined the term "vitamine." Funk had been born in Warsaw and trained in Berne, Paris, Berlin, and London. He had then spent the war in New York working with pharmaceutical firm H. A. Metz & Company to sort out the manufacture of important products such as Salvarsan and adrenaline that had been imported from Germany. While there, he had also produced the first vitamin supplement to be approved by the AMA as an ethical product. After the war, he had returned to Warsaw to head the Rockefeller Foundation–funded National Health Institute. In 1928, Funk moved to Paris to work half time with a large pharmaceutical company while spending the other half of his time pursuing a dream of setting up his own research establishment, which he called "Casa Biochemica." He had been interested in the sex hormones for some time and now wanted to throw himself into the study of the male hormone.[64]

Harrow saw a golden opportunity for collaboration. Funk had expertise but needed private funding for his independent laboratory in France. Harrow could work on the chemical problem as well in his laboratory in New York. And Benjamin not only had the clinical side of the work covered but possessed many valuable contacts with wealthy businessmen, some of whom were his patients. Together, Harrow, Benjamin, and Funk devised a plan to attempt the isolation of the male hormone. In July 1928, it was hellishly hot when Harrow traveled to Paris to meet with Funk. He reported back to Benjamin with great excitement that Funk had already started work on the testicular hormone and had even arranged for a full-time clinical assistant to do operations and injections. He was enthusiastic about their prospects. For one thing, money went a lot further in France than it did in America, he suggested. "I confess that without Funk our chances of success become far more remote: & I for that matter, I can't think of anyone aside from Funk who could tackle the chem. work," he wrote. "I think we are terribly fortunate to be able to come in at this stage."[65]

Benjamin courted three of the rich men of his acquaintance: Harold McCormick of International Harvester; August Heckscher, a mining magnate; and Jules Bache, the head of one of the top brokerage houses in the country. Benjamin explained to them that in the fight against age, the leading science was moving away from using surgery. Instead, the ambition now was to prepare an active principle of the gland that could be given by hypodermic injection. He told them that the product of the female sex gland had been successfully isolated in recent years, but the male principle had not as of yet. He further added that he, Harrow, and Funk offered to freely contribute their labor to the work but required funds for research expenses. By the summer of 1928, Benjamin had successfully convinced all three investors to contribute $5,000 each to form the Hormone Research Corporation and to fund Funk's work for a year and a half.

McCormick, for one, was already well acquainted with rejuvenation. In 1922, just after a divorce and before a new marriage, he had undergone a testes transplantation by a Chicago surgeon for a reported sum of $50,000. The woman he went on to marry was none other than opera singer Ganna Walska, the widow of Joseph Fraenkel, the man who had introduced Benjamin to glandular science. (Since Fraenkel's death in 1920, Walska had also married and divorced the carpet tycoon Alexander Smith Cochran.)[66] Despite Walska's apparently modest talent—she was reportedly once pelted with rotten vegetables by an audience after straying off key too often—McCormick lavishly supported her career with thousands of dollars in voice lessons and even arranged for her to have the leading role in a Chicago Opera performance. (Orson Welles claimed her story was the inspiration for the character of Kane's second wife, Susan, in *Citizen Kane*.) The connection of McCormick and Walska with rejuvenation went even further. In 1927, newspapers reported that Walska was applying for a license to open a string of beauty parlors in Paris in the heart of the Champs-Élysées quarter in partnership with monkey-gland surgeon Serge Voronoff. The salons were to be funded with capital of 1,500,000 francs (almost $60,000) and would offer perfumes, powders, and lotions alongside glandular rejuvenation surgery.[67]

In France, Funk selected a two-acre plot in Rueil-Malmaison, a suburb on the outskirts of Paris, and began construction of his Casa Biochemica. There, he envisaged building laboratories, animal facilities, a residence for his young family, three houses for his married assistants, and another three for those who were single. Funk, a slight man with a gentle, boyish appearance, was hesitant with strangers but possessed a charm that emerged when he was among friends. He tended to have astringently opinionated views, not only in areas of which he was clearly a master but even on topics such as music or women's fashions in which his mastery was somewhat less clear. Over the next few years, Casa Biochemica would become very much a family affair. Funk's four-year-old daughter, Doriane, helped to tend the animals in the colony, though she became attached to the cats and hid them from her father when one or two were slated for adrenal operations. When Funk declared that he planned to get rid of the spotted cats and keep only the ones that were completely black, the resourceful Doriane painted the spotted ones with black ink. Funk worked long hours but came home for meals with his wife and children and returned to the lab in the evening. He loved talking as he worked, usually thinking aloud several steps ahead of himself. Meanwhile, the ash of his cigarette would grow longer and longer, though it was never allowed to fall into the beakers full of his precious solutions.[68]

In the 1920s and 1930s, endocrine researchers explored many sources from which to extract hormones, from organs salvaged from slaughterhouse animals to placentas collected at maternity hospitals to the urine of pregnancy. Funk decided to change tactics: instead of trying to obtain the male hormone from testicles, he began to use to urine from young men, which was obviously a far more plentiful and easier-to-obtain source. Benjamin came up with the idea that they collect urine from the male students at City College. In this period, biochemists were devising better methods to isolate the hormones, but once the substance had been purified, it was critical to have a physiological test that could evaluate whether it performed a clearly defined function in a living animal. Extracts of the testes could be assessed on capons, that is, roosters that had been castrated when they were young so that their combs and wattles degenerated. When an active extract of the testes was injected into such birds, their combs and wattles developed once more and their overall appearance improved. When treatment was stopped, the birds soon reverted to their original appearance.[69]

By the summer of 1929, Funk's laboratory and family residence had been completed, but it was becoming apparent that everything was taking more time and money than expected. Funk traveled to the United States to attend the International Physiological Congress in Boston on 19–23 August. The congress, for the first time held outside of Europe, was an event of major consequence bringing together more than 1,600 participants from forty-one countries. Many of the greatest physiologists in the world were in attendance, the most honored of whom was Ivan Pavlov. Some arrived together from Europe on a specially arranged steamship, and others came from as far as China and Japan. There were four to six simultaneous sessions per day, with presentations lasting only ten minutes each, as well as live experimental demonstrations. A number of endocrine breakthroughs were announced, including Doisy, Veler, and Thayer's crystallization of female hormone from pregnancy urine. Voronoff reported that some of his testicular grafts had shown effects lasting for five years. More directly relevant—and more worrying to Funk, Harrow, and Benjamin—was the report of the University of Chicago team of Fred Koch, Carl Moore, and Thomas Gallagher that they had obtained an extract of bull testicles that caused comb growth in capons.[70] The next day Funk wrote Benjamin from his hotel reporting that Koch's demonstration had received much attention. Because he knew Koch's picture and story were likely to hit the daily papers, Funk urged Benjamin to come to Boston and arrange for reporters to cover his own talk as well, "in that I should get at least the same attention," he insisted. "It is important that we should not be put aside."[71]

Funk made his presentation before a large audience, announcing that he and Harrow had managed to obtain an active male hormone from the urine of human males. The *New York Times* featured Funk in its report on the congress the next day, proclaiming "Isolation of Hormone Offers Rejuvenation by Means of Injections, Funk Says." Funk exhibited roosters with combs erect and wattles filled out. He explained that just four to five days after beginning injections of the extract, the combs and wattles of castrated birds looked improved, and by the end of four to six weeks, these capons looked virtually the same as uncastrated roosters. The newspaper announced that Funk's method "would be applied clinically to humans by Dr. Harry Benjamin of 239 West Seventy-Fifth Street." Benjamin, who attended the demonstration, was quoted as saying the new treatment looked very promising.[72]

When it came to the matter of clinical testing, Benjamin enthusiastically offered to be first in line. According to Benjamin's recollection, Funk almost fainted as Benjamin injected himself. Fortunately, the only ill effects that Benjamin felt were a terrible soreness and bruising at the injection site because of impurities in the preparation.[73] At the close of the meeting, Funk decided to stay on in the United States for a few more weeks to try to raise additional funds. He found to his disappointment, however, that the amounts raised were still far from what he felt was needed. For another year and a half, Funk continued his work in France, and Harrow attacked the same problems in New York. Meanwhile, Benjamin tried to balance the books and manage the expectations of the investors. Funk and Harrow worked at purifying the hormone extract so that it was safe for clinical use and at scaling up production to industrial levels. They had to deal with many practical problems, from arranging for a regular supply of large quantities of urine to creating the facilities in which to treat these huge volumes.

The next year, Benjamin spent July to October 1930 in Europe, where he had a full schedule of activities. He spoke at Albert Moll's Second International

Congress on Sex Research in London (where he also saw a tailor and had shirts made), visited his mother in Berlin, and then presented at Hirschfeld's Congress of the World League for Sexual Reform in Vienna in September. In between, he went to see Funk in Paris and met with potential pharmaceutical partners for their venture in Cologne. For several months, the collaborators worked to make arrangements for the commercial manufacture of the hormone with one firm near Paris and another in the United States. Tempers began to flare, though, as Funk's demands for funds grew more pointed. Funk felt sure the project was very promising. Indeed, in his more than ten years of manufacturing experience, he was certain that extracting male hormone from urine was the "easiest and cheapest" product he had ever seen made, requiring only a small outlay of funds and yet, as a luxury item, having the potential of being sold at a good profit.[74] He felt stretched, however, between his own research and dealing with problems at the factory. Both Funk in France and Harrow in New York had been able to produce small numbers of ampoules of the male hormone, but the activity of the product was not reliable. At the end of October 1930, Benjamin reported the results of his clinical tests, saying that their product was certainly purer than before and no longer produced pain and discomfort as their earlier product had, but unfortunately thus far, there had been no discernible endocrine effect.[75]

Funk, though, began to propose a second line of inquiry. Other endocrine researchers had begun to find links between the sex hormones and the anterior pituitary gland. The anterior pituitary is the forward-facing lobe of the pea-sized pituitary gland that rests below the base of the brain, and there was growing evidence that it had a role in controlling the activity of the sex glands. As a scientist, Funk recognized the importance of trying to work out the complex interactions among the different glands and hormones. Benjamin, on the other hand, was appalled at Funk's idea. He begged Funk to see things from the perspective of the investors. The work on the male sex hormone had not been completed, and now Funk wanted money to start the new project before even delivering on the first.

Indeed, Benjamin was having difficulties with his money men. McCormick, though initially willing, had grown wary of the attention drawn by the project and now backed out, having perhaps been burned by the scrutiny he had received in the press years earlier with his testicle transplant. Benjamin explained to Funk that McCormick had decided he did not want to have anything to do with "medicine for profit" and declared, "I can hardly express my admiration for him adequately."[76] Bache was more willing, however, and even made a trip in 1929 to see Funk's facility in France. Benjamin found him a charming and intelligent man who he was sure could appreciate all that Funk might tell him. He warned Funk, however, not to discuss finances. He explained that "Bache is a business man of the highest type and tremendously wealthy." He speculated that Bache might even help them in the future "on a much larger scale by possibly endowing an institute etc." but warned that Bache needed first to be impressed with the seriousness of their endeavor and its importance for medicine and to be shown actual successes before anything more could be proposed.[77] In New York, Benjamin, Funk, and Harrow were even treated to an elegant dinner at the Bache mansion and to a viewing of its fabulous art collection, which would one day grace the walls of the Metropolitan Museum of Art. (Bache, a renowned collector, had just paid $250,000 for a small Holbein portrait and $600,000 for a Raphael.)[78] Bache could not, however, be induced to contribute any more funds to their project. Harrow would later reflect that Bache was a practical man interested in practical results. Bache just wanted to know, "When will this stuff be ready for rejuvenation?"[79]

By October 1930, Benjamin was worrying that "if we cannot begin to sell anything within the next three months, we might just as well quit." He was sure that they would not be able to raise any further funds. In early 1931, the collaboration of Benjamin, Funk, and Harrow finally fell apart, dissolving into heated denunciations over money. Benjamin was irate that Funk had angered their investors by making direct appeals to them, and he reported to Funk that Harrow was also furious at his minimizing of Harrow's contributions to the scientific work. In a letter drafted to Funk—which at Harrow's suggestion was left unsent—Benjamin railed, "This is our last friendly communication. . . . Everybody here is united in considering your actions and character disloyal, rotten or insane, the reason why an unwillingness exists here to continue an association with you."[80]

In this failed venture, Benjamin, though regarded by Morris Fishbein as on the questionable margins of medicine, had also managed to put himself tantalizingly close to the cutting edge of hormone research. Harrow and Funk published a number of papers together on this work, and later on insulin, but in the meantime, it would be left to other research groups to achieve the isolation and manufacture of the male hormones.

Funk continued his research on vitamins and worked with Rousell Company until 1936. In 1939, after the invasion of Poland by Germany, Funk returned to New York, where he worked for the US Vitamin Corporation and, with its help, set up the Funk Foundation for Medical Research in 1947. Today, he is best remembered as a pioneer in the study of vitamins. Harrow continued his career as professor of chemistry at City College. In 1955, he wrote a biography of Funk in which he called him "one of the original minds of our time."[81]

———

This unsuccessful enterprise must have come as a personal and financial blow, especially because Benjamin had already lost money as a result of bad investments in the crash of 1929, though he certainly was not alone in doing so. As a private practitioner with no institution or salary, his attempts to augment his practice with other related financial ventures were no doubt important to his comfort and security. As the Great Depression deepened, Benjamin bemoaned his straitened circumstances, which meant he would not be able to make his usual visit to Europe.[82] Later in life, Benjamin claimed that money had never meant a lot to him.[83] But this is only partly true. Instead, it seems Benjamin was rather like his father, Julius, whom he described as a man who liked living as a millionaire even though he wasn't one. Despite these ups and downs, his practice was graced by strange and wonderful windfalls. Once, he gave a one-hour consultation to a wealthy patient, and when asked what the fee was, Benjamin told the man to send whatever he wanted; a check for a thousand dollars arrived shortly after.[84] Whatever his financial situation, he continued to mix with the rich and famous. Benjamin spent a lot of time with the banker and philanthropist Otto Kahn, who was sometimes called the "King of New York"; Kahn was known as a great patron of the arts, especially the Metropolitan Opera. Benjamin felt quite a blow when Kahn died suddenly in 1934.[85]

What was it that helped Benjamin's practice survive and attract such an elite clientele? In reality, Benjamin's therapeutic armament—his rays and masks, procedures, pills, and injections—formed only part of his appeal. Decades later, Gertrude Atherton continued to send referrals to Benjamin. One of her colleagues, a literary man in his midfifties, wrote back to her raving for pages about his experience. He explained that he had been just about ready to "cash in" when he had made his way to Benjamin's office. He was greatly relieved when Benjamin told him he was in amazingly sound condition for someone his age. He went on his way feeling much better having had, as he described it, "some hormone injections (I don't know what they are)" to build up his resistance. He thanked Atherton heartily, explaining, "Just his approach is enough to make one feel better. He doesn't scare the life out of you the way some doctors do."[86] This was the face Benjamin showed to his patients, and perhaps to his colleagues as well—at least, when they were in agreement with him. As one associate would later put it, "Harry Benjamin elevated courtesy to the point where it became personality. You could sense that his beautiful manners were not the result of training, but rather grew out of a deep caring for other people."[87] Benjamin's European charm may have enchanted his patients at first meeting, but what seems to have held them was a sense of his sincere concern and genuine warmth, which made him a clinician of first order. As patients described it, when Benjamin spoke to them, they felt really seen as a human being, heard, cared for, and understood. There were perhaps times when Benjamin wondered how effective his glandular treatments actually were, but on the whole, his ministrations seem to have been offered with a sincere belief and compassionate manner that impressed patients, whether rich and famous or not. And perhaps it was this feeling of being seen and cared for that was as much a part of his therapeutic success as the glandular treatments.

Chapter 8

Wanderer between Two Worlds

Through the 1920s until 1930, Harry Benjamin traveled to Europe almost every year, carrying back with him to America the ideas and practices he absorbed in Berlin and Vienna. Historian Erwin Haeberle would dub him the "Transatlantic Commuter." Benjamin would call himself a "wanderer between two worlds."[1]

The sexual freedoms of Weimar Berlin have been made famous through such works as the musical *Cabaret*, which was itself drawn from the Berlin stories of Christopher Isherwood.[2] In March 1929, Isherwood made a brief visit to his friend W. H. Auden, who was spending a postgraduate year in the city. In his memoir, *Christopher and His Kind*, Isherwood acknowledged that he was drawn to Berlin by his hunger to meet young men. By November, Isherwood moved there, taking up residence next door to the Institute for Sexual Science, in a room rented from Magnus Hirschfeld's sister. Other famous visitors to the institute included French writer André Gide and filmmaker Sergei Eisenstein, while writer Walter Benjamin, philosopher Ernst Bloch, and the communist member of parliament Willi Münzenberg lived for a time in the adjoining house.

Isherwood spent the next few years gathering the materials that would go into his portrait of the denizens of Berlin's cafés and clubs as the city fell under the shadow of Nazism. Isherwood was invited into the social life of the institute, and he recalled lunch as "a meal of decorum and gracious smiles," presided over by a dignified, silver-haired woman whose bearing seemed to guarantee that here, sex would be "treated with seriousness." The staff and guests gathered each day, and though Hirschfeld himself rarely ate with them, he was represented by Karl Giese, his secretary and longtime partner. Isherwood was shocked to realize that one of his fellow guests, whom he had taken to be a woman—and who was related to as a woman by the others—was someone who had been assigned male at birth. Before this, Isherwood had harbored stereotypes of transvestites as "loud, screaming, willfully unnatural creatures," but he was shaken out of his assumptions by seeing this person, who was quiet, natural, and accepted by the others.[3] Isherwood had thought he had shed bourgeois notions of respectability, but his experiences at the institute unnerved him, revealing to him his own latent puritanism. He could only giggle in nervous embarrassment as Giese and a friend took him for a tour of the institute's museum, complete with its displays of whips, chains, high-heeled boots for fetishists, and lacy underwear worn by Prussian officers under their uniforms. There was a gallery of photos of everything from the sexual organs of hermaphrodites to portraits of famous homosexual couples. Isherwood had until then behaved as if homosexuality were a private way of life that he and a few friends had discovered, but now he was "brought face to face with his tribe." He was forced to acknowledge a connection with these strange others, and initially he did not like it. In time, however, he grew to honor Hirschfeld as a heroic leader of this tribe. He would also realize that like everyone else who entered the world of the institute, he became something of a specimen, subject to diagnosis and classification by Hirschfeld. (Hirschfeld declared him "infantile.")[4]

Since the mid-1920s, the questionable gland preparations of earlier years were increasingly replaced by powerful new hormone products with demonstrable pharmacological effect and legitimate therapeutic value. Advances in the isolation of the estrogens in the 1920s had made it possible for pharmaceutical firms to manufacture products that had discernible results in physiological tests in the laboratory. They could be shown to affect the female reproductive system and were offered in therapy for the treatment of menstrual disorders. From an early stage, the dream of using hormones for contraception was among the goals of physiologists.

Eugen Steinach's work continued to be highly respected. He would be nominated for the Nobel Prize eleven times, by an impressive and multinational list of nominators from several different scientific and medical disciplines.[5] Beginning around 1923, he also worked with researchers at the pharmaceutical firm

Schering in Vienna on the development of synthetic estrogen products. Schering would launch the first orally active estrogen product Progynon in 1928. Progynon was initially made from ovarian extracts, then placentas, and later the urine of women late in pregnancy.

Steinach sent Gertrude Atherton Progynon pills,[6] and she would take them for the rest of her life. Over the next decades, her correspondence with Benjamin would regularly contain a reference to how many "Progynons" she was taking, how many she had left, and whether he might get her some at lower cost. By 1934, she was taking four a day, at $3.50 a bottle. "Would you send me more progynon?" she asked. "I really think that was helpful."[7]

Ties between laboratory scientists and the pharmaceutical industry were intricate and deep. Hormones of therapeutic value were discovered one after another through the 1920s and 1930s, but their discoverers needed to collaborate with pharmaceutical firms to bring these products to market. In 1930, James Bertram Collip, the Canadian biochemist on the insulin team, worked with the Montreal firm Ayerst, McKenna, and Harrison to develop an orally active estrogen product from placentas called Emmenin. As a result of this collaboration, Ayerst went on to develop Premarin, a form of conjugated estrogens from pregnant mare urine. Whole new firms such as Organon in the Netherlands were established to develop hormone products.[8]

Much of today's scholarship on Hirschfeld's institute focuses on its pathbreaking work in the scientific study of homosexuality and transgender identity. It is, however, important to remember that the work of the institute covered a broad range of questions about sex. Hirschfeld and his colleague Bernhard Schapiro carried out studies of male hormones and male sexual dysfunction including premature ejaculation, erectile dysfunction, and underdeveloped genitals. In the late 1920s, Schapiro collaborated with the company Promonta/Hamburg in the study of a hormone preparation called Testifortan for the treatment of erectile dysfunction and Praejaculin for premature ejaculation. Testifortan was an organ compound that included freeze-dried pulverized anterior pituitary glands and bull testicles. Testifortan, with a small change to its formula, became a greater financial success when it was marketed by a Berlin entrepreneur as Titus-Perlin (Titus Pearls) both in Germany and around the world.[9]

Benjamin was eager to try these products and, in January 1928, wrote to Hirschfeld about getting a further supply of Testifortan tablets and ampoules because he found he had the opportunity to treat several patients with it.[10] He was, however, all too aware of how questionable testicular extracts were in general, well into the mid-1930s. In a lecture he gave in 1933, he explained that many male hormone products were practically useless in the clinic, though they continued to be used frequently for "old age," which he acknowledged "is only too often nothing but a polite designation for sexual deficiencies." Similarly, he knew "rejuvenation," at least in English, was almost always used to refer to the restoration of sexual function. He admitted that he found reports of occasional good results not at all convincing.[11] By the late 1920s, however, significant work was done on the male hormones with definite progress in the development of biologically standardized and tested products. Adolf Butenandt would successfully isolate a crystalline androsterone from 25,000 liters of male urine in 1931, and Ernst Laqueur and his team would isolate a crystalline hormone from the testicle in 1935, giving it the name testosterone.[12]

At Hirschfeld's Institute for Sexual Science, Benjamin continued to be exposed to new ideas in sexology. Hirschfeld had in 1910 defined transvestites as belonging to a category distinct from homosexuals. Indeed, many of the male transvestites he knew had an erotic attraction to women. Hirschfeld came to realize, however, that some individuals strongly wished not only to cross-dress on occasion but to actually change sex. He considered these individuals to have an extreme form of transvestism.

There is evidence that, by the late 1920s, individuals—including a number of Americans—were receiving medical interventions to change sex at various centers in Europe. These interventions included both hormone therapy and surgery. Florence Winter (pseudonym) visited Berlin and consulted with Hirschfeld about the possibility of female-to-male surgery. When Hirschfeld agreed to arrange for the procedure, he warned her that afterward, she would not be either man or woman.[13] She ultimately decided against surgery, opting to live as a man for many years, and then returned to Chicago to live as a lesbian. Another American, Carla Van Crist (pseudonym), grew up in Berlin and San Francisco as a boy and then worked as a female impersonator. She recalled visiting Harry Benjamin in New York, who advised that she consult Hirschfeld. (Benjamin himself did not remember this meeting.) At the institute, she had surgery in 1929 or 1930 and worked as a receptionist until 1933.[14]

Hirschfeld's housekeeper Dora Richter (known as Dorchen) would become the first person known to undergo complete genital transformation. Richter, assigned male at birth, had cross-dressed in childhood and had been repeatedly arrested for dressing as a woman until a judge wrote to Hirschfeld for advice. Hirschfeld invited Richter to the institute and offered surgical treatment, which Richter welcomed. In 1922, Richter underwent castration. For many years after, she would work as a domestic and a demonstration patient at the institute. In 1931, she had additional procedures to remove her penis and have a vagina surgically constructed under the care of Hirschfeld's associates, gynecologist Ludwig Levy-Lenz and surgeon Erwin Gohrbandt.

Institute staff member Felix Abraham wrote the first scientific report on human sex-change surgery, documenting the genital procedures on two male-to-female subjects, one of whom was Richter. The patients were described as "homosexual transvestites." Abraham argued that the surgeries—castration, amputation of the penis, and creation of a vagina—had been imperative because they saved the patients from self-mutilation. Levy-Lenz also recalled that such patients were the most grateful he ever had.[15]

Publicity surrounding these surgeries reached a high point in the early 1930s with the story of the transition of Lili Elbe. Elbe (then living as a man) was an artist from Copenhagen, living in Paris with wife Gerda Wegener. A friend introduced them to the gynecologist Kurt Warnekros, who was the head of the women's clinic in Dresden. Warnekros in turn sent them to see Magnus Hirschfeld. In March 1930, Hirschfeld diagnosed and conducted psychological tests on Elbe, and she received the first of four surgeries, an orchiectomy (removal of the testicles), performed by Erwin Gohrbandt at the institute. Later, Elbe went to Dresden, where under the care of Warnekros she received additional genital surgeries and the transplantation of ovaries. She died of complications from the final surgery, a vaginoplasty, in 1931.[16]

After her death, a semi-fictional book documenting her transformation was translated into several languages and became widely read. The English translation, *Man into Woman*, was published in Britain and the United States in 1933, with an introduction by Norman Haire. Individuals who recognized something of their own struggles and desires—people who might have previously identified themselves as "inverts," sexual intermediaries, transvestites, or homosexuals—now saw the possibility that medicine might play a role in their attaining the physical characteristics that they desired. This book would become a key vehicle for transmitting to a popular audience the idea of medical procedures to change sex.[17]

What is intriguing about Elbe's narrative is that her story reflects a very different conceptualization of her lived experience from what might be recognized by transgender people of today. Elbe thought of herself as two distinct people inhabiting the same body, a man named Andreas and a woman named Lili. She conceived of the medical procedures as a means of killing off the man. Even more intriguing is the fact that Elbe experienced the transplantation of ovaries as a rejuvenation. She was not only becoming a woman; she was becoming a *young* woman with a fresh start in life because she had received a young woman's ovaries.[18] Elbe's narrative may be as much an expression of the ideas of glandular rejuvenation of her time as a presage of the transsexual narratives of midcentury.

There is not much direct evidence of how Benjamin's experiences in Berlin translated to his own medical practice in New York during the 1920s and 1930s. Benjamin would no doubt have been familiar with the Institute for Sexual Science's atmosphere of openness to sexual minorities and gender-variant people, though he seems to have had only a minimal engagement with these issues himself. In his correspondence with Hirschfeld, he acknowledged receipt of Hirschfeld's publications such as the latest of his multivolume *Geschlechtskunde* (Sexology) and expressed his appreciation for the work but said little that was substantive regarding the contents.

In March 1930, Hirschfeld referred Ernest F. Elmhurst, a homosexual activist, to Benjamin. Elmhurst was eager to set up a homosexual reform organization in New York, a "movement of inverts," as he described it. Years before, in Germany, Elmhurst (then known as Ernst Klopfleisch) had made an unsuccessful attempt to turn the Kurhotel in Altenau in the Harz Mountains into a summer gathering place for "inverts," and now having spent seven years in New York, he felt he had sufficiently studied the psychology of Americans to believe there might be an opportunity to do the same in the New World. He suggested they might set up a large club building similar to a YMCA or an athletic club, on the water or in the mountains, where inverts could claim a place in the world. Elmhurst noted that the only opportunity to reach inverts then was at the very successful costume balls. He thought that by distributing cards among the guests at such a dance, he could announce the formation of his organization. Elmhurst visited Benjamin a number of times and Benjamin seemed to want to oblige Hirschfeld, but he felt he had to dampen Elmhurst's enthusiasm for the plan with his assessment that it was "practically unrealizable." In his opinion, an "honest and open association of inverts" was still impossible in America. Benjamin suggested instead that Elmhurst begin more modestly, by bringing together a small group of like-minded people.[19]

In their correspondence, Benjamin and Hirschfeld often complained of the prudery they perceived in US society, and Benjamin obviously felt that, faced with this puritanical attitude, a fully public organization was unrealistic at that time. What Benjamin may have been unable to appreciate, or was perhaps unaware of, was that there already existed a lively demimonde that included semipublic organizations such as Paresis Hall, a gay bar and center of homosexual life in New York, and the Cercle Hermaphroditos, housed in the hall, which since 1895 had served as the first known informal organization in the United States concerned with social justice for transgender people. This group, however, did not seem to have any lasting influence or inspire any successors.[20]

Hirschfeld's commitment to combining science with activism clashed with the approach of psychiatrist Albert Moll. Moll was a bitter opponent of Hirschfeld who argued that sexology should be developed along strictly scientific lines, with the aim of objectivity unmarked by advocacy. Benjamin thought of Moll as a typical German professor who was abrupt, opinionated, and very Prussian, a real "stuffed shirt." While Hirschfeld's sexology congresses brought together researchers and reformers, Moll organized a rival series that was more conservative and focused on science. Benjamin, however, managed to straddle both these worlds, speaking at Hirschfeld's original meeting in 1921 in Berlin and again in Vienna in 1930 as well as at Moll's congresses in Berlin in 1926 and London in 1930, presenting papers on the problems of geriatrics and potency. These sexology meetings allowed Benjamin to meet many of the leading researchers in the field of sexology, including the biologist Oscar Riddle, who later became both a friend and a patient; F. A. E. Crew, an Edinburgh University sex research scientist; and Herbert Lewandowski, who wrote about the sex habits of people in antiquity and in foreign cultures, with whom he corresponded for decades. Benjamin became good friends with Norman Haire, the Australian-born London-based sexologist whom he considered "brilliant and courageous." Margaret Sanger, the great birth control advocate, quizzed Benjamin about what endocrinology might have to offer to prevent pregnancy. She was envisioning something like "the Pill," but that was still many years in the future. Benjamin tried to help organize a meeting of the World League for Sexual Reform in Chicago in 1933, but the plans failed to materialize. During these years, the focus of the meetings would shift; the goals of legal and social equality for homosexuals were increasingly sidelined in favor of issues surrounding eugenic birth control, abortion, and sex education. The league would disband in 1935 as a result of a clash of interests between middle-class liberal reformers and revolutionary Marxists.[21]

———

At this point, none of Hirschfeld's major publications were yet available in English. In 1928, Benjamin was sure this was because of the prudery of US culture, though he held out hope that if the works could be published in Britain first, a US publisher might be willing to take them on and introduce them, though "only in limited circles."[22] Two years later, Benjamin tried to arrange a meeting between Horace Liveright and Hirschfeld. Benjamin urgently recommended to Liveright that he publish Hirschfeld's massive five-volume *Geschlechtskunde* and was disappointed when the meeting failed to materialize, despite Liveright's efforts to see Hirschfeld. A few years later, Benjamin wrote Hirschfeld in alarm that an unauthorized, abridged translation of the first volume of Hirschfeld's *Sexualpathologie* had been published by Julian Press in 1932 with "a most atrocious translation, utterly impossible."[23]

In his correspondence with Hirschfeld, Benjamin referred to Liveright as "my friend, the well-known New York publisher," despite his ongoing lawsuit. (He had assured Liveright that he was really targeting Morris Fishbein but was required to name Liveright Inc. in the suit because Fishbein, in Chicago, was in another jurisdiction.) What Benjamin did not know was that by this time, Liveright was losing his hold on the publishing company he had established. Liveright had been channeling money into his Broadway productions, most of which were flops. By late 1930 he was forced out of the company, and in May 1933 the company declared bankruptcy. Liveright, who had transformed the face of publishing, would die broke that September.[24]

———

In 1933, *Fortune* magazine called the study of hormones "the most important field in medical research." It noted six products that were already "of definite and immediate utility to the man-in-the-street and the physician-in-the-office"— thyroid extracts, pituitary hormones, adrenaline, cortin, estrin, and insulin.[25] Benjamin's practice rode on this swell, though ironically it would be the very success of endocrinology that would bring an end to the rejuvenation work that had launched his career.

Endocrinology had emerged as the quintessential modernist enterprise, marked by a faith in science to engineer everything from the physical shape of the human body to the moral fabric of an entire society. Along with psycho-analysis, endocrinology offered the possibility of unearthing the urges and moti-vations that lay beneath conscious understanding and of charting the pieces of an increasingly fragmented self. In laboratories in Europe, in North America, and around the globe, hormone research was a flourishing field of study, promis-ing a chance to understand the workings of mind and body at a chemical level. In clinics, endocrinology became a fount of powerful, effective new products that served to treat not only a range of specific glandular diseases but, increasingly, a broad swathe of human ills.[26]

Aldous Huxley tapped this fascination with hormones and, with a pessimis-tic slant, explored how these new technologies might be used by a regime to engineer its citizenry. In his 1932 dystopia, *Brave New World*, Huxley imagined embryos manipulated with placentin, thyroxine, and other organ extracts, and female embryos purposely made infertile by treatment with male hormones. In the novel, all citizens are required to take monthly treatments to stimulate their adrenals so that they can experience the livening effect of fear and rage without disrupting society.[27]

More specifically, the study of the hormones brought a new light to the understanding of biological sex. Steinach's work of 1912–16 had been striking in showing that male characteristics could be triggered in a female animal by the transplantation of testes, while female characteristics could be created in male animals by the transplantation of ovaries. Even more remarkable, when in 1916 he transplanted both male and female gonads into animals that had been castrated at a young age, he was at times able to create specimens that displayed both male and female physical and psychic characteristics.[28] The ovaries had been thought to be the source of the "female hormone" and female qualities, while the testes had been thought to be the source of the "male hormone" and male qualities, but new complexities emerged as biochemists entered the field in the 1920s and 1930s. Biochemists developed techniques to work not only with proteins (which include hormones such as insulin) but with lipids as well, allowing them to make headway into understanding the sex hormones, which belong to a class of lipids called steroids. Once they had determined the actual chemical structure of individual sex hormones, it became apparent that there were in fact more than one "female hormone" and one "male hormone." It also became clear that the so-called male and female hormones were actually closely related molecules. As steroid molecules, estrogens and androgens are composed of four linked rings of carbon atoms. The various forms of estrogens and androgens differed only by small groups of atoms attached to this basic structure, so that for example a small tail of one oxygen atom bound to one hydrogen atom (a hydroxyl group) was all that differentiated testosterone from estrin. One male researcher of the day was said to have quipped, "There but for one hydroxyl group go I."[29]

As chemists learned more, it became clear that so-called male hormones were produced in "normal" female bodies and so-called female hormones were produced in "normal" male bodies. The most vivid illustration of this was the fact that the most abundant source of estrogen turned out to be the stallion. Steinach had thought of the male and female hormones as antagonistic in function, so that the presence of the "female hormone" would counteract the function of the "male hormone" and vice-versa. The biochemists of this period began to challenge the notion of the female and male hormones as opposites. Not only were these hormones shown to play important physiological functions in the bodies of the so-called opposite sex, but at times, and in normal processes, one might be chemically transformed into the other. Researchers also learned that the ovaries and testes were not the sole location where these hormones were produced; they were manufactured in the adrenal glands as well. It became apparent that it did not make sense to think of these hormones as "male" and "female" at all.[30]

In November 1930, Hirschfeld left for a lecture tour in the United States, funded by speaking fees as well as by royalties from Titus Pearls. He hoped that it would give him a rest, a visit with family members who had emigrated, and a chance to extend his research.[31] Thanks to the efforts of Harry and Gretchen, his first stop was in New York, where Hirschfeld spent many hours in their home. When it came time to give a seminar in Benjamin's office, Hirschfeld's heavily accented English proved to be a problem. Benjamin begged him, "Dr. Magnus, please speak German." He explained, "At least some people will then understand you. If you speak English nobody will." But it was to no avail. Hirschfeld pushed ahead in English, and the seminar was a complete failure.[32] However, their mutual friend George Sylvester Viereck, a German American journalist, supported Hirschfeld and published many interviews with him in American newspapers, describing him as the "Einstein of sex."[33] In the English press, Hirschfeld was promoted as an expert on marriage, and it was only in German-language papers that Hirschfeld's more radical work on homosexual rights was described. In his six weeks in New York, he met with writers, artists, reformers, scientists, and physicians. He also conducted fieldwork for his ethnographic research in Harlem, in bathhouses, and at night court.

While in the United States, Hirschfeld began to extend his plans to a world tour. Before Hirschfeld departed, Benjamin gave him a routine physical examination and expressed concern about his diabetes.[34] Benjamin and Hirschfeld parted for the last time at a splendid dinner given in Hirschfeld's honor in Chicago by their mutual friend Max Thorek. Thorek also tried to dissuade Hirschfeld from going to Asia with predictions of diabetic coma and gangrene if he were not able to take care of himself.[35] Hirschfeld's travels took him through the Midwest and then to California where Benjamin sent him one last letter begging him, for the sake of their long friendship, not to go through with his plans to travel around the world, as he was sure that Hirschfeld would have trouble sticking to the careful diet and lifestyle he needed to stay healthy as a diabetic. Hirschfeld, however, could not be persuaded and he continued on through Mexico before journeying to Japan and China.[36] Thankfully, the dire consequences his friends feared did not come about and Hirschfeld was to survive his journey. In Shanghai, he met twenty-four-year-old Li Shiu Tong, a medical student who became his disciple and companion. After stops in the Philippines, Indonesia, Singapore, Ceylon, India, Egypt, and Palestine, Hirschfeld and Li arrived back in Europe in 1932. With Li's help, Hirschfeld wrote up and published the details of his tour and ethnographic observations in his book *Men and Women: The World Journey of a Sexologist*. As he had traveled, friends wrote to him of the increasingly hostile environment in Germany and warned against his returning home. Hirschfeld spent the next several years traveling in Greece, Czechoslovakia, and Switzerland and ultimately settled in the south of France as the Nazi Party came to power.

On 6 May 1933, a mob of students backed by the Nazi Party broke into the Institute for Sexual Science and plundered its library. Four days later, portions of the library holdings were thrown into a bonfire, along with a bust of Hirschfeld. In Paris, Hirschfeld watched the book burning in a newsreel at the cinema. Months later, the remaining books, furniture, and materials were sold at auction, and all the staff and even Hirschfeld's sisters were turned out of the house. The government stripped away Hirschfeld's German citizenship as well as the royalties for Titus Pearls, leaving him with few resources. Hirschfeld dreamed of continuing his research elsewhere but was never able to find the support. He continued to correspond with Benjamin about a return to the United States, but despite Benjamin's considerable efforts and reports of Hirschfeld's improving ability to lecture in English, plans for a lecture tour fell through.[37]

Hirschfeld died in exile in Nice in 1935 at the age of sixty-seven. His papers and personal effects and the burden of continuing his life's work were left to his two closest disciples and companions, Karl Giese and Li Shiu Tong. Giese fled to Czechoslovakia and lived in difficult circumstances, unable to access Hirschfeld's estate. He died by suicide in 1938. Li continued his studies in Zurich and at Harvard and then returned to Hong Kong in 1960. In 1974, he immigrated to Canada and died in Vancouver in 1993. From the notes he left behind, it seems he hoped to write about Hirschfeld's teachings but never did so.[38]

By the mid-1930s, Benjamin had built up a practice serving a who's who of the rich, powerful, and famous, though those who were less wealthy found their way to his office as well. Gretchen continued to support Harry's practice in many practical ways. On one occasion when Harry was in Europe for several months, Gretchen wrote to Max Thorek to explain that she was scrambling to have painters in to do some work while she also assumed the secretary's job and then the nurse's job as the office staff took their vacations in turn.[39] In 1934, Benjamin moved his office from West Seventy-Fifth Street to 791 Park Avenue. By then, both his mother and brother were living with them, and Gretchen found the large apartment too much of a burden; Harry also decided he wanted to separate his home from his office.[40] Three years later, he bought a co-op at 728 Park Avenue, at Seventy-First Street. There, along a stretch of boulevard where doormen tended the canopied entrances to stately apartment houses, he would remain for the next two decades, welcoming his patients to a twelve-room suite of offices. Dominating the waiting room was a life mask of Goethe at the age of eighty.[41]

Whatever success Benjamin experienced in his practice, he could not let go of his sense of injury against Morris Fishbein, and he refused to let his lawsuit die. Attorneys for both sides went to court time and again on numerous pleadings and appeals until 1934. At length, Benjamin hinted through his lawyers that he would be willing to drop the lawsuit if he were allowed to present his side of the story in the AMA journal. Fishbein replied tersely that the *Journal of the American Medical Association* would "under no circumstances" publish a manuscript by Benjamin.[42] (A colleague concurred, jotting a quick memo saying, "Dr. Fishbein, I would not desecrate the [journal].")[43] In September 1935, Benjamin's long, sorry case against Liveright and Fishbein drew to a close. The defense insisted that if there had been any libel, it was very slight and fell under fair comment. The appellate court agreed. Benjamin finally consented to withdraw the case.[44] Fishbein had been proved right in thinking that he had nothing to worry about. In his relentless pursuit of quackery, he would be sued more than thirty times for a total of $40 million, but in all those years, he did not lose a single suit.[45]

As outraged as Benjamin might have felt, in many ways, his status as an outsider to the medical profession suited him. He continued his interest in the science of sexology and in social reform, always leaning in the direction of greater sexual liberty. In general, he had little use for the hypocrisies that he felt pervaded American social discourse. He consorted with social reformers and was unafraid to thrust himself into the limelight. When the nation was rocked by the 1931 Seabury investigations revealing that crooked police officers, judges, and bondsmen had been extorting money from prostitutes under the guise of fighting venereal disease, Benjamin was fired up with indignation and wrote an article for a medical journal that he titled "For the Sake of Morality." He argued that it was fruitless to defend against venereal disease by trying to suppress prostitution; such laws were hypocritical and unrealistic and did great harm to society.

Benjamin collaborated with Albert Ellis, the American editor of the *International Journal of Sexology* who had an office nearby at 56 Park Avenue. In later decades, they collaborated on articles about prostitution. Benjamin was one of the few professionals at the time to advocate for the rights of sex workers, risking his professional reputation in order to be a counselor and friend to them and to fight against their persecution. Ellis consulted with him on a number of occasions when he had to testify in court about the public distribution of nudist magazines or the rights of homosexuals and other people who were being prosecuted because of their sexual preferences. Ellis found Benjamin to be a source of sound advice as well as helpful in his clinical work. Benjamin always took the side of sexual liberty. Ellis suggested that Benjamin might have been the originator of the use of sexual surrogates in therapy, long before William Masters and Virginia Johnson famously introduced the practice in the 1970s. He recalled that Benjamin had a number of extremely shy and inhibited young male patients who desired sexual contact with women but were too panicked to follow through. According to Ellis, thanks to Benjamin's contacts with sex workers, he was able to arrange with some to "date" these men and actually show them what to do with a woman.[46]

Benjamin also became friends with gynecologist Hans Lehfeldt, whose office was two blocks away. Lehfeldt was an early proponent and practitioner of family planning, famous for his research on intrauterine devices and for inventing the cervical cap. They began to exchange patients. A friend and schoolmate of Lehfeldt's, Martin Gumpert, became Benjamin's subtenant. A writer and poet as well as a physician, Gumpert debated the morality of euthanasia with Benjamin in *The Nation* in 1950. Benjamin argued, "It seems inconceivable that in a happier world of the future no provision should be made for putting out of their misery persons suffering from an excessively painful and incurable disease. We shall have to find some legal way to accord to human beings the relief we accord to animals." Gumpert, just having returned from witnessing postwar trials in Germany, countered that euthanasia might be "humane and merciful as an idea" but "inhumane and dangerous as a practice."[47]

Benjamin was a close friend of Judge Ben Lindsey's, a nationally famous reformer who with Wainwright Evans wrote *The Companionate Marriage* in 1927. The idea of companionate marriage was considered daring at the time because it described marriage as an equal partnership cemented by sexual love rather than by childbearing or property relations. It advocated sexual and psychological equality for women and argued that couples should be able to choose to use birth control to delay having children until they had been married for several years and that those without children should have access to easier divorce.[48] Lindsey, a short, round-headed man, was a dogged fighter who took his message to lectures, magazines, and the radio waves. One evening, he and Benjamin were having dinner at the Algonquin Hotel when Lindsey brought up the fact that the Episcopal bishop of New York City was intending to discuss companionate marriage from the pulpit of the Cathedral of St. John the Divine the next day. A few years before, the bishop had denounced companionate marriage from the pulpit as "not marriage at all, but simple harlotry." Lindsey told Benjamin, "I am going there tomorrow and if the Bishop criticizes my book, I won't say a word; but if he attacks me personally, I shall answer right back." Benjamin warned him that such a step might prove risky, but his warning had no effect. Since Lindsey also announced his intention to be at the sermon in a letter to the bishop as well as on the front page of the *New York Times*—declaring that he might "'rise up' and retort to [the] bishop"—four uniformed police officers were assigned to the cathedral. That Sunday, 7 December 1930, the bishop stood before the assembled and declared Lindsey's book "one of the most filthy, insidious and cleverly written pieces of propaganda ever published in behalf of lewdness, promiscuity, adultery and unrestrained sexual gratification" and equated Lindsey's views with free love. As the bishop closed his sermon, Lindsey leaped from his seat onto a table, waving his arms and shouting, "Bishop Manning, you have lied about me!" Pandemonium broke out as members of the congregation cried, "Throw him out." Lindsey was finally rescued from the wrath of the crowd by being taken to the relative safety of a police station. Days later, Benjamin accompanied the judge to court, where the magistrate rebuked Lindsey for his behavior but dismissed the charge of disorderly conduct for lack of a complainant.[49]

A 1935 *Esquire* article titled "Rejuvenation" shows how the popular presentation of reactivation therapy changed over the years to encompass advances in hormone science.[50] The author argued that while Gertrude Atherton's novel *Black Oxen* might have been greatly exaggerated, now, twelve years later, it might be closer to truth than it had been when the book was first published. The author explained that further refinements had been made in the Steinach procedure of vasoligation that now allowed several successive reactivations to be done. For women, the original stimulation of the ovaries by X-rays had been supplanted first by diathermy and more recently by the use of ultrashort radio waves. These techniques were further supplemented by the use of the greatly improved and highly concentrated female hormones, which had since become available. The author noted with anticipation the recent reports that a male hormone, androsterone, would be commercially available very soon. This meant that a "nonoperative" Steinach method would become available for men as it had been for women, and these new methods could be used in combination with vasoligation and ultrashort waves. The article also described the use of reactivation on not only glandular but "psychic impotence" in men by creating a "masculinization" that helped to break down mental inhibitions. It also suggested that the same treatments helped on occasion in certain forms of homosexuality, "especially when the patient really wishes to be cured" and where psychoanalysis had failed.

Through the Great Depression, some patients looked to endocrinology with a new urgency. For some of the weary, graying, and impotent, Benjamin's practice offered a glint of hope. One blustery day in December 1935, a middle-aged man arrived from Long Island at Benjamin's medical office on Park Avenue. A former lecturer and writer, he had developed pernicious anemia that had played havoc with his physical and mental health. Despite taking all the liver and iron remedies that had been prescribed for him, he found his abilities sorely diminished and was ready to make almost any sacrifice to restore himself to the vitality he had once enjoyed. While in the waiting room, Harold Walker (pseudonym) leafed through an *Esquire* article describing the Steinach treatment and Benjamin's work. He noted that there was a special shelf of Gertrude Atherton's books there as well. When he was asked if anyone had referred him, he mentioned Atherton's name and found that it seemed to work like magic. Everyone in Benjamin's office treated him in the most wonderful manner. When Benjamin asked whether Walker knew Atherton personally, he blurted out "yes," even though in truth he had only written to her to ask for her doctor's name after having read about her experiences in the newspaper. (Walker later wrote to Atherton, confessing that he had thought he might be permitted this white lie, having read so many of her books that he felt he did in fact know her.)

Benjamin proved to be "kindness itself" and took great pains to get to the bottom of his patient's problems. He ordered many tests, and when Walker returned two days later to learn the results, Benjamin explained that his troubles were glandular in origin and prescribed a course of treatments with shortwave ultraviolet rays followed by a Steinach operation two or three weeks later. He explained to Walker that he believed that by these means, his health and activity would be greatly restored. Benjamin bent over him as he received his radiation treatment and asked whether he would be writing to Atherton before Christmas and, if so, to please convey his sincere regards and compliments of the season.

Walker's income had been badly depleted since 1929, so he was grateful that Benjamin offered him therapy at half his usual rate. The monthlong course of radiation, three times a week, would be billed at $150 instead of the usual $300, while the operation would cost $250 instead of $500. A further $100 would be due for various tests and for the hospital, making the complete fee $500. (In 1935, this would have been about a third of the average annual income and just slightly less than the price of a car.) Benjamin also offered the option of paying monthly installments, to which Walker agreed only reluctantly. He usually preferred to pay in advance. He felt "a torture of hope" as he waited for the results. After his first treatment, he wrote to Atherton that he felt somewhat better already. As for the ultimate outcome of his treatments, we know nothing further, though

Atherton assured Benjamin, "He has the greatest faith in you and that is half the battle."[51]

———————

Through these years, Benjamin continued to spread his gospel of rejuvenation. He coined the term "gerontotherapy" and was very proud that it was formally included in the twentieth edition of *Dorland's Medical Dictionary*. In April and May 1937, he made one more visit to London, Paris, Berlin, and Vienna.

Avies Platt was an art mistress at Wellingborough County High School for Girls in Northamptonshire, and in April 1937 she made her way to the Grafton Galleries in London to hear Benjamin speak at a meeting for the Sex Education Society. She had already had long meetings with Benjamin's colleague Norman Haire, whose country cottage was near where she lived. She had poured out her worries to Haire and through him exchanged letters with Benjamin in New York. She was deeply troubled about her lover, whom she referred to as "MM." He was an older man who was experiencing impotence, and Platt hoped he would seek medical treatment for it. In her correspondence with Benjamin, she had found him to be unconventionally kind, with a desire to help. Before the lecture, as Haire shepherded Benjamin to the front of the room, Platt had a brief opportunity to introduce herself to Benjamin and was pleased to find him as sympathetic in person as he had been in their correspondence.[52]

That evening, Benjamin spoke of his goal of adding life to one's years rather than years to one's life. Platt listened admiringly, taken by Benjamin's quiet assurance, scientific understanding, and hope for humanity, a utopian vision featuring the fellowship of nations and the conquest of old age. "Life, after all is not important," Benjamin declared; "only living is."[53]

In her early forties, Platt was striking and dramatic, with fine features and a tumble of raven curls. As Benjamin spoke, she perched on the thin gilded chair, absorbed in thought until she became conscious of a powerful force among the listeners behind her. She turned to meet the gaze of a gaunt, aristocratic-looking man with "strange, otherworldly eyes." In the discussion that followed the lecture, one man scornfully asked what possible connection there could be between rejuvenation and the love that poets had spoken of through the ages. In answer to this, one woman rose from the audience to announce that she had herself been rejuvenated; she had done this solely to benefit her health but had found to her surprise that she had fallen in love and, to her even greater amazement, that her love had been returned. And this, she declared, was the answer to the man's question. After the meeting broke up, Platt was one of the last to leave. The spring evening was cool and refreshing after the stuffiness of the hall. All the fashionable cars had departed when she, in her evening dress, was left struggling to crank up the engine of her old Singer.

"I'm sorry, I'm afraid I am not much good with those things," came a voice from the half shadow. It was the man from the lecture, distinguished and motionless.

"That's all right," she replied. "Please don't apologize, I'm used to it."

The place was deserted by the time the motor spluttered to a start. Platt learned that she and the man had both been invited to a party in Benjamin's honor, hosted by Haire at his Harley Street home. She offered the stranger a lift. They rode in silence until he asked whether she was connected with the arts and she replied that she was.

"And may I know the name of my kind chauffeur?" he continued.

Platt told him her name and asked his in return.

"Yeats, W. B. Yeats," he said. "I am a poet."

So stunned was she at this revelation that she promptly lost her way in the London streets. When they finally arrived at Haire's residence, they were ushered through to a room ornate with chinoiserie, wreathed in smoke, and abuzz with conversation. Yeats stayed by her side the entire evening, speaking quietly and directly. Benjamin was at the center of attention most of the time, but when the crowds around him thinned, Platt took the opportunity to greet him and discreetly ask whether her lover MM had visited him in New York as he had claimed. To her great disappointment, Benjamin replied that MM had not sought him out. Platt realized with a shock that MM had lied to her. Benjamin was gentle and sympathetic, trying to soften the blow by explaining that shame and concealment were a common part of this psychophysical condition. He agreed to see her again. (Benjamin's diary entry for that evening says, "Yeats Irish poet," and two days later there is a note of an appointment with "Miss Platt" at twelve.)[54] After the party, Platt ferried Yeats to the Athenaeum Club. She became more and more astounded by "a mystical torrent of words" that poured forth as Yeats praised Benjamin's lecture and spoke admiringly of the Steinach operation and its tremendous effects. She realized with a start that he could only be speaking from personal knowledge.

"Do you mean you yourself have had the operation?" she asked incredulously.

"Yes, I am sorry; I thought I had made that clear," he replied.

Platt was staggered by the thought that not only was she driving the greatest living poet, but she had, as she put it, "a Lazarus beside me," living proof of the Steinach operation in one as if raised from the dead. All that Benjamin had spoken of that evening seemed revealed as scientific fact.

Yeats continued, "I regard it as one of the greatest events, if not the supreme event, of my life."

He recalled that when he had come out of the anesthetic, he had felt something akin to the sudden rush of puberty but at a time of life when this rush could be made intelligible.

"I felt life flowing through me," he explained.

Before the operation, he could scarcely walk across the room and was prostrate with exhaustion when he tried to write. But now, he was completely cured, he said. In fact, he believed that what he had written since had been some of the best work in his life. When they arrived at the Athenaeum on Pall Mall, they continued to sit talking in her car at the curb. Yeats gently suggested that they meet again, either in Dublin or in London, but Platt was so caught up in thoughts of her lover MM that she failed to understand or follow up on Yeats's invitation. Finally, they said their farewells. He took her hand and held it even through the open door of the car. It was dawn as she drove home.

When she later described these events to Haire, he was astonished that she would have forgone the chance to have the great man as her lover. Why else would Yeats have told her his secret? Over the years that followed, she would have many occasions to reflect with a mixture of regret and gratitude on Yeats and the brief interval in which their lives touched. At his memorial a few years later, she was overcome with emotion. The poet, rejoicing that spring evening at Harry Benjamin's words, had honored her with his revelation. She was sure that for Yeats, the Steinach operation had been no mere physical or sexual rejuvenation but a "re-creation, a reassembling of himself," that was inextricably bound up with his endless search for truth and beauty.[55]

Benjamin met with Platt two days later, and after that, he had one more appointment: a visit with Havelock Ellis. This would be one of the most cherished experiences of his life. Ellis was a pioneer in the study of sex who challenged Victorian morality on subjects such as masturbation and argued that sex should be pleasurable for women as well as men. His 1897 book, *Sexual Inversion*, was the first English-language medical text on homosexuality. He, like Hirschfeld, identified transgender identity as a phenomenon distinct from homosexuality, in 1913 proposing the term "eonism" for it, named after the French diplomat, soldier, and spy the Chevalier d'Éon, who lived to age forty-nine as a man and then after that lived more than thirty years as a woman in the court of the empress of Russia. Ellis welcomed Benjamin to his home for tea. By this time Ellis was seventy-eight, rather slender, and Benjamin thought quite beautiful looking, reminding him of the great Indian poet Rabindranath Tagore, whom he had met just a year before in Steinach's office. They spoke at length on many subjects in sexology, and Benjamin found the older man engaging, cordial, and "typically British." Ellis had just been sent some newspaper clippings about the police raid and closing of burlesque houses in New York.

"How stupid can they get," thundered Ellis, "to close up a perfectly good safety valve. Unbelievable!"

Ellis prepared and served the tea himself and Benjamin was charmed, but after an hour or so he worried that he might be outstaying his welcome and prepared to make his leave.

"No, please stay a while," Ellis asked graciously; "we may not meet again."

At the end of that golden afternoon, Ellis waved from the garden door of his house as Benjamin made his way to the underground station. Benjamin thought Ellis was the wisest man he had ever met and that there was "something divine about him." He would always carry that image of the saintly "Darwin of Sex" with him, as they indeed never met again. Ellis would die two years later.[56]

As hormone products became more numerous and more potent, perhaps as challenging a task as learning about the chemistry and physiology of hormones was determining what physicians and scientists ought to do with that knowledge. Saving children with diabetes from imminent death by treating them with insulin was a clear triumph. Tending patients stricken with hypothyroidism was a great advance. But almost as soon as these treatments succeeded, practitioners began to dream of doing more. If the person with dwarfism caused by pituitary deficiency could be helped, could not children of shorter stature—though hormonally normal—be helped to grow taller? Why could athletes not be made faster and stronger? Why couldn't criminals be prevented from committing further crimes? Perhaps male homosexuals could be "masculinized" and female homosexuals "feminized"? Could physicians find new ways to affect social behavior and shape the future of humanity?[57]

Like all technologies, hormone therapies can be a double-edged sword that can serve for good or ill. Their long-term consequences can be difficult to foresee. What is even more complicated is that often those doing ill are convinced they are acting for the greater good. Through the early decades of the twentieth century, eugenic ideas were popular among both conservative and progressive reformers. Negative eugenics sought to improve society through birth control and sterilization to prevent reproduction of people considered to possess undesirable traits. Positive eugenics sought to encourage reproduction among individuals with desirable characteristics. For some theorists such as Louis Berman, hormone therapy offered a third alternative: eugenics in which individuals were not simply selected for or against, but actually made better in themselves and able to pass along their improved traits to their offspring. An endocrinologist could function as something of a creative engineer of this enhanced version of humanity.[58] Berman's utopian vision included setting up special centers where the endocrine status of individuals, especially pregnant women and infants, could be checked and adjusted as needed; he also proposed creating a central authority in every country to research psycho-endocrinology.

Benjamin said little of his views of birth control and eugenic sterilization, though he, like most of his sexology colleagues, was interested in eugenics. He attended the Third International Eugenics Congress when it was held at the Museum of Natural History in New York in 1932 and was impressed by its beautiful and carefully prepared exhibition.[59] Like many fellow progressives, he noted with concern that the availability of birth control methods might lead to their being used primarily by those of higher income, intellect, and education—"the very ones who should have children." But he also recognized that "sterilization for human betterment" was faced with the fundamental problem that no one definitely knew which of life's ills were inheritable and which were not. He doubted that sterilization laws would fulfill what their originators envisioned. In his book manuscript of the early 1940s, he wrote, "In any event, it should be practiced not in the spirit of fanaticism (as in the 'New Germany') but on the basis of further studies in the laws of heredity."[60]

During the 1930s and 1940s, the mass media presented many sensationalized stories of sex change that brought the possibility of medical intervention to the attention of individuals who had a sense of cross-gender identity and were looking for solutions to their predicament. Reports of surgical interventions, such as those done in Europe on Lili Elbe, tended to blend together the experiences of people whom we would today consider intersex with those we consider transgender. In stories of sex change, the individuals were often described as possessing both male and female organs; the surgery was characterized as a means of "correcting" where nature had made an error. Other sensational stories described situations in which sex change was supposed to have occurred spontaneously. The dilemma for many Americans who found themselves drawn to these stories and who perhaps saw in them a possible solution for their own problems was that it would have been difficult to find US physicians disposed to provide the treatments described. Surgeons were unwilling, or felt unable, to provide a surgery in which healthy tissue was removed. On the other hand, there seem to have been a number of physicians willing to quietly offer hormones. In 1941, newspapers reported that Barbara Richards had spontaneously begun to transform from a man to a woman, but reading beyond the headlines, one could learn that she had been receiving female hormone injections to "stabilize her condition."[61]

We know very little of any contacts Benjamin might have had with gender nonconforming individuals in these years, but one very significant engagement was with Otto Spengler, who was introduced to Benjamin through Hirschfeld in the 1920s. Spengler was the German-born owner of a press clipping bureau. A tall, lean man with long, thin red hair that he kept rolled up under his derby hat, he eagerly attended the lectures during Hirschfeld's visit to New York in 1930. At these events, he shared details of his private life with anyone willing to listen and invited them to visit the site of his home and business on Third Avenue. He was pleased to be pointed out as an example of a typical transvestite. Sometime in the 1920s, Spengler went to Benjamin for treatment. Benjamin intuited there was something "extremely unusual" about Spengler and sensed that he cross-dressed at home. He later asked Spengler about this and learned he had been right.[62] Spengler had indeed been the inspiration for Hirschfeld's 1910 book on transvestism. Spengler's biography had been presented at the New York Society for Medical Jurisprudence in 1913, where it was the first case history of a transvestite to be presented in the United States. The biography was subsequently published in the *New York Medical Journal* by Bernard Talmey in 1914.

In 1925 or 1926, on a bid to become more feminine, Spengler reported that he "went through rejuvenation, the American Steinach operation" at the age of fifty-two. What was intriguing about this was that by "Steinach operation" he did not mean the vasoligation that Benjamin would have been performing on men but the X-ray irradiation of his testicles to make him sterile, an adaptation of the X-ray treatment of ovaries that Benjamin was then using on women. Spengler also later asked Benjamin to provide him with Progynon. He reported that he took "a great deal" of them, which to his great delight, produced a mild enlargement of the breasts.[63]

In 1938, Spengler wrote Gertrude Atherton a letter praising *Black Oxen*, "which thrilled me very much." Moreover, he told her that they had something in common: both of them had received Roentgen rays from their "mutual friend" Dr. Benjamin, though Spengler clarified that he had received his not for the purpose of rejuvenation but for feminization. He explained to Atherton that he belonged to "the class of Transvestites" and that Hirschfeld had credited him with inspiring his book. In particular, he hoped that Atherton would send him a copy of her new book, *Can Ladies Be Gentlemen?*, and suggested she might follow up with a sequel, *Can Gentlemen Be Ladies?* In exchange, he offered her the services of his clipping bureau for her reviews, as well as a photograph of himself posed as Queen Louise in the style of the painting by Gustave Richter.[64]

Atherton's book—actually titled *Can Women Be Gentlemen?*—was not actually about transvestites as Spengler seems to have hoped. It was instead a lively collection of essays dealing, among other questions, with whether women could possess gentlemanly qualities. (Atherton argued that there were actually very few differences between women and men other than sex, and any differences in virtues and moral failings were due to cultural circumstances.) Atherton was rather astonished by the letter and sent it to Benjamin with a scribbled note asking, "Is this a man, a woman, or a lunatic?" Benjamin joked that Spengler was "somewhat of a lunatic" but explained more seriously that Spengler was really a person of decent character, a married man with several children, and that he was a transvestite. He said that Spengler dressed in women's clothes and noted to Atherton that "the condition is considered the very first stage of homosexual tendencies." Benjamin told Atherton she didn't have to answer Spengler's letter, as he was likely to see Spengler someday and would clarify his mistake to him. He reminded Atherton that he had warned her that the title of her book was likely to attract attention from transvestites, and now "here you have an example," he said. "There are thousands of them in all countries." When he later wrote to tell Atherton that Spengler had sent him press clippings from his bureau, he used scare quotes in "Mr." Spengler, though whether this was in gentle ridicule or respectful acknowledgment of ambiguity—or perhaps a little of both—it is difficult to tell.[65]

Benjamin's encounter with Spengler gives us an intriguing glimpse into his evolving thought on sex and gender and his very pragmatic approach to treating his patients in the 1920s and 1930s. Despite Hirschfeld's 1910 work distinguishing transvestism from homosexuality, Benjamin continued to hold the idea that transvestism was an early stage of homosexuality. He also seems aware that transvestites existed in considerable number throughout the world. In the clinic, he was willing to use and adapt the tools at hand to serve his patient's needs and requests, however unusual they might have seemed. Spengler clearly understood the treatment in terms of making him more feminine. Benjamin, though, may have been considering X-ray irradiation and female hormones as a means of making his patient feel calmer and more comfortable.[66] The two goals were not inconsistent. What is clear, however, is that there was a real continuity between Benjamin's work in rejuvenation and his work with transgender patients decades later.

When Germany annexed Austria in March 1938, Eugen Steinach and his wife were safely away on a lecture tour in Switzerland. Two-thirds of the Vivarium staff were Jewish and were dismissed on racial grounds; many would go into exile and several to concentration camps. The founder, Hans Leo Przibram, and his wife escaped to the Netherlands but were captured and deported to Theresienstadt; Przibram died there and his wife took her own life the next day. The Vivarium's legacy was obscured and the contributions and efforts of its investigators ridiculed. Although the Vivarium continued to exist for several more years, its heart was destroyed in 1938. In 1945, the building was burned to the ground by Allied bombings. After the war, the pioneering work of its researchers was almost completely erased from official histories, and the once internationally renowned institution was almost forgotten.[67]

Steinach and his wife were granted residency in Switzerland, and Steinach kept hoping that he would be able to continue his research in the United States, but many efforts made to bring him to America failed. In September 1938, his wife died by suicide. Benjamin wrote Gertrude Atherton that, "with Austria no longer being a civilized country, I doubt very much whether I shall go to Europe this year at all."[68] Benjamin never saw Steinach again but continued to write faithfully. Gretchen managed a visit to Steinach in Zurich in 1939, just before the war, and he seemed to her still a gracious host and loyal friend, but she knew he felt greatly frustrated.[69]

Benjamin had become an American citizen in 1921, but as late as 1931, when his practice was poor and his income small, it seems he still harbored the hope that he might finally return to Berlin for good.[70] Until 1933, his sympathies were with the Weimar Republic. But his transformation from a German into an American was made complete by his horror at what he described as "the revolting demonstration of the Nazi brand of the Furor Teutonicus" (the legendary ferocity of the Teutons). With the rise of Hitler, Benjamin felt that he would have to go back almost to Goethe's time to find the Germany of which he could be proud.[71] Berlin had been the world center of sexology, but Benjamin watched in despair as, he would one day say, "this whole hopeful science fell victim to Nazi barbarism."[72] From 1921 to the early 1930s, Benjamin had seen himself serving as a bridge between the Old World and the New World. After the collapse of sexology in Berlin and Vienna, he was left one of a small number of surviving links to a once flourishing and avant-garde intellectual tradition.[73]

Chapter 9

Changing the Body to Match the Mind

Faddism and self deception is easy in the border fields of scientific medicine and critical faculties must be ever present and awake. On the other hand, the narrow minded scientist without imagination may add valuable tools but will hardly help medicine, or any other science, to progress.

—Harry Benjamin

In 1933, Harry Benjamin began to turn his eyes away from the Old World toward the wide expanses of the New World. That autumn, he opened a second practice in California, and almost every summer thereafter, and some years in winter, he and Gretchen would trade New York's gray canyons for the waving palms of Hollywood and the gabled roofs of San Francisco. Benjamin found to his delight that prices out west were a third less than they were in New York and the climate the most beautiful possible. While New York summers could be unspeakably hot ("a hell," he wrote Eugen Steinach), in San Francisco, the weather the whole year round seemed to him like "autumn in Vienna."[1]

That first year, Harry and Gretchen journeyed by rail on the new luxury train "the Aristocrat" with its solarium lounge car and matching Pullmans in pearl green. Other years, they motored their way across their adopted land, with Gretchen always behind the wheel of their broad-beamed Pontiac.[2] From Charleston and Lexington to St. Louis and Salt Lake City, they crossed and recrossed the United States, exploring it as they went. They stood on the battlefield where Custer fell. Amid the tall pines of Wyoming, they visited Buffalo Bill's hunting lodge. Did it recall for Harry the memories of his five-year-old self meeting the frontiersman long ago in Berlin? One trip, they detoured north to Canada to take in the dusty spectacle of the Calgary Stampede and the splendor of Lake Louise, where they hiked to a tea house high in the Rockies.[3]

Harry and Gretchen seem to have had a companionable partnership, and to the outside world, Gretchen was a model physician's wife and helpmate. When they were apart from each other, their letters were warm and affectionate. But the complexities and compromises of a marriage can be opaque to an outsider. As his closer friends would put it delicately, Harry had an "active romantic life" outside of marriage. One colleague called him a "female magnet."[4] He continued to be attracted to actresses and chorus girls. For a time, he saw patients in Los Angeles and mixed with the rich and famous. Jean Harlow's initials appear in his address book, and colleagues would recall that he later reminisced about "dating" her.[5] When Magnus Hirschfeld joked that he should take care to avoid the casinos of Agua Caliente, which might be a little "too caliente" for him, Benjamin assured him he need not worry: "Hollywood women interest me much more than roulette."[6]

Harry and Gretchen never had children, and Harry would say he had been too selfish to want any. In his bleaker moments, he thought it would be the greatest blessing not to have been born.[7] On the whole, it seems that Harry and Gretchen's partnership was framed on his terms, and as in other parts of his life, Benjamin knew what he wanted and usually got his way.

When Harry and Gretchen arrived in San Francisco, their first social call would always be with the city's famous literary daughter, Gertrude Atherton. Atherton and Benjamin remained friends for decades, dined, and attended the opera together. Atherton introduced Harry and Gretchen to "the right groups of people" from her circle of literary, social, and political connections—the mayor and his wife were at the dinner party on their first arrival—while Harry continued to prescribe hormones and vitamins to keep her vital and productive. He remained an attentive friend to her and her entire family, with cards, notes, or a bottle of her favorite Benedictine at birthdays. She continued to write about her reactivation and at the age of eighty-eight was still at work, finishing her fifty-sixth book, *My San Francisco: A Wayward Biography*.[8]

Benjamin came to love San Francisco. He found the city truly cosmopolitan, with remnants of its gold rush history giving it "an indefinable charm and flavor."[9] He was popular among its society ladies, but away from the living rooms of the wealthy, he reveled in the segments of San Francisco that still bore the whiff of the Barbary Coast. On his first visit there, a physician from the Department of Health took him on a tour of the town's brothels, ranging from the cheapest at three dollars a visit to the most expensive at fifteen dollars. He was impressed at how the women cooperated with the health officials so that there were rarely cases of venereal disease in these houses. He found that the majority matter-of-factly paid off the police, but he felt that on the whole it seemed to all run smoothly. Even the sailors who frequented the cheaper houses could feel safe from being robbed. In time, Benjamin began to serve the health needs of the sex workers at two of the biggest brothels in the city.[10]

Over the years, Benjamin's family members had joined him in the United States. His mother and sister had spent the Great War with him but had returned to Germany, Bertha in 1921 and Edith in 1922. In May 1926, they arrived back in New York along with Kurt Seelig, a fellow German whom Edith had married in Berlin. The Seeligs settled in the United States, naturalizing in 1932, and together with Bertha moved to Manhasset on the North Shore of Long Island, where Kurt worked as a fur dealer.

From his side of the Atlantic, Benjamin watched in dismay what he called "the Hitler-betrayal of German culture."[11] Of his immediate family, Harry's brother, Walter (who used the surname Benjamin-Benjar and later simply Benjar), remained in Berlin the longest, working as a stockbroker like their father. At one point, he was a neighbor of Friedrich Franz Friedmann. As things worsened in Germany, even he could no longer remain. His wife, Emmy, arrived in the United States in October 1932, and Walter followed in December 1933. In 1937, their cousin Max Louis Benjamin, a lawyer, came with his wife and family, and they too named Harry Benjamin as the relative they were joining in the United States.

As the world plunged into world war for the second time in his life, Benjamin became increasingly convinced of the moral and logical superiority of the American model of governance. In 1941, he said with hope, "If forty-eight states were successful in forming a 'nation by design,' why cannot—at some future time—all the present nations unite to a 'world by design.' Every birth means suffering and bloodshed. Maybe such a 'world by design' will be born out of the agony of the second World War," he wrote.[12]

He continued to be a faithful friend to Steinach. In 1931, when it was Steinach's seventieth birthday, Benjamin reminded Hirschfeld that he might want to send a telegram of congratulations.[13] In 1939, Benjamin took on the enormous tasks of meticulously revising a terrible, anonymous English-language translation of Steinach's autobiographical book, *Sex and Life*, and shepherding it through to publication. When the book failed to attract reviews in major papers or achieve many sales, Benjamin sent calm reassurances to Steinach of its significance. In 1941, Benjamin busied himself contacting press outlets to put out pieces marking Steinach's eightieth birthday.[14]

During the war, Benjamin's practice slowed down even more. He and Atherton corresponded about their relatively minor wartime privations, for him New York's frigid temperatures and the shortage of coal ("We may have to live at the office if things do not improve at the apartment") and for her an ongoing servant problem, with her "Chinese" having been claimed by military service. Benjamin explained that he now realized how many of his clients had come from out of town, and with fuel restrictions, this clientele was lost "for the duration." "But somehow we shall struggle through," he declared in 1943. "I am not ready to grumble and complain like some of my friends. We might as well complain about the weather. As long as the picture on the various fronts look fairly bright, I am satisfied whatever the restrictions and sacrifices of the home front might be."[15]

Benjamin himself was now in his midfifties. Midlife would be for him a time to ruminate on the path his life had taken and the accomplishments he could claim. In 1941 his musings took a literary turn, and he began work on a manuscript titled "The Winter of Our Discontent," which he intended as an explication of glandular reactivation for the ordinary person. It mixed practical advice on how to grow old "gracefully and sensibly" with a discussion of the concepts of gerontotherapy. As he explained, gerontotherapy did not aim to prolong life but rather to extend the "autumn of life" and minimize the "winter."[16]

Using large swathes of autobiography, he described attempts to combat old age, delineating the history of the Steinach operation through the lens of his own early encounters with glandular science. He reflected on his happy childhood, the turns of fate that had caught him mid-ocean in World War I, his inspiring evenings with Joseph Fraenkel, and his introduction to Steinach. He was now also able to think about his experience with Friedmann and the turtle serum with a detachment born of three decades of life experience. He posited that Friedmann had a "psychopathic personality" and was therefore "incapable of an unselfish act," harassed as he was "by his own infantile impulses." Thirty years before, Benjamin would have cursed the day he had met Friedmann, but now, having seen Germany's travails play out, he described the misadventure with the words of Mephistopheles in Goethe's *Faust*, who identifies himself as

> Part of that Power, not understood,
> Which always wills the Bad, and always works the Good.

Friedmann had played this role in Benjamin's story and in doing so might very well have saved Benjamin's life and that of his entire family. And if he were to ever meet Friedmann again, Benjamin wondered, how would he feel? "I would feel like blessing him and thanking him from the bottom of my heart for what he has done to me, and then—I may feel like breaking his jaw!" he decided.[17]

Benjamin continued to see himself as hemmed in on one side by quacks and charlatans and on the other by orthodox medicine. He said, "It was not in my nature to keep silent when my work . . . was unjustly attacked and willfully distorted" and noted that he "neither minced words nor did I pull any punches." He still bristled at every word of Morris Fishbein's 1927 essay and more than twenty years later fired off a letter protesting the fact that Fishbein had recently mentioned his name in a lecture he had delivered on notorious "quacketeers."[18] (Fishbein, described by *Time* magazine as "the nation's most ubiquitous, most widely maligned, and perhaps most influential medico," would be forced to retire from the AMA the following year as a result of political infighting.)[19]

Above all, Benjamin explained that he trusted his readers to have self-knowledge. He mused that many books about proper living gave well-meant advice that essentially came down to a call for moderation in sex, alcohol, tobacco, diet, and exercise. But defining what that moderation really looked like required common sense. And only the individual could really understand what happiness meant to himself or herself.

> Let nobody interpret these remarks as an advice to renounce pleasures. . . .
> Proper living is as much a matter of the mind as of the body. Therefore I say
> this: if an extra highball or an extra cigar adds to your mental comfort and
> satisfaction, to your feeling of happiness, by all means have both, even at
> the risk of doing some harm physically. This harm is problematical anyhow

and the authorities often disagree. But nobody can disagree as to the state of your own happiness. And if you are at all an intelligent observer you will know better than anybody else (including your doctor) where and when and how much of a physical harm is done.[20]

When it came to trying to publish his book, he approached his literary friends for assistance. Gertrude Atherton said she didn't really know how to advise him about finding a publisher, though she thought the subject matter was sure to interest many. She recommended he use a "light touch," saying, "Most of you scientists, no matter how entertaining in conversation, become heavy-handed and dry when writing."[21] When at the end of 1941 Benjamin had completed a chapter outline, introduction, and the first three chapters, Somerset Maugham agreed to try to pitch the book for him to Doubleday, Doran & Company. (Do we perhaps catch a glimpse of Harry Benjamin in Maugham's 1943 novel, *The Razor's Edge*, in the doctor who comes to see his seventy-year-old patient "twice a week to thrust into an alternate buttock a hypodermic needle with the fashionable injection of the moment"?)[22] Maugham wrote to Benjamin, "I think I may say that I have boosted it in no uncertain way and got them all excited. Now it only remains for you to write a very good book," adding, "If you want a word of advice it is not to be flowery, rhetorical or jocose."[23]

To Benjamin's disappointment, Doubleday declined his manuscript, though Maugham assured him it had received serious consideration. He had learned, however, that it was felt to be "acrimonious" and difficult for a lay reader.[24] Benjamin continued to retouch his manuscript for over eight years, sending it out to other readers. "I think your manuscript is TERRIFIC! . . . I couldn't put it down again until I'd read every word," said one enthusiastic reader who promised to send it along to a publishing colleague.[25] In the end, though, he could find no publisher for his book, and his carefully typed drafts were left to yellow in his files.

At the beginning of 1944, Benjamin suffered a serious health setback: he lost one of his kidneys and almost died of infection as a result of a stone. This illness caused his friends great concern, and his recovery required several months. At the same time, he and Gretchen became greatly concerned because their letters to Steinach began to be returned unopened. In May 1944, Harry and Gretchen anxiously sent a telegram to Zurich. It was then that they learned that Steinach had died on 14 May. He had been eighty-three. Benjamin would write a tribute to the man to whom he had been a faithful disciple for over twenty years, his article being "the only kind of monument" that he could make.[26] He called Steinach a scientist who had dared to "penetrate the primeval forest of human prejudices and sex taboos" and had thus added immeasurably to human happiness.[27]

At the close of the war, the horrifying truth of the Nazi regime came to light as the Allied forces liberated the concentration camps. The eugenic principles, so different from those dreamed of by Steinach and Paul Kammerer, had resulted in the brutal murder of up to 6 million Jews, Poles, Serbs, Roma, homosexuals, and people with disabilities. The Berlin of Benjamin's birth was carved into four by the occupying forces.

By the late 1940s, Benjamin's approach to endocrine treatments for his geriatric patients was looking more and more out of step with that of his contemporaries, and other medical experts were not afraid to say so, sometimes in scathing ways. When Benjamin published a paper describing his use of combinations of estradiol and testosterone for his menopausal patients, one critic called his methods not only questionable but potentially harmful: "Personally I would hate to inflict upon a defenseless old patient some of the god-awful mixtures of endocrines which the author suggests. . . . My own reaction to this paper was that it represents a throw-back to the joy-riding, empirical, gun-shot type of 'gland treatment' which we thought had been pretty well discredited. I hope that the author will not mind if I do not recommend his article to my confiding clients."[28]

Atherton, though, faithfully continued taking Benjamin's hormones until her final days, reporting to him, "I take your hormones regularly twice a day. I am sure they are doing me some good."[29] Her biographer, Emily Leider, says that Atherton "elevated Dr. Benjamin to divine status, making him the high priest of a new religion," and if so, then Atherton's faith was surely rewarded in that almost all press accounts of her in her later years mentioned her striking glamour, youthfulness, and capacity for work.[30]

Life itself was beginning to exhaust Benjamin. The winter of 1947–48 felt like one of the worst in thirty years. At one point, both he and Gretchen had their mothers living with them. He wrote to Atherton, "We are allright, but between my patients, my accumulated reading, my lectures and the two mothers at home, I haven't got a very easy life."[31] The Christmas of 1947 was particularly strenuous, and he resented his sister having taken "the easy way out" by escaping to Bermuda, leaving him and Gretchen with the two elderly women.[32] His mother fell occasionally, though thankfully with no serious results, and he insisted that she use a cane with a rubber tip. With the terrible weather and having to work almost every night on some articles he had promised to write, he felt very much in need of a vacation. "Gretchen is already getting rebellious. I really don't blame her," he said, "except for having married a doctor."[33]

The close of the decade would bring to an end two important relationships. In 1948, Gertrude Atherton died at the age of ninety, more than a quarter of a century after first walking into Benjamin's office seeking rejuvenation. The following year, Benjamin's mother, Bertha—the woman who taught him to love opera—died at the age of ninety-seven. To Benjamin, who had lost his mentor, his most famous patient, and his mother in the span of five years, it must have truly felt like the end of an era.

———

During these years, Benjamin continued to make long stays in San Francisco, and when he wasn't there, he would speak longingly of it. He regarded his months there as something of a vacation and did not make any special effort to have many patients, but by the late 1930s, he found his practice quite busy.[34] In 1940, he took an office in a skyscraper in the heart of the city. The Sutter Medical Building, twenty-six stories high, offered spectacular views of Union Square and San Francisco Bay. When it was built in 1929, it was the second-tallest structure in the city and possibly the tallest one in the world designed solely for medical and dental offices. The building remains an art deco masterpiece, richly clad in terra-cotta carvings in a Mayan Revival style that consciously used the architecture of the Americas rather than motifs imported from Europe as its inspiration.[35] It was from this soaring new-world office that new prospects were to open for Benjamin. The longtime purveyor of gerontotherapy was about to have his own second act.

In the summer of 1949, Benjamin was in San Francisco staying at the Sir Francis Drake Hotel just across the street from his medical office. Alfred Kinsey, the American sex researcher, was staying there as well, taking sex histories for his pioneering studies of human sexuality. Kinsey, a zoologist who had begun his career studying the biology of gall wasps, had turned his systematic eye to the study of human sexuality and in 1947 had established the Institute for Sex Research at Indiana University. He had gained celebrity status (and in conservative quarters, infamy) for his groundbreaking study, *Sexual Behavior in the Human Male*, in 1948, which would be followed in 1953 by *Sexual Behavior in the Human Female*.[36] Drawing on thousands of sex histories that Kinsey and his associates painstakingly collected, these two works, known as the Kinsey Reports, shocked the nation with the revelation that such behaviors as premarital and extramarital sex, oral sex, homosexuality, and masturbation were far more prevalent than previously supposed. They revealed that a wide gulf existed between social mores and actual practice. Like Hirschfeld before him, Kinsey recognized a continuum in the phenomena he observed. Together with Wardell Pomeroy and Clyde Martin, Kinsey devised the Heterosexual-Homosexual Rating Scale—commonly known as the Kinsey Scale—to reflect the data showing that individuals were not exclusively heterosexual or homosexual, nor did their desires and behaviors always remain consistent over time. The seven-point scale ranged from 0 for "exclusively heterosexual" in behavior or attraction to 6 for "exclusively homosexual," with a seventh category, X, for "no socio-sexual contacts or reactions."

Unlike Hirschfeld, Kinsey saw a continuum in personality and sexual behavior but considered male and female distinct and opposite categories. One individual he met left Kinsey puzzled. Twenty-three-year-old Val Barry (pseudonym) was unlike anyone he had encountered before. Kinsey was familiar with transvestites who wished to cross-dress, but he had never encountered individuals who actually considered themselves to *be* the so-called other sex. Kinsey asked Benjamin—with whom he had developed a friendship after meeting him several years before through the introduction of the New York obstetrician and gynecology researcher Robert L. Dickinson—to see this patient and give his opinion. In their amiable correspondence, Benjamin is called "Harry" and Kinsey is "Prok," the nickname Kinsey was affectionately called even by his wife.

Barry was assigned male at birth but had lived as a girl since childhood. She was feminine in her behavior, ideas, and interests, and she had wanted to become a girl. What is more, her family had raised her in female clothing and had even made special toilet arrangements for her at grade school. Barry's parents had been assured by psychiatrists that their bright, contented, and academically successful child should simply be left to "outgrow" what they considered a phase. When Barry reached high school and found she was unable to continue in this manner, her family had her stay at home and do women's work. She prayed constantly for a miracle that might allow her to one day marry and have a home and children. She read widely, searching for answers, and came across several books and articles that described surgical procedures that feminized men, including *Man into Woman*, the story of Lili Elbe. Barry became convinced this was the course of action she wished to take and begged her mother to help her find a doctor who would perform this procedure. When her hopes were frustrated, she erupted into severe tantrums and even violence that sent her father to the hospital. In 1948, at the age of twenty-two, she entered a hospital in Wisconsin for psychiatric evaluation. She refused the offer of any treatment such as brain surgery that her doctors thought might rid her of her desire to be female. Remarkably, thirty members of the medical staff gathered to consider her case and concluded that she should receive castration and plastic surgery. Their intentions were thwarted, however, when the hospital consulted with the state attorney general's office, which declared such surgery would constitute "mayhem"—the willful destruction of healthy tissue.[37]

In turn, Barry wrote to Benjamin in May 1949. Reading her case, he replied to her letter saying that he suspected she was a woman who "accidentally possesses the body of a man." He offered to write to Germany to determine whether the law there might permit surgery. In the meantime, he suggested that she take female hormones as well as receive X-ray treatment for "castration" and to remove facial hair. Barry and Benjamin met for the first time later that summer in his San Francisco office. Barry's mother pleaded with Benjamin, "You must do something for him. See how he looks! He looks just like a girl!" Benjamin had an intuition that Barry was not a transvestite: she did not want to dress as a woman on occasion; she wanted to live her entire life as a woman, and as far as medical science would allow, she wished to remove all the physical signs of maleness, from facial hair to the genitals she found so disgusting. But it also seemed clear that she was not an intersex person and that she was physically a "normal" male. Benjamin asked for Barry's psychiatric examination. Most psychiatrists of the day would have assumed that the best approach in a case like this was to use psychiatric measures to change the mind to match the body. Benjamin tentatively proposed something few had considered before in American medicine: that the body be changed to match the mind. Thanks to his long connection with Steinach and Hirschfeld, Benjamin was predisposed to consider his patient's experience as grounded in biology rather than in psychological disturbance. Thanks to his own keen, sympathetic gaze, he was inclined to recognize his patient as sane and to accept her expressed sense of self. And thanks to his pragmatic bent and the years he had spent wrestling with human suffering day by day, he thought it reasonable to try to do something to help.[38]

Benjamin, who for decades had used the science of the glands to make the old young again, would now use hormones to create perhaps the most striking transformation of all. Under Benjamin's care, Barry began to receive female hormones. Soon, he began to notice they were having a calming effect. But Benjamin's help was not limited to these clinical measures. He also tried to help Barry find a surgeon in the United States who would carry out the required surgeries. Benjamin wrote to California's state attorney general, Edmund G. Brown, to inquire whether there would be any legal obstacle to a sex change operation being done there. Brown initially thought that this would not pose a problem but after further discussion with another lawyer changed his mind. Benjamin objected strongly, but Brown, like Wisconsin's attorney general, issued the legal opinion that genital modification would constitute "mayhem." The mayhem statutes stemmed from a prohibition left from English Common Law, which had been intended to prevent the maiming of men who might serve as soldiers. Benjamin was outraged: "It is difficult to reconcile my common sense with the fact that statutes based on the requirements of English kings in the middle ages should still be valid."[39] Kinsey also discussed the case informally with Karl Bowman, the former head of the American Psychiatric Association and then head of the Langley Porter Psychiatric Clinic at the University of California, San Francisco, which was an important center for research on variant sexuality and gender through the 1940s and 1950s. Kinsey and Bowman concluded, though, that they could not endorse the surgery on Barry. They were concerned that the operation would leave an underlying psychological problem unresolved and at the same time take away Barry's genital outlet for sexual expression. Even Benjamin's good friend and colleague Max Thorek, who was initially sympathetic, refused to cooperate once he had consulted with his lawyer. As it turned out, no one was ever prosecuted for sex change surgery under the mayhem statutes or any other law, but historian Susan Stryker argues that this legal opinion would "cast a pall" over the efforts of transgender people to receive surgical treatment in the United States for many years and over the physicians who might have wanted to help them. Over the next decades, only a small number of operations were done in the United States, most by Benjamin's colleague Elmer Belt, a Los Angeles surgeon, and all of those done in strictest secrecy. Val Barry ultimately traveled to Sweden to receive surgery in 1953.[40]

Comparing Benjamin's work with Barry to his encounters with Otto Spengler decades earlier is revealing. In 1938, Benjamin clearly thought of Spengler as a transvestite, that is, as a man who wished to cross-dress, but he had also been willing to accede to Spengler's requests to use radiation and hormone therapy to suppress Spengler's male characteristics and boost his female characteristics. In accounts by Benjamin's contemporaries, Barry is counted as his first "true transsexual." Benjamin replied to Barry using the narrative trope of a woman trapped in the body of a man, an idea that echoes the notion of inversion going back to Karl Heinrich Ulrichs. Spengler and Barry offered fairly different accounts of their life experiences. Spengler had always desired to live as a woman and had often wished for castration. When he was not allowed to cross-dress, he felt absent-minded and restless and contemplated suicide. But Spengler had also lived, worked, and married as a man and had three children. In contrast, Barry had lived as a contented and accomplished girl from the age of three and had been supported in this by her parents. The medical profession viewed Barry's unusual childhood conditioning as having an irrevocable impact on her. Decades later, Benjamin would reflect that, in retrospect, he might have said Spengler had transsexual tendencies, but in 1949, Benjamin seemed to think of Barry's case as entirely new and as belonging to a different category than Spengler's. Barry would be the first patient he would guide toward genital surgery.[41]

The biggest change, though, was that offering Barry hormone treatment was now a relatively straightforward matter. In the more than thirty years since Steinach had painstakingly transplanted ovaries and testes the size of grains of rice into rats and guinea pigs, sex hormones and many other hormones had been identified, purified, and commercialized. Indeed, they were now big business. By 1942, a synthetic version of estrogen became available in the form of diethylstilbestrol (DES). Several versions of androgens were also available since the isolation of testosterone in 1935.

During the 1930s and 1940s, there was an exhilarating atmosphere in hormone research that generated large-scale collaborations between academic scientists and the pharmaceutical industry. The promise of finding the "master molecules" that might explain and control the phenomena of life and the prospect of bringing these hormone products to market drew many of the most talented researchers and most ambitious science-based firms to the field. During the Second World War, the American government became involved in organizing and sponsoring a concerted program to develop the hormones of the adrenal cortex in the expectation that these might serve to enhance the performance of combat pilots. Endocrinology as a medical specialty had also come a very long way from the 1920s, when young practitioners might have been worried they were risking their careers by entering a field so riddled with quackery and dangerous associations with sex. An explosion of clinical research and the growth of professional journals and societies now established endocrinology as an integral part of medicine.[42]

What is important to note, however, is that people changed gender long before the creation of a medical or scientific label and before the widespread availability of surgery and hormones. People like Lucy Hicks Anderson, the American socialite and chef, made lives for themselves without the use of medical interventions or a medical diagnosis. They often lived inconspicuously, worked, formed relationships, and contributed to their communities in their desired gender roles. Some lived in community with others like themselves, while others lived far from the urban demimonde.[43]

Gender-variant patients were few and far between in Benjamin's experience, so he had few opportunities to consider the views about gender identity that he had encountered at Hirschfeld's Institute for Sexual Science or Steinach's laboratory. Kinsey had a vast network of subjects for his research and became an important source of referrals for Benjamin. Benjamin also began to connect with a number of transgender individuals through Karl Bowman and Louise Lawrence, a pioneering transgender community organizer. Lawrence had been assigned male at birth but had been living full-time as a woman for many years. Over time, she developed a large correspondence with others across the United States who identified as "transvestite." She found others by placing personal advertisements in magazines and reaching out to individuals who had been arrested for cross-dressing in public. In time, she met Bowman and his colleagues at the University of California, San Francisco, and offered lectures to them.[44]

Benjamin gained a reputation as a sympathetic doctor among those in this network. Benjamin's thinking about Val Barry's case and that of others like her was to evolve slowly over many years, case by case. In these early years, he had no clear conceptual framework and little scientific literature and language with which to discuss the concerns of those who identified cross-gender. Benjamin listened to the voices of his patients with respect and sought to do what he could to help them, whether with hormone therapy, counseling and moral support, or referrals to others for legal help, psychological treatment, or surgery. Over time, he gained a sense of the complexity and rich diversity of the lives lived by gender-variant people.

In 1949, Kinsey referred a remarkable couple to him named Carol (pseudonym) and Christian (pseudonym). Their marriage, as Benjamin's colleagues later put it, was "a love affair worthy of a romance novel." Carol had been assigned male at birth and Christian assigned female. They had married in their birth gender roles but then had their marriage annulled when they each changed sex. They then remarried in their new gender identities, Carol staying at home to keep house while Christian became the breadwinner. Benjamin became a sympathetic counselor to them both, overseeing their hormone treatments and offering emotional support and medical advice. He helped them connect with Elmer Belt, one of the few surgeons in the United States then doing genital-reassignment surgery, who operated on Carol in 1956.[45]

Sexual identity was still cast in the framework of a male-female binary. Like Carol and Christian, one could opt to change from a man to a woman or from a woman to a man; there were only two options. But other patients had a more challenging time figuring out who they were and what they wanted, and they presented a more complicated picture. In 1951, Benjamin met a thirty-five-year-old male machinist named Frank (pseudonym) who wished to become a writer. Frank had strong cross-gender feelings but vacillated about whether to "give in" to those feelings or to continue to fight them. Benjamin worked with Frank on a weekly basis for a year and a half, trying to understand what was underlying his concerns. Benjamin wrote, "Beyond listening to him, I don't see what I can do for him. I try to give him better balance to make better decisions. . . . The poor fellow is really in a terrible emotional turmoil." Frank ultimately decided not to have any hormones or surgery, and Benjamin referred him to his psychologist colleague Albert Ellis. In 1972, Frank returned to see Benjamin again and explained that after twenty years of considering the matter, he had decided against a sex change. Benjamin framed Frank's journey as one of vacillation and confusion but was forced to recognize that not all journeys were alike.[46]

Louise Lawrence, elegant and dignified, became an important collaborator and influence on Benjamin's thinking. Historian Joanne Meyerowitz describes her as a "one-woman social hub." Through the course of many years, she taught Benjamin much about her experience and served as a valued sounding board for his ideas. They introduced each other to their contacts, and Lawrence introduced Benjamin to several of his earliest patients. Lawrence, an artist, had lived the first half of her life as a man, marrying twice and having a daughter while secretly cross-dressing. When her second marriage ended in divorce, she decided to attempt to live full-time as a woman as she had always dreamed. She moved to another city and successfully sold her paintings while managing a small apartment house and offering services in remodeling and decorating.

While she considered herself a champion of transvestites, she moved freely among several different communities, attending gay drag parties, working with the homophile movement, and associating with the gay female impersonators who performed at the nightclub Finocchio's. She had experimented with homosexuality while living as a man and continued to socialize with lesbians and gay men. In the 1950s, her efforts to bridge these social groups was unusual.[47]

In letters between Benjamin and Lawrence, they bandied about ideas on terminology and treatment and considered more profound efforts to get at the heart of the condition they were beginning to define. Benjamin spoke of his patients' deep desire to change sex, saying, "We lack a proper scientific term for it. I would describe it as an 'obsessive urge to belong to the opposite sex.'" Lawrence postulated that gender is a learned role, citing a recent psychological study of children reared from birth as the opposite sex. When these individuals were later apprised of their biological sex and given a choice of gender role, three-quarters of them chose to revert to their biological sex, but one-quarter chose to remain in the gender role in which they had been raised. Benjamin was not convinced but respected her viewpoint. "If the theory of a learned gender role satisfies you, fine, stick to it," he said. His thinking, though, as always, was shaped by a fundamental belief that sex, gender, outlook, and behavior were rooted in biology: "I cannot believe in its exclusiveness because I am biologically oriented. A living brain has to exist to learn anything, to have any feeling, thought or emotion, and brains are very complicated instruments and very different in different people." Lawrence appreciated Benjamin as one of the few medical professionals who really understood these issues.[48]

Benjamin also began to work with Virginia Prince, a chemist, transvestite, researcher, and well-known figure at the center of a large network of cross-dressers in Southern California. She emerged as a spokesperson for a view of transvestite identity, though one that explicitly excluded homosexuals and transsexuals.[49]

In New York later that year, a newly discharged army private was in despair and confusion. Christine Jorgensen (then living as a man) had combed books and magazines to search for a clue to her experience. A recent popular book, *The Male Hormone* (1945) by science writer Paul de Kruif, proved eye-opening. Since his collaboration with Sinclair Lewis two decades before, De Kruif had published the enormously best-selling *Microbe Hunters* (1926), which inspired a generation of research scientists to enter the study of microbiology and immunology. In *The Male Hormone*, De Kruif made the tale of the 1935 discovery of testosterone as exciting as a detective story. The promotional blurb on the cover promised readers "a gleam of hope for prolonging men's prime of life." The author's personal account of using testosterone bore faint echoes of Steinach's rejuvenates twenty years before, but his was now an experience legitimized by decades of research, backed by powerful new commercial hormone products, and equated with any other hormonal disorder. He promised, "So, no different than a good diabetic child who knows that insulin every day makes the difference between living and dying, I'll be faithful and remember to take my twenty or thirty milligrams a day of testosterone. I'm not ashamed that it's no longer made to its old degree by my own aging body. It's chemical crutches. It's borrowed manhood. It's borrowed time. But, just the same, it's what makes bulls bulls."[50]

For Jorgensen, just twenty-one years old, midlife struggles were a distant concern, but what intrigued her was De Kruif's explanation of the role of sex hormones in determining maleness and femaleness. De Kruif elaborated, "Chemically all of us are both man and woman because our bodies make both male and female hormones, and primarily, it's an excess of testosterone that makes us men or an excess of female hormones that makes us women."[51]

Reading this book felt like an epiphany for Jorgensen, who had been struggling with feelings of sexual attraction to men and the sense of not being a real man. Jorgensen became convinced she was suffering from a hormonal imbalance. Inspired by a more serious scientific book, probably *Hormones and Behaviour* (1948) by Yale professor Frank A. Beach,[52] Jorgensen made an appointment to meet with its author to try to pursue this hypothesis. Beach was conducting pioneering studies of the interrelation of hormones, neurological factors, and environment in shaping the sexual behavior of rats. These studies would be considered the foundation of modern behavioral endocrinology. But Jorgensen was disappointed. The professor did not offer any hormone tests or any other support and instead referred Jorgensen to a psychiatrist who in turn recommended psychoanalysis to remove "feminine inclinations."[53]

Jorgensen rejected this suggestion. She did not want to be more masculine, nor did she want to live as a homosexual man. She was determined to gain a better understanding of human physiology, and though she had worked as a photographer, she now decided to train as a medical technician. Dr. Joseph Angelo, the husband of a classmate, helped Jorgensen procure estradiol. (Perhaps to protect Angelo's identity, Jorgensen gave an alternate account of how she first obtained the hormones: she said that she had taken a bus to a distant part of town where she could not be recognized and convinced a pharmacy clerk that she was a student who needed materials for a research project. She walked out with one hundred tablets of high-potency estradiol.)[54]

By the early 1950s, Benjamin was finding his practice winding down. One side effect of the mass marketing of hormones and the growing acceptance of endocrinology was that more practitioners were able to prescribe hormones and fewer patients sought the reactivation treatments he offered. At the same time, Freudian psychoanalysis had exploded in popularity so that sexual difficulties that might have previously brought a patient to Benjamin's door were now laid out on the analyst's couch.

Benjamin met Virginia Allen at a medical meeting in Atlantic City in 1950. Allen and her husband, a doctor, had met and spoken at length with Benjamin to compliment him after a lecture he had given on psychosomatic illness. When she and her husband relocated to New York City two years later, she called on Benjamin to renew their acquaintance. He did not let on that he couldn't remember who she was but, with his ingrained courtesy, took her to lunch. Soon after, he invited her for drinks at the Sulgrave Hotel. He explained to her that he was now sixty-seven and since he felt he had only a few years left to him, he wanted to spend them quietly in a retirement practice.[55]

"My patients are retiring me," he explained a little sadly. He wanted to move from his beautiful office at 728 Park Avenue to smaller accommodations on East Sixty-Seventh Street. "Would you like to come help me wind it down?" he asked her.

In the dim of the cocktail lounge, Benjamin whipped out his throat flashlight to inspect a tray of canapés, then turned its bright beam on Allen.

"It would be fun, working together, don't you think?"[56]

Dazzled, she agreed. She began to work for him as his secretary, first part-time and later full-time. Before long, she became an indispensable part of his life.

Allen got down to work sorting and packing files and setting up the new office. As Benjamin recalled, their days consisted of "coffee breaks occasionally interrupted by a patient." Allen noticed a few medical records off on their own, and they looked strange to her as the files bore both a man's name and a woman's name. She asked Benjamin what they were. Benjamin sighed. He explained that they were the records of his patients who dressed as, or felt themselves to be, the other gender.

"Not very much is known about them."

Allen was intrigued.

"Why don't we do something with them, since we have so much time?" she proposed.

Oddly, given his eventful career, Benjamin described himself as unambitious and as having always been lazy. He had found it difficult to sit down to write because he usually preferred being with people.[57]

Benjamin nodded. "Yes, that may be very good. They are sad people and deserve help, but they make everyone, even other doctors, so nervous and uncomfortable."

Now, the autumn of his life had finally given him the leisure to delve more deeply into the rich loam of his experience.

"Bring the records in here and we'll go over them."[58]

Chapter 10

Defining Sex in the Atomic Age

Every hour—every day—we encounter something new
Electric this—atomic that—a modern point of view
Now anything can happen—and we shouldn't think it strange
If oysters smoke cigars—or lobsters drive imported cars
For we live in a time of change.
—Christine Jorgensen

On 12 February 1953, Christine Jorgensen gracefully descended the stairs of a Scandinavian Airlines plane at New York's Idlewild Airport. A crowd of 350 was waiting. Despite the long flight from Denmark, Jorgensen looked radiant, swathed against the chill in a long nutria fur coat with matching cap, her elegant gloved hand raised in greeting. A New York City police sergeant and several Hearst public relations people bundled her into the terminal where, according to one report, she had a few minutes to enjoy a cigarette and down a Bloody Mary before striding into the press room that was wreathed in smoke and ablaze with newsreel lights. She had a smile worthy of a movie star.[1]

It had been thirty months since Jorgensen had gone off to Denmark to seek medical help and now returned, renamed Christine. The hormones that Jorgensen had acquired in New York had begun this transformation. Initially the amounts taken were too small for much effect, though Jorgensen felt refreshed and noticed a greater sensitivity in her breasts. In Denmark, Jorgensen had been able to convince endocrinologist Christian Hamburger and psychiatrist Georg Stürup to experiment on her for free, administering hormones by injection and by mouth. Month by month, the hormones effected a slow, steady trans-formation. Within a year, Hamburger noted that Jorgensen's testosterone pro-duction had diminished, her libido had declined, and there was a darkening of pigmentation around the skin of her nipples and genitals. Jorgensen felt more at ease "psychically" and able to work on photography with greater vigor and inspiration. She described the changes she perceived for herself: "skin clear and smooth, body contours definitely more feminine." She reported to friends, "Of course I am my old self inside only much happier."[2] Soon, she felt she had reached the point of no return. Stürup concluded there was no benefit to fur-ther psychiatric treatment and, given Jorgensen's insistence on having surgery, sought approval from the attorney general of Denmark to allow two genital sur-geries.[3] The American ambassador to Denmark, Eugenie Anderson, promised to handle Jorgensen's case herself, and in May 1952, the State Department issued a new passport under a new name, chosen in honor of Dr. Christian Hamburger.

Just before her return to the United States, the *New York Daily News* broke the story of her transition with the front-page headline "Ex-GI Becomes Blonde Beauty." Reporters were sent to Copenhagen, and a clamor of publicity ensued. Jorgensen signed a deal with Hearst for an exclusive story series to be published in the Sunday newspaper supplement *American Weekly*. Hearst agents carefully managed Jorgensen's arrival on the tarmac, and over the next five weeks the public read her story lavishly illustrated with photos of Christine at home with her parents and out on the town dressed in smart suits. These were shown in contrast with photos of the man she had been. Whatever the prurient interests of the press and the crude jokes that circulated at her expense, her story also evoked sympathy and praise as a tale of courage. Jorgensen's transformation became the top story of the year for the *New York Daily News*.

By the spring of 1953, she had become a celebrity. The former private from the Bronx was now dining at the Waldorf Astoria with the likes of Irving Ber-lin, Samuel Goldwyn, Cole Porter, and Truman Capote. She was also inun-dated with letters from hundreds of individuals who found in her story the first glimpse of hope for their own struggles with gender identity. She felt bound to answer these desperate messages asking for help and was overwhelmed. But among these letters, Jorgensen found one that offered to help her instead; it was from Harry Benjamin.[4]

In 1953, Benjamin was sixty-eight years old and had lived long enough to see his old nemesis, tuberculosis, beaten back. By the beginning of the decade, physicians could safely and effectively treat tuberculosis using a trio of drugs: streptomycin, para-aminosalicylic acid, and isoniazid. At the peak of the sanatorium era, there had been over 800 institutions across the United States providing 136,000 beds. A decade later, almost all were closed.[5] They had become obsolete. The days when the Waldorf Astoria lobby had been jammed with members of the "White Plague Army"—whom Benjamin had been so powerless to help— must have seemed a lifetime away. Benjamin had also lived to see his early faith in the importance of the endocrine glands vindicated. The Wednesday evening conversations in Joseph Fraenkel's office had been speculative. Now, endocrinology was an integral part of medicine, with research and clinical journals and professional associations.

Medicine was on a triumphant run. During the war, scientists had figured out how to manufacture penicillin on a large scale. Now, 1953 would usher in the first tests of the Salk vaccine for polio and the discovery of the molecular structure of DNA by James Watson and Francis Crick, a development that would transform biology. No mountain seemed too high, no goal beyond human reach, for good or ill. (That year would also see the creation of the hydrogen bomb, the next generation of lethal weapons.) The DNA discovery would mark the start of a robust new research enterprise to delineate the genetic influences on life, one that would dominate the life sciences for the next half century. The genes would now take the place that hormones had held in the cultural imagination as the keys to understanding and controlling the fundamental aspects of life.

But for Benjamin, ordinary life was now becoming increasingly trying. He faced growing health problems. "Don't envy me living in New York," he told one English correspondent. "It is sometimes my modern conception of Hell, impossibly overcrowded, the people rude and overwrought nervously, the air full of poison and the climate abominable." He conceded, however, "There are indeed many concerts and many good shows but you try to get tickets and stand in line and then get lousy seats at a price often way above that of the box-office."[6]

He had not given up his hopes for gerontotherapy, and he continued keeping up with the literature and being attracted to ideas on the margins of medical respectability. After one trip to Zurich, he gave an interview saying he was impressed with the live cell therapy pioneered by Dr. Paul Niehans in the 1930s. Niehans, a leading glandular transplant surgeon, used the injection of embryonic animal cells to arrest aging. He counted Pope Pius XII, Charles de Gaulle, Konrad Adenauer, and Somerset Maugham among his patients.[7] (Though now discounted by medical authorities, this therapy continues to be offered in private clinics around the globe.)

⸻

On 12 February 1953, the same day that Jorgensen arrived at Idlewild Airport, members of the British Everest expedition sailed from Tilbury Docks in London on their way to assail the world's highest mountain. Months later, journalist Jan Morris (then living as a man) and mountaineer Michael Westmacott made their way across the notorious Khumbu Icefall, laced with crevasses and towers of ice, down the slope of Everest from 22,100 feet. At twenty-six, Morris looked dashing, handsome, lean, and angular with a shock of wavy hair, keen eyes, and an emphatic nose. Although a novice to climbing, the young reporter had shown stamina, fortitude, and good humor, following the veteran climbers three-quarters of the way up the mountain, all the while sending off lucid dispatches describing the frostbite, avalanches, and sheer audacity.

But on this day, Morris and Westmacott had made the risky decision to begin their descent late in the afternoon.[8] They carried with them a message they thought might well be the story of the century. The glacier was thawing and their carefully marked route was now streaked with icy rivulets. At each step, the ravenous snow swallowed their legs, at times up to the thigh. As the last light blinked out over the horizon, they lost their way. Morris floundered. One crampon broke and was left a flapping impediment. A toe smashed so violently the nail fell off. The hand wielding the ice ax shook with fatigue. Enfolded by exhaustion, Morris asked Westmacott to untie the rope between them.

"I think I'm going to stop here for a bit, and get my breath back," Morris said, with forced lightness. "I'll just sit here quietly for a minute or two. You go on Mike, don't bother about me."

Westmacott was but a vague shape in the dark at the other end of the rope. There was a pause.

Out of the night came Westmacott's reply: "Don't be so ridiculous."[9]

At length the companions staggered into the safety of base camp. At first light, Morris handed a note to a trusted runner. It was a message specially coded to outwit rival journalists. Decoded, it read, "Successful ascent. Hillary, May 29. Tenzing. All well."

The *Times* had its scoop. In London, Morris's message was relayed to Queen Elizabeth II the night before her coronation, and on 2 June 1953, the conquest of

Everest was announced to the crowds lining Pall Mall to greet their new monarch. Cheering and dancing erupted in the streets.[10]

Mutual friends arranged for Benjamin and Jorgensen to meet for the first time at a dinner party at the home of the actor and author Tiffany Thayer and his wife, Kathleen. Benjamin liked Jorgensen right away; she seemed honest to him.[11] Jorgensen later visited him at his office, where he examined her, and they had a long chat. Writing to Alfred Kinsey, Benjamin suggested that Jorgensen might provide a most valuable history for Kinsey's research; he speculated that she might be one of the very few cases in which a radical operation could succeed in helping her "to a reasonably happy life for the future." He hoped to do some hormone assays on her and expected to see her fairly regularly but wanted to wait until his initial tests were completed before beginning any endocrine treatment. At any rate, he felt she was still too distressed by the "'Frankenstein' publicity" she had been facing.[12]

Jorgensen and Benjamin soon began a fruitful correspondence and collaboration. She and her mother had been trying in vain to reply to the mountain of letters she had received as a result of all the press coverage. Jorgensen asked if she could refer patients to him, and when he agreed, she felt huge relief. "The deluge fell onto poor Harry's shoulders," she admitted.[13] On one occasion, Jorgensen drove Harry and Gretchen out to her home in Massapequa for an afternoon and evening with her family. Benjamin recalled the occasion fondly and remembered that he was particularly impressed by the love and support Jorgensen had from her "charming, lovable mother, her good-looking sister, and a father whose eagerness to understand Christine's problem was truly admirable." This, he remarked, was unfortunately very different from what many of his patients experienced, who faced ignorance, prejudice, and cruel rejection just when they most needed love.[14]

In a year that saw the conquest of Everest, the crowning of a new queen in Britain, and the end of the Korean War, Christine Jorgensen garnered thousands of lines of press. The media made much of the fact that she was an ex-GI, playing up the before and after of her transition. It was a Cinderella story with a twist, a magical transformation that at the same time did not disrupt the gender norms of a conservative postwar America. With her high heels, tailored suits, and glittering gowns, Jorgensen cultivated a feminine ideal of beauty and glamour. She also always took care to minimize any discussion of her sexual life.

Jorgensen's story symbolized many things in the public arena. For some, it was a heroic tale of can-do spirit; for others, it seemed like individualism run amok. For some, it was about the power of science to accomplish previously undreamed of feats; for others, it triggered anxiety about a Frankensteinian science, reaching where human ingenuity had no business going.[15] Jorgensen also found that a small portion of her mail was hostile. Some writers were upset at the challenge she posed to traditional morals; others were angry that she shed a bad light on those who were already facing discrimination. Most gay men loved her and found her inspiring, but some felt she was a betrayal to them. Some worried her example meant that they too would have to undergo the knife to "normalize" their same-sex desires. But for the large majority of writers, including many who were not sexual or gender minorities, her story of triumph over adversity was an inspiration. For Benjamin, the connection with Jorgensen might have felt like a re-spinning of the story played out in the press with Gertrude Atherton three decades earlier. Jorgensen expressed the hope that, by weathering the storm of publicity, perhaps someday, for some other Christine, there would no longer be any sensation and that her story would be seen as perfectly unremarkable.[16]

One of Benjamin's most helpful suggestions to Jorgensen was that she begin to set up networks of support for those who wrote to her. Thanks to her celebrity status, she became something of a postal clearinghouse for transgender people. Benjamin and Jorgensen helped many people in a number of practical ways, such as answering legal questions about how to get identification papers that matched their chosen names and gender. Benjamin also played the role of medical adviser. In 1954, when vaginoplasty (the surgical construction of a vagina) became legal in the United States, he along with Dr. Joseph Angelo oversaw Jorgensen's next surgery.

Recognizing that she could not escape the glare of publicity and needing the money, Jorgensen decided to capitalize on her newfound fame by creating a nightclub act complete with dance, music, and short dialogues. She played on her sex change with clever songs that she wrote herself. She opened with show tunes like "Getting to Know You" and then built an inspiring narrative of how an individual can overcome adversity. She sang about how, in the atomic age, science made anything possible and change was the order of the day. Finally, she closed with the uplifting anthem "You'll Never Walk Alone." At the peak of her fame, she was able to command $12,500 for a week's appearance at the Orpheum Theater.[17]

One key development was the emergence of the notion of "gender" and "gender identity" in the mid-1950s and early 1960s in the work of John Money and his associates Joan Hampson and John Hampson at Johns Hopkins University, as well as psychiatrists Robert Stoller and Ralph Greenson at the University of California at Los Angeles. Gender, the lived experience of masculinity or femininity, was distinct from biological sex, which was constituted by chromosomes, hormones, and anatomy. Gender referred to an individual's subjective sense of being masculine or feminine, what previous theorists had tried to describe as a "psychological sex" or what Karl Heinrich Ulrichs had tried to suggest when he talked about a feminine soul in a male body. Gender identity, or one's internal sense of being a man or a woman, was differentiated from sexual orientation—whether one had an erotic attraction to members of the same or other sex. Gender identity—a subjective experience of gender—was also distinguished from "gender role," the social behaviors associated with men or women.[18]

Money's work emerged from his efforts to understand and work with intersex infants and children, that is, children born with ambiguous biological sex. During the 1950s and 1960s, physicians following Money's theories about how to treat intersex individuals carried out a set of practices that would later come to be seen as cruel and mistaken. Parents were not informed of the intersex condition of their children because physicians thought this would lead to anxiety and confusion about how to raise them. Instead, the physicians took on the responsibility of deciding whether a child should be surgically altered and whether that child should be reared as a girl or a boy. For example, Money suggested that a child with male reproductive organs but whose penis he considered too small would not be able to function properly as a boy and that the child would be better off surgically altered and raised a girl. The terrible aftermath of these practices would come to light only in later decades thanks to the activism of intersex individuals and their families. The concepts of gender and sex that were developed became useful in describing transsexual individuals as well, that is, people who were unambiguously one sex in a physical sense but who had an internal feeling of belonging to the other sex.[19]

Benjamin's contribution to the treatment and understanding of transsexuality would be described by his colleagues Leah Cahan Schaefer and Christine Wheeler as the sum total of his previous interests and knowledge: "an accident for which he was totally prepared." Indeed, it was his grounding in early twentieth-century European sexology that had given him the conceptual framework, the belief that male and female are two ends of a spectrum. His decades as a gerontologist had taught him compassion for those who suffered and strengthened his willingness to intervene in what others might have considered a natural condition. And his work as an endocrinologist had given him a vision of the male-female spectrum as one that might be traversed and a command of the very tools with which to do so. After all, much of gerontotherapy was shaded with the manipulation of sexual characteristics—reactivation in men was linked to the recovery of sexual function and "manly" qualities of strength and vigor, while female reactivation was linked to softness, attractiveness, and stereotypical ideas of youthful feminine beauty.[20]

With the help of Jorgensen's creative and focused attention and the input of his other patients, Benjamin began to formulate the transsexual idea. Articulating the concept of transsexuality involved a complex and often uneasy collaboration between transgender people and the medical professionals who worked with them. The metaphors that they used to describe their experience of sex and gender were varied, depending in part on the imagery and language that was available to them. Lili Elbe, whose story had inspired so many, had described herself in the 1930s as being both a man and a woman sharing the same body. Her goal in seeking medical help was to rid herself of the male personality. In the 1950s, many of those who were striving to make sense of their own experience of desire and identity, and most of American physicians and sexologists, would have used the category "homosexual" to describe people like Jorgensen and Val Barry. When Jorgensen described herself to Christian Hamburger in 1950 or 1951, she called herself homosexual with "a large amount of femininity." She also used the image of "lost between the sexes." In European medical circles, the category "transvestite" prevailed, and Hamburger used that term to describe Jorgensen.[21]

In the early 1950s, as Benjamin mulled over his case notes and debated ideas with colleagues such as Jorgensen and Louise Lawrence, he used the hypothesis that those who desired to change sex had an extreme version of transvestism. Drawing on the same impulses as Magnus Hirschfeld and Alfred Kinsey in trying to apply scientific order to this phenomenon, he developed a diagnostic scale with categories Transvestite I, II, and III, in which Type III was a person who sought medical help to change sex.

Although Hirschfeld had used the term "seelischer Transsexualismus" (psychological transsexualism) as early as 1923 to refer to what he called a "true transvestite," English readers generally date the appearance of the term "trans-sexual," used in the sense we now understand it, to the work of the physician David Cauldwell, who in 1949 coined the term *psychopathia transsexualis*. Cauld-well served as the letters editor for the journal *Sexology* from 1946 to 1959 and authored dozens of popular pamphlets for the counterculture publishing house Haldeman-Julius Publications. With an irreverent and lighthearted style, he wrote pieces that challenged moralistic, guilt-ridden approaches to sexuality. He used stories sent in by letter writers to offer answers to many popular questions. He created transsexualism as a separate sexological category, distinguished from intersex individuals, transvestites, and homosexuals. He completely rejected the idea of surgical treatment of transsexuals, arguing that it would be criminal for a doctor to excise healthy tissues and organs. He did, however, articulate the idea of psychological sex as separate from biological sex and described transsexuals as people who had the biology of one sex while having the psychology of the other.[22]

Benjamin began using the term soon after. His work with patients was char-acterized by a steady conviction that their experience of identity was rooted in biology, though he did not have any specific hypothesis or evidence as to what this biological cause might be. Jorgensen's belief that she suffered from a hor-monal imbalance meshed with his beliefs, as did her assumption that medical science could be used to correct it. In contrast, psychiatrists and psychoanalysts who interpreted the experiences of these individuals as signs of a mental illness believed that any attempt to use hormones or surgery would only be danger-ously feeding a delusion. While many American sexologists such as Kinsey believed in male and female as separate and opposing categories, Benjamin had, since his youth, held the idea that male and female were two ends of a spectrum and that every individual possesses a mix of female and male characteristics. This conception was only strengthened in his mind by his appreciation of the experiments of Eugen Steinach and later by the revelations of the close chemical relationships among the sex hormones. The male and female body were mallea-ble structures built on a fluid foundation.

Benjamin began to speak and publish on the subject of transsexuality and developed the term "gender dysphoria" to describe the condition of feeling discomfort or distress that one's sense of gender did not match one's sex at birth. In 1953, he gave his first lecture on transsexualism to the Association for the Advancement of Psychotherapy. In his 1953 article "Transvestism and

Transsexualism," he described a masculine psyche within a female body that had an overwhelming desire to gain outward recognition in occupation, dress, or sexual behavior, or a female psyche in a male body. He acknowledged that psychoanalytic interpretations of the phenomenon might have some validity and that milder cases might have exclusively psychological causes. He was, however, convinced that if there were conflicts in a person's psyche, they would produce the pronounced characteristics he saw in his clinical practice only if they found "fertile soil" in disturbances of the body's genetic or endocrine constitution. Moreover, he argued that more serious cases were not amenable to psychoanalytical interventions. In his nearly forty years of practice, he had never once seen a pronounced case of homosexuality or transsexualism cured by psychoanalysis, even when treatment was persistent and continued for years. (He acknowledged that such cures had been reported by others, though, so he could not deny their possibility.) This being the case, he argued that the best approach was to use psychotherapy to "ease tension" and work in the direction of, rather than against, the patient's male or female psyche. This could be done by using large doses of estrogen for men and androgen for women for "chemical castration," that is, to suppress the activity of the opposite endocrine function.[23]

While in some extreme cases transsexuals demanded genital surgery, Benjamin felt that such a radical step was rarely indicated and that in fact the majority of transvestites would not want it. Benjamin argued that surgery was not a guarantee of a happier life because it is only possible to transform the secondary sexual characteristics and not genetic sex and that if a patient were not well suited to this change, tragedy might ensue. Thus far, successful cases had been rare but had resulted in some reasonably contented and successful women. He argued that such a patient had "every right to be accepted as a woman and lead a woman's life" and decried as blind prejudice the attitudes that would deny to her what she was entitled to by virtue of science and by her own nature and humanity. He concluded, "Where such behavior does not intrude on the rights of others, it should be viewed in the light of science and common sense and not, as it is now done, in the twilight of prejudices and misconceptions." Moreover, he pointed to the fundamental question of how and where physicians should intervene. In the case of transvestites, he suggested, "instead of treating the patient, it would frequently be wiser and more constructive to 'treat' society, educationally, so that logic, understanding and compassion might prevail." After all, what really needed changing? Was it the individual, or was it society itself?[24]

For Benjamin and his collaborators, one of their central preoccupations was figuring out how to determine who was a "true" transsexual. This was of critical importance to them because it would indicate which individuals could be candidates for medical transition. For Benjamin, the characteristic that was key to identifying a true transsexual was the unshakable internal sense of belonging to the other gender and with it an urgent desire to change sex. This urgency was so profound and desperate that many of his patients had considered suicide. Typically, he thought, true transsexuals had always known they were in the "wrong" gender from childhood. But in his practice, Benjamin began to meet increasing numbers of people who did not share this classic narrative. Some wavered; some changed their minds. Some wanted to live as the other gender without medical intervention; some wanted to use hormones but not surgery. Moreover, the publicity surrounding Jorgensen brought to the fore even the basic question of how to define a man or a woman. In questions of law, this had not yet been sorted out. Science could be brought to bear on the question but did not provide definitive answers. Was sex determined in the chromosomes? In the gonads? In the hormones?

In correspondence with his colleague the surgeon Elmer Belt, Benjamin grappled with the question of who should receive treatment. In these early years, practitioners like Benjamin and Belt had to muddle their way through these deliberations using only their intuition and their still-limited clinical experience. It was not obvious to them who should qualify for treatment, and the possibility of making terrible errors hung over them. One of their earliest decisions was to require that patients have a psychiatric evaluation. Typically, Benjamin referred patients to Belt, who then sent them to psychiatrist Carroll Carlson for assessment; they did not ask Carlson to determine whether the patients were transsexual but whether they were mentally well enough to make their own decisions. Clearly, Benjamin's and Belt's own sense of what men and women should be like played into their opinions. Historians of transness have elucidated the fact that trans people often had to "perform" gender to their doctors in order to prove themselves "real" transsexuals and worthy of medical transition. More recently, historian Beans Velocci has shown that Benjamin's and Belt's conclusions were often based not only on whether candidates fit the category of a true transsexual but whether they would be able to "pass" to observers after they transitioned. Although having an unshakable internal sense of belonging to the other gender was a necessary condition of access to surgery, in practice Benjamin also weighed whether, in his view, a trans woman would make a convincing woman. Would strangers read her as a woman, and would she be able to find employment? A small, delicate individual might pass, but he thought a large, bulky one might not. If the post-transition patient were to find she could not pass, these practitioners feared she would come to regret her surgery. In February 1960, Belt wrote to Benjamin, "Each of us will probably die by getting shot by some patient like E. V.," a telling half-joke that conveyed his sense of anxiety about how their decisions might not only affect the well-being of their patients but bring lawsuits or even violence upon themselves if patients regretted their transitions and turned on them.[25] Their caution, which would later come to be codified in the Standards of Care, perhaps drew as much from the need to protect physicians' interests as it did the wish to ensure a successful outcome for the patient.[26]

Pioneering plastic surgeons would, over the course of the next decades, develop more and more refined techniques for the removal of organs and the reshaping of new ones. For some transgender individuals, a surgical transition, usually requiring several operations, was the ultimate goal, the signature of what it meant to be transsexual. But for individuals who identified as transsexual in 1950s America, there were few surgeons willing to provide the operations. Denmark's government, after the surprise attention received after Jorgensen's transition, quickly changed its laws so that only Danish citizens could be treated. For some Americans, having enough money to travel for an operation seemed as unlikely as a fairy tale. In drastic circumstances, some sought the help of disreputable "chop-shop" surgeons akin to back-alley abortionists, and some even literally took matters into their own hands, carrying out their own kitchen table castrations that doctors could then attempt to clean up.[27]

Hormones, however, were more readily accessible. Sympathetic physicians could be found who were willing to prescribe hormones for transvestites and transsexuals. And it was hormonal treatments that held the potential to make subtle, gradual changes that made an individual not only look different but feel different. For a transsexual woman, it could mean a greater calm and a softening of the hard edges of a male body. For a transsexual man, it could provide a lowering voice, more abundant facial hair, and increased libido. Before Benjamin, there had been physicians in other parts of the country or in Europe who saw an occasional transgender patient. Some were willing to provide the treatments these patients sought. But it would be in Benjamin's clinic that the largest number of them found a physician sympathetic to their condition, and as a result, it was here that the most significant pool of clinical data on transsexuality would be created.

In her definitive account of the history of transsexuality, historian Joanne Meyerowitz explains that for anyone interested in transsexualism in the 1960s, "most roads led to Harry Benjamin." Benjamin, by then in his late seventies and early eighties, was at the hub of overlapping networks of sexologists, physicians, psychologists, and transgender activists.[28]

In 1961, Ira Pauly, a young psychiatry resident at the New York Hospital-Cornell Medical Center, was called to consult with a patient who had spent several days in the urology ward. The patient sported a full beard and spoke with a low voice. After some discussion, Pauly realized that his patient wanted to have his ovaries, fallopian tubes, uterus, and vagina removed. Pauly was fascinated. He knew almost nothing about transsexualism and discovered that the literature on the subject was scarce. Fortunately, there was an extensive historical library at the hospital, so with the discipline and relentlessness befitting a former starting center for his varsity football team, Pauly plowed through the old tomes to find the few clues he could. Most of the relevant articles were in German and French, and not being able to read these languages himself, Pauly carried out the dusty volumes one after another, asking three or four of his French- and German-speaking patients to translate the articles and then painstakingly write the text out by hand.[29]

There were only a few case studies, one from Sweden, another from Denmark, and a few from Germany and France, but when he got to the US literature, he found one brief article in an obscure journal by Harry Benjamin. It gave Benjamin's address, which Pauly realized was just five blocks away. Pauly dialed his number and was put through to Benjamin immediately. When Pauly explained that he wanted to learn more about transsexualism, Benjamin invited him to visit the following day when he was to have his weekly Wednesday afternoon transsexual clinic.

Benjamin was warm, gentle, and hospitable even to this perfect stranger. He asked Pauly to lunch and then welcomed him into the sanctum of his private practice, allowing Pauly to meet with several of his transsexual patients, who with equal generosity allowed the young resident a glimpse into their lives. In a single day, Pauly's familiarity with transsexuals was increased, as he put it, by about "1000%." Benjamin carefully summarized each patient's life history and shared his wealth of clinical experience. Pauly, open and friendly, had chosen psychiatry precisely because he loved the part of medicine that involved talking with people rather than memorizing biochemical equations. As he listened and watched, Benjamin interviewed the patient, occasionally excusing himself to turn to Pauly to emphasize one point or another. Pauly was struck by how each patient received Benjamin's full attention, and because Pauly had been introduced to them as an associate of Benjamin's, the patients graciously opened up to him as well, revealing a whole new world to his view. In the months that followed, he continued to attend Benjamin's weekly clinic, learning at the side of the master and seeing, in his estimate, "more transsexual patients than any psychiatrist in North America. Or for that matter, in the world."[30]

Although Pauly had studied with renowned academicians at UCLA, Cornell, and the New York Hospital, Benjamin taught him something that he had never learned from his professors before. Pauly had never met anyone who cared about his patients in such a deep way, as if they were his family. He saw that Benjamin's patients were totally at ease with him. In his four years of medical training, he had always been taught the importance of cultivating a professional distance from his patients, but Benjamin showed him that this did not have to be the case. Benjamin's approach came to epitomize for Pauly the ideal doctor-patient relationship, one marked by "comfort, intimacy, and caring."[31]

In order to appreciate how striking this approach looked, it is important to understand how transsexuals were regarded by most other professionals of the day. Psychiatrists in particular saw transsexuals as mentally ill, and often as irritating and hostile. In medical literature, transsexuals were frequently described in very deprecatory terms. In clinical practice, doctors who were accustomed to being addressed with deference were put off by the urgency with which many transsexuals demanded treatments that strained the limits of conventional medicine. They perceived transgender individuals to be angry and impatient and often found their insistence annoying. Even Benjamin had qualms about some of his patients, writing in one 1969 publication about the "selfishness, unreliability and questionable ethical concepts" he had encountered with some of the transsexuals he had worked with.[32] Additionally, even the few doctors who worked regularly with transsexuals could be condescending and antagonistic. One spoke of them as "a real pain in the neck." Robert Stoller described some

transsexuals as "dissatisfied" and "exhibitionistic and unreliable"; Elmer Belt
referred to some of his patients as "queers" and "nuts."[33] Those transsexuals
who found the courage to make their way to Belt's clinic often felt treated in a
condescending and rude manner by his staff; one found her confidential records
laid out on the business manager's desk like "a best seller." At other institutions,
transsexual patients were made to feel like exotic specimens. At one hospital,
staff from many other departments lined up to have a look at one patient as he
arrived for his hysterectomy.[34]

Pauly realized that many of his contemporaries thought that giving hormones to patients and helping them transition to the other sex was unethical.
Moreover, any physician willing to treat these patients was considered by many
to be "equally crazy." It became apparent to him that Benjamin was just about the
only physician around who felt comfortable doing this. And it was in the positive
results that he achieved that he found his justification. Pauly gained a great deal
of face-to-face clinical experience over the following six months and found that
the patients uniformly reported being happier after their gender transition. In
1963, Pauly decided to write the first systematic review paper on transsexualism.
He pored over the literature obsessively to collect one hundred case studies and
to statistically correlate the subjects' family history and genetic characteristics.
Benjamin also allowed him to see some of his patients on his own so that he
could collect information for his own case reports. Although the paper was
rejected by the first two journals it was sent to, it was ultimately published in the
Archives of General Psychiatry in 1965. Pauly was delighted when, in the months
following its publication, he found stacks of reprint requests waiting for him
from psychiatrists, surgeons, and endocrinologists from around the world. He
ended up sending out about a thousand copies of his paper and with this one
publication became known in the field. He would go on to be one of the handful
of psychiatrists who supported sex-reassignment surgery.[35]

The patients who underwent sex-reassignment surgery in those days were
truly pioneers, given the rudimentary and experimental state of the surgical
techniques. The surgery and postoperative procedures could be extremely painful. Some patients also wondered at the rough, unsympathetic treatment they
received from Elmer Belt and his son, Bruce Belt, a urologist who practiced
with his father. Transsexual women who underwent genital reconstruction
faced months of painful dilations after surgery to keep their newly constructed
vaginas from closing. Transsexual men sometimes found their newly created

penises failed to take. Grafts shriveled and turned black, infections raged, and ugly scar tissue formed. Patients were sometimes left with painful problems with urination or new parts that did not look or work as they had hoped. Among practitioners themselves, there continued to be considerable disagreement and critiques of the new diagnosis and procedures. Benjamin tried to warn his patients of the limitations of surgery: "Please . . . do not expect either one-hundred per cent success, or one-hundred per cent happiness. There is no such thing," he advised. He urged his patients to take only small, gradual, and carefully considered steps.[36]

In the decade after Everest, the journalist Jan Morris (living as a man) became a distinguished foreign correspondent, covering the trial of American spy plane pilot Francis Gary Powers in Moscow and the execution of Nazi Adolf Eichmann in Israel. Morris had been a firsthand witness to wars, riots, and revolutions. As husband to Elizabeth Tuckniss, Morris would father five children. To friends, Morris had always seemed both disciplined and carefree, at ease in the company of soldiers and adventurers. But this air of cool self-possession had hidden a profound torment, one that had driven Morris to doctor after doctor and even to contemplating suicide.

In 1964, wearied by this daunting struggle, Morris made one more trek, this time to the office of Harry Benjamin in New York. Benjamin's accent reminded Morris of a Viennese psychiatrist from the movies and his appearance seemed that of a "white gnome" who was "white-haired, white-jacketed, white-faced," and too small for his desk.

"Sit down, sit down—tell me all about yourself," Benjamin said.

Morris was disarmed by his warmth.

"You believe yourself to be a woman?" Benjamin probed. "Of course, I perfectly understand. Tell me something about it—take it easy, take it easy—now, tell me, tell me . . ."

For the first time, Morris felt truly understood. In this teeming metropolis, a firm hand appeared at the other end of the rope.

Benjamin identified Morris as a transsexual and explained to Morris's great relief that no true transsexual had ever been "persuaded, bullied, drugged, analyzed, shamed, ridiculed or electrically shocked" into changing his or her conviction that he or she had been born the wrong sex. Benjamin advised

Morris to exercise caution, however, and not to rush into any decision but to try to continue to live as a man. Changing the body must be only a last resort, he insisted.

"Stick it out. Do your best. Try to achieve an equilibrium, that's the best way. Take it easy!"

Morris agreed to try.[37]

━━━━▬▬

For the whole of his career, Benjamin had operated as a private practitioner, pursuing his other interests in his own time, with his own funds. His travel to Europe, attendance at conferences, and speaking to many audiences were all paid out of his own pocket. He admitted to a colleague that he realized only late in life that he might have asked for speaking fees for the many times he was invited to give a talk. He never did. Benjamin lived lavishly when the money was coming in but was not particularly successful in storing up in the years of plenty what he might need for the years of famine.

In 1962, Reed Erickson came into his life. While most of Benjamin's patients had been transsexual women, Erickson was a transsexual man who would become one of the most significant influences on Benjamin and on the nascent study of transsexualism. Erickson, born to a wealthy family that had made its money in lead-smelting, had been assigned female at birth. In the 1950s, Erickson, who was then living as a woman and a lesbian, joined the family business and also started a new company that manufactured stadium seating. In the years after meeting Benjamin, Erickson went on to have a hysterectomy in New York in 1965 and then a mastectomy at Johns Hopkins in 1966. In gratitude to his doctors, Erickson created the Erickson Educational Foundation (EEF) in 1964, funded completely from his own fortune. The EEF sponsored research into "areas where human potential was . . . limited by adverse physical or mental conditions or because of public ignorance or prejudice" in an expansive, counter-cultural model of activism that was strikingly different from later modes that emphasized liberal reform and civil rights.[38] The EEF promoted investigation into many esoteric subjects—hypnosis, lunar cycles, interspecies communication, hallucinogenic mushrooms, and telepathy—but a chief activity was financing research of transsexualism and providing support to transsexuals. The impact made by the foundation was huge. Over the course of the next thirteen years, it spent an estimated $2.4 million. At a time when other funding bodies were rarely willing to sponsor exploration in this field, the EEF paid for clinical research, conferences, and symposia and supported scholarly publications on transsexuality. The foundation funded the publication of pamphlets for public education and worked with journalists to arrange interviews for print, television, and radio. It organized presentations for medical audiences as well as for colleges and churches, and it created a service to refer transsexuals to doctors. The EEF truly helped to transform transsexuality into a medical specialty and gain recognition as an important social issue.[39]

Erickson, an engaging though somewhat eccentric individual, lived a colorful personal life with four marriages, two children, and a pet leopard. He moved between homes in Los Angeles and Mexico, eventually building an opulent custom home called the "Love Joy Palace Ashram" in Mazatlán. A savvy investor, he built a fortune estimated at $40 million from oil found on properties he had acquired in the Baton Rouge area. Erickson thrived on interacting with innovative people and using the power his wealth afforded him to fund their efforts. He wanted to invest in the future of humanity, and he viewed his grants as seed money for projects to build the social conditions that would allow human beings to flourish.

Recognizing that for most transgender people, the hope of changing sex was just a distant dream, Erickson threw the weight of his money into creating the social and professional conditions that would make it possible for others to follow in his footsteps. He felt strongly that progress could best be made by cooperating with doctors who were supportive of transsexuals. He sought to fight ignorance by generating reliable scientific knowledge and then using this knowledge to fight prejudice. He envisioned a world in which transgender people would be able to use their talents, contribute, and live fully.[40]

Benjamin had already been involved in efforts to bring associates together. In 1950, he had participated in a preliminary meeting of fellow sexologists to discuss the founding of a professional society. This attempt initially failed, possibly because of opposition from Alfred Kinsey, who was mistakenly concerned it might rival his own Institute for Sex Research, but in 1957 Benjamin became one of the charter members of the Society for the Scientific Study of Sex, along with Albert Ellis, Henry Guze, and Hans Lehfeldt. He was an enthusiastic proponent of the society, and many of the early meetings of its board of directors were held in his office. As Lehfeldt recalled, this in itself was a courageous act, as sexology had not yet become an accepted part of medicine. This network of sexologists was so small and closely knit that they could easily just pick up the phone to talk to each other.[41]

Through the early 1960s, Benjamin gathered together a loose community of physicians and psychologists who were sympathetic to sex change. This included gynecologist Leo Wollman, with whom he shared his practice, sexologist Robert E. L. Masters, endocrinologist Herbert Kupperman, and psychologists Wardell Pomeroy, Ruth Rae Doorbar, and Henry Guze. In 1964, this association was formalized with the creation of the Harry Benjamin Foundation, thanks to funding by the EEF, which provided a minimum of $1,500 a month for three years. Benjamin began to outline an ambitious program of research. With his patients serving as research subjects, he and his associates completed thorough endocrine, neurological, and psychological evaluations before and after transition, with the goal of not only evaluating the success of their therapies but trying to fathom the genetic, hormonal, or neurophysiological factors that might be responsible for transsexuality. Benjamin remained staunch in his faith that there was an underlying biological cause for cross-gender identities; he began to think that it might have something to do with the hormonal environment before birth, though he had not identified any clear mechanism.

The members of the Harry Benjamin Foundation met regularly in Benjamin's office in New York to discuss their research. Benjamin and his circle were not always taken seriously by academic sexologists. None of them were affiliated with university programs, and Benjamin himself had no advanced training in psychiatry. Some of his cohort pursued interests in counterculture subjects such as psychic phenomena and the use of psychedelic agents. Masters experimented with LSD on transsexuals and determined that none of the individuals they had identified as "true" transsexuals ever changed their minds about their gender identity as a result of an LSD experience. Robert Stoller of the UCLA Gender Identity Clinic thought there was a hint of quackery about Benjamin and worried that he did not always publish in the most reputable journals. He politely declined Benjamin's invitation to sit on his board.[42]

In 1964, Renée Richards (then living as a man) nervously made her way to Benjamin's office. At six feet two inches, lean and athletic, Richards cut a striking figure as befitted a former Yale tennis captain. Richards was a lieutenant commander in the US Navy as well as a prominent eye surgeon with a $75,000 a year practice. Raised "a nice Jewish boy" in New York City, Richards had married a model, fathered a son, wore pinstriped suits, and piloted fast cars and a plane. For eight years, Richards had made weekly visits to one of the top Freudian analysts in New York, lying on a couch enveloped in clouds of cigar smoke but succeeding only in becoming more and more confused. Finally, having had enough, Richards announced she was quitting and going to see Benjamin. Her analyst warned that terrible consequences would ensue.

Nonetheless, Richards found the courage to walk into Benjamin's office at East Sixty-Seventh Street between Park and Madison Avenues and sit uneasily in the waiting room filled with transsexual patients at different stages of transition. Benjamin met Richards with a warm handshake and escorted her to a chair opposite himself. Benjamin, by now small and balding, peered at his patient through thick glasses. At first, Richards thought Benjamin seemed like a regular "old fuss-budget," a typical old-world practitioner in a long white coat, but she soon found her anxiety dissipating.

Benjamin gently probed. "How long have you had this problem?"

"As long as I can remember."

"Yes, that's right, that's what transsexual patients say," Benjamin replied.[43]

Benjamin started treating Richards that day. Richards, a fellow physician, was intrigued by what she thought was the ingenious way Benjamin administered the hormone shot. It was not like anything she had seen a physician do before: Benjamin slapped her at the site of injection so that she felt the slap and not the needle.

A few years later, Benjamin was pressured into giving her up as a patient. According to Richards, the pressure came from her family and others who felt that Benjamin should not be treating a fellow physician. Richards then spent years on what she called a "wild goose chase," traveling to Europe and to Casablanca to seek the help of other experts. In Paris, she sought out the famous transgender entertainers who performed at Le Carrousel. The glamorous Coccinelle and Bambi, who were initially female impersonators and later transitioned to women, served as inspiration to many transgender people in the United States who were looking for role models. Richards had a twenty-minute conversation with Bambi that gave her hope that a surgical solution might be available if she really wanted it. As she roamed the world, she became more and more convinced that there was no one who understood transsexualism as well as Benjamin.[44]

As Virginia Allen recalled, Benjamin's gerontology patients grew increasingly uncomfortable sharing his waiting room with people in various stages of transition. Over time, they left his practice. Benjamin now focused more and more on his transgender patients. As before, Benjamin's involvement in his patients' lives did not end at the office door. He provided counseling, moral support, and very practical help. For two to three months every year, Benjamin had his practice in San Francisco, where he became integrated into circles of transvestite and transsexual social networks. He socialized widely and was an inveterate connector of people, introducing colleagues and clients to each other. Don Lucas, head of the San Francisco Mattachine Society, part of the homophile movement for gay rights, remembered Benjamin taking him to Christine Jorgensen's show and introducing him to her. Benjamin's sense of his role as a physician and a researcher followed very much on the model he had seen exemplified by Hirschfeld decades earlier, in which treatment and study were linked with advocacy and educational, legal, and practical support.

━━━━

Aleshia Brevard was from a small town about forty miles outside of Nashville.[45] She had grown up as a boy during the 1930s in genteel poverty on a sprawling farm. She twirled circles to tunes on the radio with her grandmother's crocheted shawl buttoned around her waist, living in a little world of imagination where she could be Veronica Lake. As Brevard grew up, she became increasingly aware that something was not right and that she wasn't like the other boys. In her early twenties, she arrived in Los Angeles and lived as a femme gay man in velour, oversized shirts, and stovepipe pants. One night, she was taken by her gentlemanly boyfriend to San Francisco to Finocchio's, a nightclub world-famous for its female impersonators. Located in the North Beach area, amid the cafés and bars of the Beat poets, Finocchio's was popular with tourists as well as many Hollywood celebrities. In an era of segregation, it was also notable for its mixed-race audience and for being a mecca for the gay community.

Brevard had never seen a drag show. The master of ceremonies noticed her sitting ringside and pointed her out in his patter, saying, "Ladies and gentlemen, this is one of my star pupils—won't you stand up, darling?" Brevard gingerly rose.

"Isn't she beautiful?" the emcee drawled.

This was the first time Brevard had ever been called "she." It was a moment of profound recognition. In the days that followed, Brevard ran out to rent a velvety outfit from a costume shop and arranged for photos to be taken. She was allowed to audition at the club and, under a hastily given stage name, was shoved onstage as "the long-stemmed American Beauty Rose Lee Shaw." Brevard had no act or any particular talent, so she did her best, dancing and posing to the swoops of her favorite tune. Fortunately, Stormy Lee, Finocchio's resident stripper, took an interest in the young newcomer and persuaded the owner to hire her despite her lack of experience.

"Don't worry, I'll teach her," Stormy told the owner; "she's beautiful, and if you don't hire her, somebody else will, and you'll be very, very sorry."

Stormy was several years older than Brevard and took her under her wing. Stormy had grown up as a very effeminate boy in Annapolis. Her parents had taken her to a doctor who had attempted to treat her with male hormones. It had done nothing but make her hairy. "Oh, poor thing, electrolysis was a nightmare for her!" recalled Brevard. Brevard also wondered whether, if she herself had not come from such a "backwater" in Tennessee, her parents might not have attempted the same with her, and she felt grateful that she had managed to avoid such an experience.

At night, performers had to be careful to remove their makeup and "powder down" before leaving the club. Brevard would wind her long hair up under a sailor's skullcap. Harassment by police or violence from strangers was an ever-present threat. After work, there was no community for transgender people except on the margins of the gay world, in the windowless dives in the Tenderloin district. Just a mile or two from Gertrude Atherton's Pacific Heights, the Tenderloin was a world away, the haunt of sex workers, drug addicts, and merchant seamen. Brevard wrote, "If you are gender imperfect, it is always to your advantage to know who's on your blind side. Keeping one's back against the wall becomes a survival instinct. On the streets, awareness can save your life when violence suddenly erupts around you—or is directed at you."[46] She remembered, "We were so illegal, everything was so underground." Finocchio's was the one place she found complete acceptance. Donning gowns and eyelashes, she could truly be herself. It was in the outside world where she always had to put on an act and where she so desperately tried to avoid being noticed.

Within the community of female impersonators, there was a sharing of knowledge about makeup, costumes, padding, and electrolysis. One night as they were at the bathroom sink taking off their makeup, Brevard saw Stormy pull out a little purple pill and asked what it was.

"Premarin," Stormy explained. "It makes your boobies grow."

Like their Parisian counterparts Coccinelle and Bambi, the Finocchio performers also shared an underground knowledge of hormones.

"Give me one," Brevard asked.

She popped it. The next day, Stormy telephoned Harry Benjamin to make an appointment for her. Brevard prepared for her visit with a great deal of care and then made her way to Benjamin's beautiful office at the Sutter building. She was amazed by its spectacular view of San Francisco Bay from the twenty-second floor. There, Benjamin carefully examined her and was particularly excited to discover that the pattern of growth of her pubic hair had such a feminine appearance. He felt this might be a significant finding for his research. Unfortunately, Brevard had to disillusion him with the admission that she had shaved just for the visit.[47]

As Brevard remembered it, "Harry led me through the maze to my day of deliverance."[48] Benjamin usually asked his transsexual patients to live in their desired gender for a time before making a medical transition, but he exempted Brevard since she had already made such a convincing success of it onstage. As she transitioned, however, Brevard felt less and less content having to wear male clothing in her life outside the club. She was too well known as a professional female impersonator to be able to go out in public as a woman, but she chafed at these limitations, knowing that really living the day-to-day existence of a woman was very different from swanning about in sequined gowns. As she ventured beyond gay bars to dance with merchant mariners in the Streets of Paris club, Benjamin provided her with a letter to carry at all times to explain her medical condition in case of arrest.

Frustrated, she increased her oral doses of Premarin and Provera (progesterone) and doubled her injections of estrogen. The Premarin, as Stormy had promised, soon gave Brevard an impressive cleavage and soft curves. "The physical changes could not happen fast enough for me," Brevard recalled. "Nausea, emotional fluctuations, and hot flashes were minor side effects, considering the physical results. A sore, burgeoning bosom was a wonderful daily reminder of the miraculous changes occurring in my body." Onstage, with her long, shapely legs and voluptuous figure, she was promoted as Marilyn Monroe's double, singing "My Heart Belongs to Daddy." One night, Monroe herself came to catch Brevard's performance, though she slipped out right after the act. For Brevard and many of her colleagues, it was very important to always be in the company of a handsome, attentive man—"like a purse, you must have one hanging on your arm," she said. She had a string of boyfriends, some from high society. In time, she began going out to elegant dinners in makeup and dresses.

Brevard recalled that Benjamin really "went to bat" for her, setting up a meeting with a psychiatrist and a lawyer. He even telephoned her parents back in

Tennessee to explain to them what was happening to their child. But, she said, "even though Dr. Harry Benjamin, the world's leading authority and originator of the term *transsexual*, telephoned them and explained, they still didn't understand."[49] She couldn't blame them, though. She was determined to undergo genital surgery, and when she went to visit the surgeon Elmer Belt, she selected her outfit carefully. She was disappointed to find herself condescended to by the nurse and treated coldly. In contrast, Benjamin took Brevard and two other transsexual patients out to elegant lunches. Through him, she learned to sip the sweet, spicy Dubonnet that was Benjamin's favorite aperitif. Benjamin in his cheerful, if chauvinist, manner, liked to refer to his transsexual women patients as "His Girls" or HGs, as opposed to "Real Girls" or RGs. Of the many professionals working in the field, he was generally regarded as the most sympathetic of the lot, a genial if sometimes somewhat patronizing old-fashioned physician. Zelda Supplee, director of the EEF, thought of him as a "cute little devil."[50]

At the time of her transition, Brevard did not care much for the broader theoretical questions surrounding transsexualism. She just wanted her problem to go away. "I simply wanted my emotional and physical pieces aligned," she said. "As far as I was concerned, scientists could label me any way they wanted. . . . What we needed were not words to identify us but rather the technology to free us." Benjamin told her he suspected that her condition derived from a hormonal problem while she had been in the womb. This suited Brevard. "My misery was not something I'd caused. . . . I was the product of a biological accident, and that could be corrected. Dr. Harry Benjamin was my liberator." Among those in the circle of HGs their chief goals were "womanhood and anonymity," and their greatest hope was that once they had quietly had their surgeries, they could disappear into a "normal" existence. They braved these procedures not really knowing what the long-term physical and psychological consequences might be. "Few of us cared," Brevard later recalled. At the time, there were simply no answers to how such invasive surgery would affect their life spans or what the risks might be. Brevard remembered that the small handful of fellow transsexuals she met were caring, feminine, and nurturing. They all felt proud to be among Benjamin's select few. "We had all taken the same painful journey to reach this point." Later, many would follow in their footsteps, but in 1962, she believed they were quite alone.[51]

Benjamin continued to be connected with many of the leading sexologists of the day. When his old friend Norman Haire visited from England, Harry and Gretchen hosted a party for his sixtieth birthday. Haire suffered a heart attack during his stay in New York and ended up in the hospital, but Haire and Alfred Kinsey had a decided wish to meet each other, so Benjamin took Kinsey to Haire's hospital room, and for half an hour the three were able to converse. Haire would die in 1952, shortly after returning to the UK.[52] Kinsey too died of heart problems in 1956, at the age of sixty-two. He had probably done more than anyone to bring the science of sex to public awareness.

Once settled into what was supposed to have been his quiet "retirement office," Benjamin began writing his first book, *Prostitution and Morality*, which he worked on with sexologist Robert E. L. Masters. Masters did much of the field research (at times posing as a client) while Benjamin provided the clinical heft with his many years of experience and several publications on the subject. Benjamin had long been known as a friend and counselor to many sex workers, and when he had been approached to write this book, he found he could not resist the opportunity to produce a work based on common sense and science rather than on what he saw as the usual "sanctimonious platitudes and prejudices."[53]

Benjamin could see the clear connections between his interest in sex work and transsexualism, as he had come to know a number of transsexuals and transvestites engaged in sex work. The book provided a broad survey of prostitution, including its historical, legal, and social aspects, and explained the experiences and motivations of prostitutes, pimps, customers, and madams. The authors identified several different types of prostitutes, including a "new type," the transsexual who was in the process of transition, whose appearance made it difficult for them to find other work and who had a strong incentive to earn money required for the expensive procedures. Most of these, Benjamin noted, were from a poorer socioeconomic and educational background. Of the 108 female transsexuals he had in his practice in 1963, 44 had surgical transition, and the remainder wished to do so. Of these, about 15 were making their living with sex work while another 15 were labeled "promiscuous and/or part-time prostitutes." He noted that of the 44 who had completed their transitions, about 12 were married and leading happy "normal" lives. Most of the remainder of his patients wished to be married. Benjamin concluded that in almost every case, whether they engaged in sex work or not, these individuals, some of whom he had followed for up to twelve years, were happier and better adjusted in their desired gender.[54]

More generally, Benjamin and Masters argued that prostitution rendered a service to society and was not in itself degrading or immoral. Interestingly, Benjamin conceptualized sex work in terms of fantasy: "Prostitution thrives on man's capacity for imagination," he posited, and the prostitute who was able to "create the illusion of an ideal sex partner" had really done something for a man's mental health, no matter how fleeting that illusion might be.[55] Prostitution was, however, useful rather than desirable, the authors concluded. They believed that regulation of prostitution and treating it in a rational and positive way would reduce the harm associated with it, but they urged women who had any other options to get out of prostitution. Benjamin and Masters were not particularly optimistic that their ideas would be well received but trusted that time and reason stood on their side. Their vision of an ideal future was one that allowed free, loving, sexual relationships for women and men, married or unmarried, and they argued, "The struggle to achieve that idea must never be abandoned."[56]

The work on the book was demanding. When Virginia Allen became frazzled with the endless retyping of drafts and at one point complained that she could not continue, Benjamin joked (in a comment that reflects much about the gender dynamics of their relationship as well as Benjamin's own complicated feelings about women and sex work), "Keep typing, or I'll dedicate this book to you!"[57] The book was published in 1964 and was one of the first medical texts to publicly advocate on behalf of sex workers. Benjamin was now seventy-nine. In the book's introduction, he explained that he had reached the stage of life where he had nothing left to fear. He knew his opinions were widely shared among medical colleagues, but as some had told him themselves, they felt unable to say this openly because of concerns for their jobs or for the sensibilities of their wives and daughters. "Having no job that could be endangered, and no daughters, but a wife of a superior mind, I had no such handicap," Benjamin declared.[58]

For the very same reasons, the time was also right to pull together all that he had learned about transsexualism since he had first met Val Barry a decade and a half before. A lifetime of experience had equipped him with the scientific vision and clinical insight he needed, but it was the fearlessness of age that would give him the courage to tread where so few others were willing to go.

Chapter 11

The Transsexual Phenomenon

In 1966, transgender activist Louise Ergestrasse strode into the office of Elliot Blackstone, the sympathetic liaison for San Francisco's police department with the gay community. She dropped a book on his desk with a triumphant thud and demanded that he do something for "her people." The book was *The Transsexual Phenomenon* by Harry Benjamin.[1]

The Transsexual Phenomenon was the first major text to define transsexualism in clinical terms and to argue for compassionate treatment for transsexuals. It was a landmark work that influenced a generation of transsexuals and the health professionals who worked with them. Benjamin credited the courage of Christine Jorgensen, her willingness to be public with her story, and her brave Danish physicians for the significant change in public awareness of transsexuality. Moreover, Jorgensen's own hard work in trying to understand her experience and her readiness to serve as a conduit for others had created broad sympathy for transsexuals and early sparks of acceptance.

At a dense 286 pages, the book ranged over the entire field of study. A 16-page supplement of photographs was also available upon request but only to medical and psychological professionals. It began with a survey that disentangled transsexuality from homosexuality and transvestism. Benjamin described the "heart-breaking anguish" felt by transsexuals, observing that "there is hardly a person so constantly unhappy" as the transsexual before a sex change. These individuals, he said, were vulnerable to self-mutilation and suicide. Benjamin admitted that the causes of transsexuality were still unknown, though he favored endocrine and genetic explanations rather than psychological ones. He discussed surgical and nonsurgical treatments as well as legal issues. In the appendix, Benjamin presented the most recent of his data from 193 transsexual women and 27 transsexual men. Other appendices were contributed by colleagues. Journalist Gobind Behari Lal wrote on the broader religious and cultural context of ideas about the complementarity of the sexes. UCLA psychiatrist Richard Green wrote on the historical, mythological, and cross-cultural aspects. Robert Masters presented four autobiographical statements and three biographical sketches of transsexuals.[2]

In trying to make sense of the wide variation he saw in his case studies, Benjamin devised as a "working hypothesis" a six-point scale he called the Sexual Orientation Scale, which echoed the Kinsey Scale and before that Magnus Hirschfeld's sexual intermediate types. At one end of the Sexual Orientation Scale was the person who only occasionally cross-dressed, and at the other end was the "true" transsexual who experienced a high-intensity desire to change sex and what Benjamin called "total 'psycho-sexual' inversion." Since it was clear from his own practice that "the mind of the transsexual cannot be adjusted to the body," he argued that, "it is logical and justifiable to attempt the opposite, to adjust the body to the mind."[3] To have believed otherwise would have meant being left with therapeutic nihilism—a conviction that treatment was not possible—a view that Benjamin had rejected all his life.

While the book was primarily about transsexuals, he also addressed the nonsurgical management of transvestites. He noted that most transvestites wanted nothing from the medical profession, preferring to be left alone. Instead of desiring treatment for themselves, they wanted society to be "treated educationally" so that a more tolerant attitude would be fostered.

The response to the book was sudden and tremendous, thanks to prominent articles in the *New York Times* that November. Benjamin wrote to a cousin, "We are drowning in letters and telephone calls. The publicity . . . actually was nationwide and quite unexpected."[4] The book caused what historian Susan Stryker calls a "sea change" in the popular and medical perception of transgenderism in the United States.[5] For Benjamin and his associates, it would prove key to their being taken seriously by academic audiences. Even Robert Stoller, who had hesitated in joining Benjamin's board, now acknowledged that Benjamin had not only "a good heart" but lots of very good clinical data. Stoller agreed to be the first speaker when the Harry Benjamin Foundation organized its first serious scientific meeting in 1967. The proceedings of the meeting were presented as a preliminary report to the New York Academy of Sciences and published in the academy's *Transactions*.[6]

The impact of *The Transsexual Phenomenon* was also felt immediately and powerfully in clinical services. Again, Erickson Educational Foundation funding was key. Within a year, a gender identity clinic was opened at Johns Hopkins University, which was the first university medical center to provide gender-reassignment surgery. In setting up the clinic, the Johns Hopkins team worked closely with the Harry Benjamin Foundation. John Money recalled that, without Benjamin's evidence of successes with hormonal and surgical therapies, the Johns Hopkins program would not have been possible. The opening of the program was a source of great satisfaction for Benjamin as it was a vindication and an institutionalization of his many years of lonely advocacy for a group of patients who had until then been ridiculed or despised by the medical establishment.[7]

Within a short span, several other prestigious academic institutions followed suit, the earliest of them basing their protocols explicitly on the findings of the Johns Hopkins Gender Identity Clinic and the Harry Benjamin Foundation. Organizers sent many visitors to observe Benjamin and his associates. The University of Minnesota Medical School opened its program in 1966, Northwestern University Medical School in 1967, and Stanford University and the University of Washington in 1968. By the end of the 1970s, there were some fifteen to twenty major centers across the United States that conducted sex-reassignment surgery and more than a thousand individuals who were treated at these university-based clinics.[8]

One significant outcome of the emergence of university-based gender-reassignment clinics was that academic physicians and psychologists became the gatekeepers to transsexual treatment. The rules by which they guarded the gates became standardized into medical protocols. The cautious clinical approach that Benjamin and his colleagues had developed patient by patient was codified, with minor local differences, into a Standard of Care that was shared among institutions. In general, individuals seeking transition were required to have a full medical and psychological assessment to screen for mental illness. They were then required to live for a year in their chosen gender before they were allowed to proceed to surgical treatment. Physicians were anxious not to provide treatment on demand to someone who might later come to regret the decision, especially when it involved potentially painful, dangerous, and life-altering surgery. But inevitably, the social and cultural prejudices of the gatekeepers fed into these decisions. Professionals noted that some transsexuals were quiet and calm and had lived with their sense of gender disjunction all their lives. Others were loud, demanding, and flamboyant. Physicians tended to prefer working with the former group, favoring these whom they felt were likely to have a better outcome, by which they usually meant settling down to a quiet, "normal" life.

These early experts believed they needed to define what a "true" transsexual was in order to determine whether an individual should be allowed to undergo medical transition. One norm they applied was heterosexuality. They assumed that, after transition, the individual should be sexually attracted to the other sex, and there was no room in their conception, for example, for someone who had lived and married as a man to still be attracted to her wife after transitioning to become a woman. Another part of their calculus was the likelihood that the person would be able to "pass," that is, to be correctly viewed by observers. For male transsexuals, a growth of beard and lowered voice from hormone treatment typically meant they would be recognized as men by observers. For female transsexuals, those with smaller, delicate features were seen as more likely to succeed in their transition than taller, bulkier individuals. The emphasis was on how the individual would be perceived by others rather than on how they would feel inside.[9]

Benjamin's thought about these issues evolved as he met more transsexuals and wrestled with a reality that was far more complex. When Renée Richards first visited Benjamin, Benjamin performed a detailed physical examination and ordered a battery of biochemical and psychological tests. Psychologist Wardell Pomeroy, Benjamin's colleague, was worried about Richards's psychological profile because Richards did not appear to be attracted to men. That meant that after transition, she would not be likely to succeed as a "normal" heterosexual woman. Benjamin decided he was not concerned about this, as he was beginning to realize that what would come to be called "gender identity" and "sexual orientation" were not always tied in ways that fit heterosexual norms.[10] These medical gatekeepers also soon learned that the networks of transgender people were agile and effective in distributing information. Those seeking reassignment soon arrived with practiced narratives, having learned how to tell physicians what they wanted to hear and omitting those facets of their story that did not comfortably fit the model.[11]

To professionals, *The Transsexual Phenomenon* served to put transsexualism on the agenda of every sexology program. It became the textbook that taught many physicians and therapists their first lessons about the subject. Although Benjamin described a spectrum of gender nonconformity, the clinical approach for the next decades would focus on those who were considered good candidates for "sex reassignment," that is, to transition from man to woman or from woman to man as completely as possible.

Elliot Blackstone, the community relations police officer in San Francisco, read Benjamin's book and soon established social services for transsexuals in the Tenderloin neighborhood, which included legal and financial assistance. Shortly after, a health services program was opened with Dr. Joel Fort as its head, providing hormones, counseling, and referrals. Fort invited Benjamin to train his staff, and in time, both Blackstone and Fort would become Benjamin's friends.[12]

But *The Transsexual Phenomenon* did not influence medical professionals only. With its easy, accessible style and detailed clinical cases, its publication became a pivotal moment for many transgender people who finally saw themselves and their experiences presented in a compassionate manner. Benjamin's book provided a way to frame their experiences and explain themselves to others. Activist groups grew up, some with new voices of protest against medical authority, something they shared with many other groups in the counterculture of the era. The interactions of transsexuals with transvestites, gay liberation groups, and feminist groups were varied. At some points, they found common cause; at others, there were painful and significant differences. Some groups of radical lesbian feminists regarded transsexual women as dangerous interlopers in women-only spaces. Other feminists who were challenging traditional gender roles worried that transsexuals were too attached to traditional ways of being men and women; in a time of unisex dressing and hippie culture, the model of womanhood presented by an older generation of transsexuals like Christine Jorgensen seemed outmoded. A new wave emerged of trans people who embraced feminism and were influenced by Stonewall and gay liberation.[13]

But in transsexual research, who was influencing whom and how proved to be a complex question. More than a decade before, Alfred Kinsey had embarked on a study of transvestites in order to fill in a gap that he had left in his 1948 study of the sexuality of the human male. When Kinsey had studied wasps, he could classify them according to his own rules. But when he applied his careful systematic study to the sexuality of women and men, he found that his subjects talked back. This was undoubtedly true as well for Benjamin in his clinical interactions with his transgender patients.[14]

Philosopher Ian Hacking argues that when theorists in the human sciences create a new category of person, a "human kind," something happens that doesn't when researchers name a new mineral, a species of fish, or a star—a "natural kind"—and it is that human beings have the ability to decide whether or not they belong to this new "kind." This recognition changes their experience of who they are. As people identify themselves as members of this new scientific category, they come to understand the experiences of their lives in light of the availability of this "human kind" and the language used to describe it. This means that in creating a new category, social scientists are actually changing the experience of the people who are classified by it, and the people who are changed, in turn, challenge and affect the way the category is defined. This is a phenomenon Hacking calls a looping effect.[15]

Benjamin drew his idea of a new human kind—the transsexual—much like Magnus Hirschfeld had defined the category "transvestite" half a century before, based on the testimony of people who came to him for treatment or whom he got to know through networks such as that of Louise Lawrence. What was excluded from his data, of course, were the experiences of people who didn't come forward, who didn't seek treatment, who didn't see themselves represented in the examples given in the medical journals or popular books, who were not part of the same networks of like-minded people and perhaps had no connection with urban queer subcultures. The kind of stories that might be missing in Benjamin's account is suggested by the work of historian Emily Skidmore, who has uncovered the lives of individuals who in the late nineteenth and early twentieth centuries were assigned female at birth but lived quiet, unremarkable lives as men, marrying women and being accepted as hardworking, contributing members of their small towns and rural communities. These trans men were neither cosmopolitan nor radical, and their stories became visible to historians only when their anatomical sex was accidentally revealed and reported in local newspapers and medical journals.[16]

Since most Americans would have learned about transsexualism through popular accounts, it is also important to consider the image of transsexuality created in the newspapers and magazines. The popular portrayal of trans-sexualism in the United States during the 1950s and 1960s was dominated by the white, middle-class, hyperfeminine example of Christine Jorgensen. It was a model that emphasized domesticity and respectability and rejected homosexuality and sexual deviance. As Emily Skidmore argues, Jorgensen's claim to the role of a "good transsexual" depended on her distancing herself from other gender-variant individuals such as homosexuals or drag queens. Unlike Jorgensen, trans women who were African American, Latina, or Asian American were more likely to be presented in the press as objects of ridicule or exotic sexual enigmas rather than as individuals who had become "authentic" women.

The present book is similarly circumscribed. In writing it, I have employed only the words of trans people who have openly written or spoken about their lives. That means that the narrative has been limited to those who have been willing to share publicly, who are often highly literate and almost all trans women. As well, it does not include the perspectives of those who did not orient their lives toward a medical diagnosis or treatment or those who perhaps did not relate to the image of transgender portrayed in the media or recognize their own experience in the definitions created by doctors. The stories here tell us how only a small number of trans people experienced their lives in this rapidly changing social environment. Moreover, it leaves out the rich complexity of trans lives beyond the clinical framework. It is far from a complete picture.[17]

In a broader view, it is important to reflect how thoroughly hormones had infiltrated the Western medicine cabinet by the 1960s. Perhaps the best-known example, and the one with the greatest social impact, was the contraceptive pill. "The Pill," which had been dreamed of decades before by birth control reformers like Margaret Sanger, was introduced in 1960. For millions of women, a daily dose of estrogen and progesterone, soon cleverly packaged in a dial-shaped dispenser, meant freedom from worry of pregnancy. Though previous generations had access to various methods of contraception, nothing before had provided the ease and effectiveness of the Pill. For the first time, large numbers of healthy young women were taking hormone products on a daily and ongoing basis. For women on the other side of the childbearing years, hormones came in the form of hormone replacement therapy for the symptoms of menopause. When hormone products such as Premarin and Progynon emerged on the market, they were initially prescribed for the treatment of menstrual disorders and menopausal symptoms such as hot flashes and heavy bleeding, and only for a short span of years. By the 1960s, however, women were encouraged to begin thinking of hormone replacement therapy (HRT) as a means of remaining "feminine forever," which was the title of a popular book by Dr. Robert A. Wilson. Wilson and his wife, Thelma, argued that HRT was not only a tool to combat menopause symptoms during the few years that a woman was undergoing menopause but a lifelong elixir to help retain youthfulness, femininity, and sexual attractiveness. In the 1980s and 1990s, these ideas would extend to promoting HRT in younger and younger women as a preventive of heart disease and osteoporosis. Marketing campaigns were aimed at women as young as thirty-five, with the suggestion that they should take HRT for the rest of their lives. By the end of the twentieth century, Premarin was the top-selling prescription drug in the world, accounting for billions in global sales.[18]

Chemists developed a large array of powerful synthetic hormones while at the same time endocrinologists gained knowledge of the multiplicity of functions played by the hormones in the body. The interactions among the hormones were dauntingly complex. Some hormones triggered cascades of other hormones; others were linked together in sensitive feedback loops. At the same time, American medicine was evolving along with consumer culture, and patients were becoming medical consumers. For many transgender people, hormones offered an accessible, relatively safe, and reversible means of exploring gender. In Louise Lawrence's circle and elsewhere, many took hormones. For some, hormones were a step toward surgical transition; for others, they were sufficient in themselves. From the beginning, Benjamin and other endocrinologists were conscious of the dangers of hormone use, namely the possibility of cancer. Benjamin often warned his patients against self-medicating and advised them to take breaks between doses. The use of hormones by transgender people was just part of a larger social acceptance of hormone use for a broad range of purposes. In the 1940s, testosterone became widely used to treat what was called the "male climacteric," or male menopause. In later decades it became clear that anabolic steroids were also being used to boost athletic performance, beginning with Russian weightlifters in the 1950s and bodybuilders in the 1960s. Hormones became a tool for self-fashioning and they were big business.[19]

During its prime years in the 1960s and 1970s, the EEF made a tremendous impact in turning transsexualism into an area of serious study. The EEF contributed to a wide range of educational and research projects as well as support for transsexual people. It promoted public lectures that introduced transsexualism to medical professionals, clergy, law enforcement officers, and students. The foundation made major contributions to research and practice, including $72,000 to the Johns Hopkins Gender Identity Clinic. It funded numerous publications, from a newsletter and educational pamphlets to major reference works such as Money and Richard Green's *Transsexualism and Sex Reassignment* in 1969 and Money and Anke Ehrhardt's *Man and Woman, Boy and Girl* in 1972.[20]

Between 1964 and 1968, the EEF provided the Harry Benjamin Foundation with over $60,000 in support. The publication of *The Transsexual Phenomenon* and EEF funding of his research gave Benjamin a new prestige. The days of EEF financing were not to last, however. Within a few years, Benjamin and Erickson would squabble over the spending of funds. Benjamin resented paying for items that he felt should have been covered by the EEF, and he disliked what he saw as Erickson's attempts to control how money was used. In early 1967, the stipend from the EEF was reduced from $1,500 to $1,200 a month, and by the fall, when the term of the original grant was over, the EEF backing of the Harry Benjamin Foundation ended. After some additional negotiations, Erickson offered the foundation a small continuing sum of $250 to $300 a month, but Benjamin refused it angrily. With faint echoes of the final days of the failed venture with Casimir Funk and Benjamin Harrow, Benjamin complained to others of Erickson's pettiness and "childish craving" to be in charge. At length, Erickson demanded that Benjamin move out of the comfortable offices that had been paid for by the EEF.[21]

The EEF also laid the foundation for a professional organization for the study of transsexualism by sponsoring the first several international symposia on gender identity. The First International Symposium on Gender Identity took place in London in 1969; the second such conference in Elsinore, Denmark, in 1971; and the third in Dubrovnik, Yugoslavia, in 1973. The fourth, held at Stanford University Medical Center in Palo Alto, California, in 1975, was named for Harry Benjamin in honor of his ninetieth birthday that year. At the fifth meeting in Norfolk, Virginia, in 1977, delegates received the surprising news that the Erickson Educational Foundation was closing. In response to this sudden withdrawal of the support that had been so critical to the development of the field, the conference planning committee immediately scheduled a business meeting to brainstorm about how to deal with the fallout. A decision was taken to found a new professional association, and a committee was created to draw up the articles of incorporation. At the Sixth International Gender Dysphoria Symposium in San Diego in 1979, the formation of the Harry Benjamin International Gender Dysphoria Association was officially approved. It would become the major organization for professionals working with transgender populations. The new association brought together endocrinologists, surgeons, psychiatrists, lawyers, and experts affiliated with the large university-based programs in transgender health.[22]

Erickson lived for many years at his Love Joy Palace in Mazatlán, Mexico, and then in Southern California. Sadly, by the time he died in 1992 at the age of seventy-four, he had become addicted to illegal drugs and was a fugitive from US drug indictments in Mexico. His legacy in promoting the recognition of transsexualism, however, was a lasting one.[23]

In the years after his break with the EEF, Benjamin moved to a succession of smaller and smaller offices. He pondered whether to stay in New York, move to San Francisco, or retire completely and live in Europe, though he admitted, "Gretchen has something to say about it too."[24]

At various junctures, he tried to pull together funding to reform his foundation under various guises, such as the "Harry Benjamin Gender Identity Research Foundation." He attempted to continue his research in tracking the psychological well-being of pre- and postoperative transsexuals to determine how successful and stable they were in their new gender roles. He also hoped to computerize the data he and his associates had obtained from over a thousand patient case histories. One of the most difficult things to do was long-term follow-up. Post-transition, subjects were often only too glad to leave a painful history behind and to quietly move into a new life. Others felt pressured by their physicians to "woodwork"—as in "go back into the woodwork"—and to leave their families and communities behind to start their lives under new identities.

At one point, Benjamin's office was no more than a tiny space he dubbed "the closet." Rather than squeezing into this space, Benjamin tried meeting with his patients in Virginia Allen's living room, only to have his consultations interrupted by Allen's young son and his friends as they arrived home from the Lycée or by the yappings of her poodle.[25] In time, Allen became what a colleague called Benjamin's "office wife," who looked after all the details of his professional life. By the 1970s, Benjamin would say that she had become much more than a secretary and was actually his research associate who also took care of all his correspondence. Benjamin called her "the much admired Virginia" and spoke of his gratitude for her intelligent and efficient help. Allen spent long hours extracting data from the files and tabulating them so that they revealed their hidden patterns. When responding to letters, Allen added her own personal words of comfort, referring the writers to resources and assuring them they were not alone.[26]

In 1969, Benjamin hired a young internist, Charles Ihlenfeld, to look after his New York office while he was away in California. Ihlenfeld, who knew nothing about transsexualism, had been warned against working with Benjamin by a colleague. He became intrigued, however, and found himself staying on after Benjamin returned. In time, Benjamin came to think of Ihlenfeld as his successor and hoped that he would be the one to whom he could pass along his practice.[27]

Psychoanalyst Ethel Spector Person became interested in studying transsexualism and Benjamin. Arriving in his waiting room in the early 1970s, she made note of the wealthy women swathed in jewels, eminent politicians peeking in for their testosterone, and showgirls who upon closer inspection revealed Adam's apples and man-sized feet. She relished the old-world charm with which Benjamin bought her a drink at a fine hotel and lit her cigarette. She described him as "perhaps the last European gentleman." Together, they spoke at length about his childhood, his love of opera, and his secret passions for unattainable women. He quoted Goethe in the original German and then graciously translated for her. Over the years, she recorded numerous interviews with him, and Benjamin eventually asked her to write his biography after his death. As a psychoanalyst, she spent much time speculating about his mentality. She was intrigued that an idea as radical as transsexualism had emerged from someone who appeared, at first meeting, an old-fashioned elderly gentleman. She soon decided that this was not paradoxical at all and that he had always been a medical maverick.[28]

Benjamin also spoke to Person about his essential sense of hopelessness about the human condition. During these years, he suffered from bouts of depression, especially as his body failed him. He told Person that he was glad he and Gretchen had never had children and that it would be one's greatest blessing never to have been born. After a life spent advocating for the marginalized, he now felt he could identify with the deviant condition, having, by reaching extreme old age, attained the status of a freak himself.[29]

In time, Benjamin influenced a new generation of professionals working with transsexuals. To many, a first meeting with Benjamin was a memorable event. Christine Wheeler, a gracious and soft-spoken psychotherapist, was then a graduate student of Wardell Pomeroy. She was taken to meet Benjamin in a crowded Irish pub. There, she felt she had "tumbled down a rabbit hole" of history. Wheeler was enchanted to hear his stories of looking down Caruso's throat and of meeting Freud, Havelock Ellis, Margaret Sanger, and other famous figures. Recalling the early days of Steinach therapy, he told her, "We were looking for the fountain of youth!" She found him elegant and old-world and discovered they had a shared love of opera. They would become close friends, sharing dinners and long conversations. In time she would herself develop a private practice with a specialty in gender disorders and would reflect on how much the direction of individuals' lives can be influenced by the people they meet.[30]

Garrett Oppenheim, a seasoned journalist, wanted to move into transsexual counseling and went to interview Benjamin when Benjamin was eighty-nine. Oppenheim was nervous that he would make a fool of himself with such a revered pioneer in the field, but within minutes, Benjamin put him completely at ease, speaking in a gentle, leisurely way about the subject. Even when asked the most far-out questions, Benjamin would answer patiently and without a hint of sarcasm. Oppenheim remembered, "A kind of magic filled the little office on New York's East Side, and I could actually feel my human insight moving up several levels. When I finally emerged onto the sunny street outside, I just stood there awhile in a state of dazzlement—not from the sun, but from the man I had just touched minds with. And I heard myself saying to myself, 'Boy, you're going to be in this field for a long, long time.'"[31]

John Money was about half Benjamin's age when they first met. For him, Benjamin seemed a living link to the early history of psycho-endocrinology, a reminder that the scholarship of his generation was founded upon the work of those in the early twentieth century.[32]

Charles Ihlenfeld knew that Benjamin was particularly sensitive if anyone should fail to give him sufficient credit and was always careful to properly acknowledge him in any paper. As Ihlenfeld put it, if Benjamin was in agreement with you, he could be magnanimous, but if he disagreed, he could be terrible. But on the whole, Ihlenfeld valued Benjamin as more than a teacher, mentor, or father figure; he was above all someone who taught him how to truly look at a patient as a person with feelings and to never lose sight of the need to take care of the patient rather than just the disease.[33]

As Benjamin grew frailer, he had to turn down more engagements and invitations to speak. "Besides," he said, in declining one invitation to Hamburg, "I am old enough now to be looked at with suspicion by the young generation who do not take too seriously what old people like myself tell them. . . . I may be wrong, but I know with what mixed feelings I myself listened to very old lecturers when I was at your age."[34] But when Benjamin was at one dinner party, guests became alarmed when the eighty-eight-year-old pulled out his flashlight and asked to peer down the throat of a fellow diner who was feeling unwell. Despite the concern of those present that he might be exposing himself to the flu at his advanced age, he remained first and foremost a physician.[35]

Gretchen too became more and more disinclined to socialize, much to Harry's sorrow. For some years, she had a little capuchin monkey for a pet. She was fond of Charles Ihlenfeld and privately revealed to him the sadnesses of her marriage.[36] Still, Harry and Gretchen had a companionable relationship, and he came to love her deeply. Even at ninety-five, he would get out of the car, walk to the other side to open the door for Gretchen, and offer her his arm in a gesture of elegance and tenderness.[37]

Christine Jorgensen said to Christian Hamburger, "Well, Christian, we didn't start the sexual revolution but I suspect we gave it a good kick in the pants!" By the mid-1970s, when the characters in the *Rocky Horror Picture Show* were singing about "a sweet transvestite from Transsexual, Transylvania,"[38] two of the most well-known transsexuals in the public imagination were Renée Richards and Jan Morris. Richards had returned to Benjamin's office in 1974 after more than ten years of fruitless searching for a solution to her predicament. Benjamin had almost retired by then and Ihlenfeld had taken over the practice. Ihlenfeld said, "Renée, you've had enough of a runaround, it's time for you to get the treatment that you need."[39] Richards underwent sex-reassignment surgery in New York in 1974. Two years later, she entered the world of professional sport, breaking into women's tennis as the first transsexual to be allowed to play. Backed by Billie Jean King and others, she took on the Tennis Association for the right to compete as a woman.

Jan Morris also went to Casablanca for surgery with the surgeon Georges Burou, who for many years was one of the few willing to operate on transsexuals. Ever an eloquent observer, Morris wrote an autobiographical account of her transition in *Conundrum* (1974). She recalled her early sense of conflict. Reading the story of Lili Elbe had given her hope, although Morris didn't recognize herself in Elbe's description of feeling like two people, both male and female. Morris had always felt like one person but "clad in an alien form."[40] Morris also worried that the artist in Elbe had never painted again after transitioning. What if changing sex affected her personality and talents?

Of Benjamin she recalled, "It was Dr. Benjamin who first called us transsexuals, and to him more than anyone we owe the unveiling of our predicament." He had an immediate grasp of her urgent desire to change sex. To change the body was what she had long prayed for, "yet to hear it actually suggested, by a man in a white coat in a medical office, seemed to me like a miracle."[41]

Morris tried to follow Benjamin's advice to live as a man for a time, especially avoiding hormones while trying to father children with Elizabeth Tuckniss. In time, Benjamin prescribed Premarin, supplemented by synthetic estrogen. Over the course of eight years, Morris would take an estimated 12,000 estrogen pills. The hormones caused a slow stripping away of masculine traits—rough skin, hair, and muscle, as well as a sense of resilience. A feeling of vulnerability emerged. And like Lili Elbe, Morris also experienced the changes as a sort of rejuvenation: "It was not merely a matter of *seeming* younger; except in the matter of plain chronology, it was actually true. I was enjoying that dream of the ages, a second youth. My skin was clearer, my cheeks were rosier, my tread was lighter, my figure was slimmer. . . . Life and the world looked new to me."[42]

In the process of transitioning, Morris experienced a new state of being as "a chimera, half male, half female, an object of wonder" even to herself.[43] And after her final surgery and having achieved her long-sought dream of changing sex, Morris could also look back with fondness at having experienced life in the body of a young man, with a body that did not sag or flag, saying, "The male body . . . when it is working properly . . . is a marvelous thing to inhabit." For sheer exuberance, she thought the best day of her life had probably been the final one she had spent on Everest, after having survived the descent with Michael Westmacott and delivered the critical news story: "How brilliant I felt, as with a couple of Sherpa porters I bounded down the glacial moraine towards the green below! I was brilliant with the success of my friends on the mountain, I was brilliant with my knowledge of the event, brilliant with muscular tautness. . . . I laughed and sang all the way down the glacier."[44]

Benjamin's work had always involved a dialectic tension between the messy, imperfect reality of medical practice and the media representations of the results in the lives of his gerontology and transsexual patients. While he tried to be frank about the limitations of his treatments, the media images were what drove new patients to his door and shaped their expectations.[45] The popular fascination with transsexual life stories was about the idea of transformation from one form to another, the seeming magic of changing completely and convincingly from man to woman or from woman to man. But perhaps, like those rejuvenated before them, part of the fascination was not so much about changing from one to another but the possibility of being both—that is, to be a woman who understands what it is to be a man, just as the rejuvenation stories tantalized with the idea of a new category of human being possessing the wisdom of age as well as the vigor of youth. In a 1967 *Esquire* article called "The Transsexual Operation," one transsexual woman described her experience like this: "I'm not anything different since my, uh, operation. I think the same, do everything the same. Except now I can see through people. I can tell at a look or a glance what's going on when I come into a room. I know what the men are thinking and I know what the women are thinking."[46]

The author of the article, Tom Buckley, interviewed many of the key experts in the field of transsexualism. He grappled with the play of image and substance in the lives of the transsexual women he met, whether secretary, bar girl, or pearl-draped matron, young or middle-aged, beautiful or plain. He called them "the great masqueraders of the world," living in the shadowland where "illusion and reality, identity and anonymity, death and rebirth, mingle and diffuse." Buckley interviewed Benjamin over several months, and his admiration never wavered. He presented a sympathetic portrait of the man he described as a "friend, defender, and medical consultant" for transsexuals. Buckley thought highly of Benjamin's rare sophistication, continental charm, sharp wardrobe, and good taste in food and wines, not to mention his life in New York and San Francisco with his vivacious blond wife. Buckley reported that Benjamin even treated many transsexuals without charge. Still "hale" and "rosy-cheeked" at eighty-two, Benjamin spoke to the reporter one afternoon while gazing at the Golden Gate Bridge from the penthouse bar, the Top of the Mark. Benjamin told him, "To me it is just a matter of relieving human suffering the best way we can."[47]

In the late 1960s and early 1970s, Benjamin made long visits to Europe again. His brother, Walter, had returned to Berlin, and his sister, Edith, had moved to Lugano, Switzerland. In 1970, West Berlin seemed to him to have become "a magnificent city," and he was very gratified to speak there at the Free University as well as at the University of Hamburg. He visited doctors and heard many great operas. Harry's relationship with Edith had been close and warm, but his letters to her are often full of irritation about Walter, and on the whole, Harry seemed glad to keep his time with Walter to a minimum. Walter had married, divorced, and remarried. Edith was now widowed. Like Harry, neither Edith nor Walter had children. In 1972, Harry, Walter, and Edith visited their father's grave in Berlin. After almost sixty years, the stone was now weathered, and there was only a faint trace of the beloved name carved there. It felt then that their papa was finally truly leaving them, and there were tears among the siblings as they parted.[48]

Harry and Gretchen had now been married almost fifty years. He had dedicated *The Transsexual Phenomenon* to her, his "companion through life" and his inspiration. He was grateful for her "insight, patience, and unfailing devotion" and acknowledged that the long hours he had spent writing the book had rightly belonged to her.[49] The two of them often spent long months apart, but when they were away from each other, he missed her. In Italy, he visited the tombs of Michelangelo, Rossini, and Galileo. He wrote to her, "If only you had been with me. Only ½ of me enjoyed the trip. The other half is you and you were not there."[50] On another trip, he wrote, "It is quite a wonderful life in Berlin." He told her that he and Edith had attended the opera—*The Flying Dutchman*—but the empty seat beside them was for his "Urm." "I do miss you *so much*. I am talking to you (perhaps also in my sleep?) ... love & love, Dien Hase (and teammate)."[51]

Benjamin remained reasonably healthy and fairly active until he was ninety. In 1975, fifty friends gathered to celebrate his birthday with a gala dinner at the Princeton Club. By happy coincidence, the Club was on the site of the old Academy of Medicine, where Benjamin had presented his first paper on Eugen Steinach in 1921. Among the guests was Abigail Van Buren, the advice columnist of "Dear Abby" fame, who had become a friend. Van Buren had written sympathetically about people and families dealing with gender dysphoria.[52]

Tom Buckley, who had written about him for *Esquire* in 1967, now interviewed him for the *New York Times*, tracing his "maverick" career. Visiting him at what Buckley described as "his modest apartment on East 31st Street," Buckley reflected that Benjamin must have been one of the last New Yorkers to receive visitors dressed in a silk smoking jacket. When he asked Benjamin the secret to long life, Benjamin conceded that the most important factor was simply the good fortune to have had long-lived parents. "The second is sensible living and having useful work to do," Benjamin said, "but at least I don't think my treatments, which I have been giving myself for the past 20 years, have done me any harm."[53]

That year, Benjamin traveled to California once more to attend the Fourth International Conference on Gender Identity in Palo Alto, which was named in his honor. While there, he took Ihlenfeld on a walking tour of his favorite sights of San Francisco. Ihlenfeld—aged thirty-seven, though admittedly tired and running a fever—was barely able to keep up with his sprightly elder. But 1975 was the beginning of the end. That year, Benjamin developed shingles of the face and was hospitalized with mild encephalitis. Early that summer, he returned to New York, never to see San Francisco again.[54]

Benjamin told Ethel Person that there were three men he revered above all others: Goethe, whose visage had long watched over his practice; Churchill, "the savior of our civilization"; and Verdi, at whose grave he left a rose (he explained, "No one has given me more pleasure").[55] Giuseppe Verdi wrote *Falstaff*, the last of his twenty-eight operas, when he was almost eighty. After a lifetime of relentlessly killing off his tragic heroines and heroes, Verdi gave his audience a comic opera rippling with joy. Winston Churchill, at the age of sixty-five, returned from years of political exile to lead his nation through the darkest hours of World War II. Goethe wrote his masterwork *Faust* in two parts. In part one, written when he was in his fifties, Mephistopheles arrives in the form of a poodle to lure the scholar Faust into a blood pact. But in part two, written when Goethe was in his eighties, Faust attains salvation. Unlike the Faust of legend, Goethe's Faust does not sell his soul; rather, he wagers that no matter what Mephistopheles offers him, he will never feel satisfied with himself; if he is wrong—if he were to experience a moment of bliss so pure that he would want to stay in it—then he would agree to forfeit his life. At the culmination of the play, Faust loses his bet with Mephistopheles. But Mephistopheles, in always willing the bad, has actually worked the good. By helping Faust to continually aspire to what is higher and better than himself, Faust has gained entrance to Heaven. The angels bear him upward, saying,

Whoever strives in ceaseless toil,
Him we may grant redemption.[56]

In 1974, Walter C. Alvarez, a medical columnist and Mayo Clinic specialist, wrote to Benjamin recalling the day many years before when Alvarez had first walked into his office. Alvarez had then made a point of seeking out physicians doing outstanding work and, as a result of that visit, had made a stimulating, lifelong friend. He would often quote Benjamin in his column in relation to healthy aging and called him "an outstanding student of sex and sex problems."[57] Now close to ninety himself, Alvarez told Benjamin, "I can say that your life, and your great kindness to the unhappy transsexuals, has given me comfort and great stimulus." He continued, "A few minutes ago I was writing a newspaper column on transsexuals and told how for years you were their only friend." Alvarez concluded, "You have lived a very good life."[58]

Chapter 12

Winter of Our Discontent

The years like great black oxen tread the world,
And God the herdsman goads them on behind,
And I am broken by their passing feet.
—William Butler Yeats

The striking redhead gazed into eyes, once twinkling, now clouded over with age. A noted ophthalmologic surgeon, she asked her patient, "Dr. Benjamin, would you like me to take the cataract out of your other eye?"

"Renée," he answered, waving aside her suggestion, "I'm going to be dead in six months."

At ninety-eight years old and nearly blind, Benjamin now found that he and his famous patient had reversed their roles. Renée Richards had returned to ophthalmology after her retirement from the world of professional tennis, and now it was her turn to play physician to the man who had helped her through her transition so many years before.[1]

Two years later, her patient was still very much alive, and she was pleased to remind him of their exchange.

"Dr. Benjamin, you know when you were ninety-eight, you said to me you were only going to live for six more months."

"Did I say that?" Benjamin wondered.[2]

I imagine he would have enjoyed that joke. Benjamin reached an advanced age, respected, beloved, and with his inherent graciousness and humor intact. As he neared one hundred, he took to telling people that the first thing he planned to do when he woke up the morning of his birthday would be to look in the mirror.

"And why is that?" his friends would ask.

His impish reply: "Because I've never seen a 100-year-old man before!"[3]

And yet the years, inexorable in their passage, claimed life's pleasures one by one, so that he often fell to despondency. "Old age often seems to me the punishment for youth," he lamented.[4] As his eyesight faded, he and Gretchen turned to books on tape or had someone read to them. When it became impossible to attend live performances, they tuned into the Saturday afternoon radio broadcast of the Metropolitan Opera, which they found a true blessing. He grumbled only about the Italian operas sung in English, saying, "This to my mind is irreverent toward the composer, illogical because nobody understands enough anyhow to follow the plot and to me personally, painful."[5] Eventually, even his hearing faded, and this must have been a particularly bitter loss. He was resigned, however, to the commonsense philosophy "to want and accept what you can have, and make the best of what you cannot have."[6] Soon, he could no longer cross a room without a cane and was always fearful of falling. He gave up social engagements and ventured out only once a month or so to visit the barber or see a doctor.

"Getting old is no fun," he told his brother, "and we all have to try to live with the 'no fun.'"[7] Walter died in Berlin at the age of ninety-three. Edith died several years later, also in her nineties.

Emily Leider, Gertrude Atherton's biographer, interviewed Benjamin when he was ninety-six. She was reminded of Tennyson's Tithonus, who was granted his wish for immortality but had tragically forgotten to ask for eternal youth to go with it. He was now tired and contemplative. When she asked him about his views on rejuvenation, he declined to answer, saying only that he thought the most important factor in a long, productive life was heredity. He was somewhat ironic and amused in recalling Atherton's vanity but on the whole affectionate and admiring of her vigor and intelligence.[8]

But even as his body fell to ruin, Benjamin continued to inspire new workers in the field with his mind and spirit. Visitors still arrived at Harry and Gretchen's apartment on Thirty-First Street. It was a cramped, drab space that Christine Wheeler likened to a tenement, but Gretchen now had so much difficulty dealing with change that Harry had to wait until she was in the hospital for a short stay before he could bring in painters for a much-needed fresh coat. Yet the humble quarters glowed with lively conversations and true feeling. Garrett Oppenheim remembered the real pleasure he felt "basking in the warm wisdom of this man who was born before electric lights or automobiles began changing the face of the earth." During their visits, Oppenheim's wife, Fae, would sit with Gretchen across the room while Garrett relaxed in a seat close to Harry, so that in that living room, "two deeply human conversations" ran "like parallel streams in an enchanted forest."[9]

Mercifully, Benjamin's mind remained sharp, and he took great pleasure in following the progress of his younger colleagues. John Money recalled, "Not a single brain cell was missing!"[10] His memory was intact, and his agile intellect continued to assimilate new ideas as well as ever. Charles Ihlenfeld found that his friendship with Benjamin helped to inspire and inform his work with elderly patients in his psychiatric practice. "It's one thing to read in textbooks that senility is *not* a part of normal aging. It was quite another experience to speak with Harry week after week and to realize that there was not one senile synapse in that marvelous head of his. . . . He didn't miss a trick!"[11]

Harry and Gretchen's circle of friends became like family to them. When Benjamin befriended a person, it was a vigorous, active kind of friendship. He faithfully collected scientific articles that he thought might be useful to his friends and saved them for their next visits. He continually generated good ideas, helpful introductions, and suggestions of new avenues they might pursue. And as visitors arrived, they would invariably be greeted warmly not with the usual bland pleasantries but with pertinent and meaningful questions about their health and current projects. No letter went unanswered; no favor, however trivial, was left unacknowledged; and when his friends were ill, they would always receive his kindly telephone call asking how they fared. These were courtesies that he did not delegate until his very final days. And even when it became painfully difficult for him to get out of his chair, he never failed to rise to greet his guests nor to walk them to the door when it came time for them to go home.[12]

Leah Cahan Schaefer and Christine Wheeler, younger colleagues and psychotherapists, inherited Benjamin's medical files and took on the mammoth task of reviewing his 1,500 cases. Visiting regularly over several years, they enjoyed spoiling Harry and Gretchen with treats, feeling a bit like Little Red Riding Hoods. Their baskets were filled with caviar, smoked oysters, sardines, cheeses, and meats. In summer, fresh raspberries and sweet cream were a special favorite. Yet, as Benjamin aged, he became less able to appreciate the subtle scents and flavors. Wheeler and Schaefer struggled to find mustards, vinegars, and other items with stronger flavors with which to tempt him. Gretchen would examine the parcel and delightedly inform Harry of the delicacies they would be enjoying for dinner that evening. Then she would retire to her crossword puzzles on the couch while Schaefer and Wheeler pulled up seats around a little card table set in front of Benjamin's favorite armchair to tell him about their new research. At times, he was amazed at their findings.

"Somehow that makes a lot of sense," he would say. "I must have known that but we just never had the staff, nor the money, nor the time to do adequate research."[13]

He came to understand how important his files would be to ongoing research. Knowing that he would not be able to attend their presentations, Schaefer and Wheeler would deliver the papers for him in his small living room with full drama, speaking as if they were at a podium. Over the years, Benjamin remained convinced that surgical reassignment was appropriate yet believed it had to be used carefully and critically. He also felt that there were some cases in which it should not be done, having seen instances where surgery had been regretted, sometimes many years later. Many transsexuals, he thought, managed well with hormones and psychotherapy alone, without surgical intervention, as long as they were allowed to live in their desired gender.[14] In 1983, Schaefer and Wheeler elaborated on Benjamin's Type IV Transsexual in an important paper that clarified the experiences of those who chose to live full-time in the chosen gender but not to have surgery. In these later years, Benjamin sometimes worried that the world was forgetting him and that his work on transsexualism would be lost. But as he heard these colleagues speak about their findings, his face lit up, knowing that the work he had begun decades earlier was being continued.[15]

In the late 1970s, the Harry Benjamin International Gender Dysphoria Association drew together the results of a decade of research to formalize the Standards of Care that became the treatment protocols for transgender patients. These standards included the requirement that the individual have a psychological evaluation and live for a period in the desired gender. The Standards of Care also included diagnostic criteria for gender identity disorder. The label of gender identity disorder became a controversial issue within the transgender community: most individuals resented having their experience referred to as a sickness or disorder, though others felt relieved to think of their condition as a medical problem that could be treated. While transgender people in the United States could then gain access to medical treatment only by submitting to the protocols, they were also in a frustrating double-bind as treatments were considered to be elective or cosmetic and thus not covered under health plans.[16] By 1980, the treatment of transgender people had become routinized. A number of the university-based programs closed or spun off to private clinics, while the protocols for managing transgender health were left to psychotherapists in private practice. As well, the success of the gay liberation movement made it impossible for the psychiatric profession to continue to label homosexuality a mental illness. In the 1980s, however, some of the liberal advances of the 1960s and 1970s seemed to be rolled back. The clinic at Johns Hopkins closed in 1979 in a cloud of controversy, and the repudiation of this program caused Benjamin great sorrow.[17]

A growing critique of the medical gatekeepers came from many directions. Psychoanalysts, who were in ascendance, continued to view reassignment surgery as feeding a delusion. Criticism also came from feminists who challenged the authority of medical professionals to define gender. Feminists were particularly critical of the gender identity clinic at UCLA, where in some periods members of its staff had interpreted the new scientific knowledge of flexible gender to suggest the possibility that transsexualism might be prevented; they had attempted early gender training of children, for example teaching effeminate boys to act in a more masculine fashion.

Benjamin's commitment to biological causation remained constant, though in later years he recognized that the mechanisms involved were much more complex. He admitted that things had changed a lot since the days in which hormones had been thought to be at the root of everything. Wheeler reflected that Benjamin's strong ties with history were both his strength and his weakness. His loyalties to the intellectual views that had shaped him in his formative years remained firm, as his loyalties—both intellectual and personal—had typically been. But these allegiances may have made him less open to the importance of psychological factors and free choice in the shaping of one's destiny.[18]

Benjamin had hopes that Charles Ihlenfeld would take over his practice. Ihlenfeld married his wife just two weeks after he first met Benjamin in 1969 (April Fool's Day, as they would always remember). As he was drawn into Benjamin's practice, Ihlenfeld found himself deeply affected by the courage and the stories of their transsexual patients. This helped him to clarify his understanding of his own sexual identity. When he came out as gay to Benjamin a few years later, Benjamin was supportive. But when later still he announced that he had decided to enter psychiatry, Benjamin was less positive. Benjamin, a lifelong skeptic about psychiatry, was particularly hurt when a newspaper article came out in which Ihlenfeld was quoted as saying that he was uncertain about the helpfulness of surgical sex reassignment and that he had decided not to treat transsexuals any longer. Benjamin felt this as a great blow. Ihlenfeld tried to explain that his remarks had been taken out of context. His point had been that transgender people often had psychological issues that did not disappear after a gender transition. These issues were understandable after a life that might have included violence and trauma, as well as the pain of being raised a gender different from the one they experienced themselves to be. As it turned out, Ihlenfeld did continue to treat transsexual patients throughout his psychiatric practice. Ihlenfeld felt that he and Benjamin managed to come to a reconciliation, and he remained a stalwart friend through Benjamin's final years.[19]

A continuing difficulty was the challenge in following up cases long-term. Postoperative life did not always turn out as transsexuals had hoped. Personal relationships were damaged; physical and sexual well-being were affected. Renée Richards would write two memoirs and be the subject of a feature film.[20] She would say that, while she didn't regret her transition, she regretted the impact that becoming a public figure had taken on her family and personal relationships. At the same time, data began to suggest that the clinical approach taken by Benjamin and his associates was largely correct and highly effective. Studies showed that patients who had transitioned very rarely regretted their decision, and the large majority were satisfied.[21]

Living to this age gave Benjamin ample opportunity to reflect. When he turned one hundred in 1985, he was feted by colleagues and friends again at the Princeton Club, this time at an afternoon reception so that it would be less strenuous for him. Months later, Ihlenfeld accompanied him to a meeting of the New York County Medical Society, where Benjamin, who had spent much of his career in the border fields of organized medicine, received a citation for his lifetime of service to his patients and his profession. In honor of his birthday, he was interviewed by the sexologist and historian Erwin Haeberle for an article in the journal *Sexualmedizin*. Benjamin was able to summon up memories of meeting and working with some of the most significant figures in twentieth-century sexology, from Eugen Steinach, Magnus Hirschfeld, and Sigmund Freud to

Havelock Ellis and Norman Haire. He could reflect on his experience with the Steinach operation and the fact that even Freud had felt his vitality had been improved and his cancerous jaw favorably influenced. Now six decades later, he acknowledged, "Today we know, of course, that these impressions were based, in part, on autosuggestion."[22]

Benjamin marveled at the changes that had occurred since his youth, when syphilis had been incurable and contraception unreliable, when views and laws against homosexuality and prostitution had been so much harsher, and when the idea of sex for pleasure rather than for reproduction, even within marriage, had seemed scandalous. Sexology had grown in sophistication, such as in the scientific distinction of types, like transvestites and transsexuals, which had greatly helped these individuals gain social acceptance. In his younger years, he had been inspired by a utopian vision of creating a freer and more humane world through science, hormones, and good sense. Now at the end of life, he felt that he had learned that "the individual can indeed make a difference" and that "a few people, through courage and hard work, have lessened the suffering of many."[23]

As Benjamin flagged, devoted friends cheered him on. When he spoke of being tired of living, his friend Joel Fort in San Francisco made him promise to stay alive until he next had a chance to visit New York. Benjamin laughingly agreed to do so. Schaefer and Wheeler teased him: "I bet you wished your mind was less sharp, then you wouldn't really know how your body was failing you!" and Benjamin would chuckle, acknowledging that was true. He was not afraid of death and spoke of it often. Ihlenfeld recalled that "he was very much alive to the end." But Wheeler also remembered existence grew increasingly difficult for him and that he became chronically depressed. His intellect remained active, containing a century's worth of knowledge, but he found his body could no longer respond to the life of his mind.[24]

As he reached 101, he told friends he knew he would not live out the summer. He was concerned only about Gretchen's welfare after he was gone and set about tidying up his paperwork. While weak and suffering from angina, he was reasonably well and still able to move about the apartment without assistance. In those final months, he was frequently in touch with his dearest friends—Ihlenfeld, Virginia Allen, Schaefer, and Wheeler—seeking their advice on one matter or another. Eventually Wheeler arranged to call him each day at eleven so that he would not have to worry when he could speak with her. Each time Schaefer and

Wheeler visited, they were reluctant to leave, and he was reluctant to let them. They begged him to stay alive until they could visit again because they still had so much to ask him. He kept assuring them that he had told them everything he could remember, but each time they asked a new question, he would proceed to share a gem they had not yet heard. Often the two women rode uptown to their respective offices with tears in their eyes, wondering whether this time would be the last.

When Garrett Oppenheim told him that he was beginning to develop an interest in past-life therapy, Benjamin didn't scoff at him. He was never caustic, no matter how strange his friends' ideas might have seemed to him.

"I won't say you're wrong," Benjamin said, "but I'm surprised that a person of your education would believe in things like reincarnation."

Benjamin felt sure that when we die, we are altogether finished, physically, mentally, and spiritually. Oppenheimer persisted: "Harry, when you cross over, you're going to look around and say, 'Garrett was right.'"

Benjamin winked and answered, "When I do, I'll send you a Special Delivery."[25]

Benjamin didn't want a funeral but agreed to a memorial service. He asked Ihlenfeld to make arrangements with the funeral home down the street. Finally, Benjamin was satisfied that his work was complete. Gretchen was away from home because she had broken her hip and was recuperating in the hospital. On 24 August 1986, a Sunday morning, Benjamin lay down on his bed and welcomed a peaceful death. Ihlenfeld, on holiday at the time, returned to break the news to Gretchen personally. She and Harry had been married sixty years, and she was bereft. Ihlenfeld looked after the cremation and several months later, on 10 January 1987, organized a memorial service at the New York Academy of Medicine. At the three-hour service, Ihlenfeld, Oppenheim, Schaefer, Wheeler, Allen, Hans Lehfeldt, Joel Fort, John Money, Walter Futterweit, and Richard Green spoke or contributed remarks that were read to the assembly. Renée Richards took the liberty of speaking on behalf of all Benjamin's patients in expressing her gratitude, saying she didn't know what her fate would have been without him. She remembered him first and foremost as a consummate physician. Christine Jorgensen, now sixty, was unable to travel from her home. In a quavering voice, she spoke via telephone link about her early days with Benjamin. She called him "a gem" and a "godsend" to her. When she died three years later, it truly marked the end of an era.[26]

Ihlenfeld and a close circle of friends looked after Gretchen, moving her to a smaller apartment and later to a nursing home after she had a fall. When she died in 1993 at the age of ninety, her ashes and Harry's were buried together on Shelter Island, where Ihlenfeld and his partner had made their home and where Gretchen had once visited with her little monkey.[27] Harry's epitaph reads "Pioneering Physician" and Gretchen's, "Wise and Gentle Friend."

Epilogue

In 1976, the year after Benjamin retired from medicine, an American athlete dazzled the world at the Montreal Olympics with five personal bests in the men's decathlon, capturing the gold medal and taking a victory lap wrapped in the Stars and Stripes. In 2015, Caitlyn Jenner stood at the front of an auditorium, swathed in a form-fitting white gown receiving the Arthur Ashe Courage Award as a trans woman. Jenner's very public declaration of her experience and *Time* magazine's declaration of "The Transgender Tipping Point" have been called part of a "trans moment" in American culture. Aided by a regimen of hormones, Jenner appeared on the cover of *Vanity Fair*, transformed like Gertrude Atherton's fictional heroine of almost a century before. She looked stunningly youthful for her sixty-five years. In the racks lining the supermarket checkout, she gives us a Madame Zattiany for the twenty-first century. To cisgender people, it may seem that transgender issues are now everywhere, but we might also recognize this as just another wave of media attention such as the one that greeted Christine Jorgensen more than half a century ago. The glamour-filled images and the stories of miraculous transformation, complete with contrasting before and after photos, are narratives that trans people might rightly view with ambivalence. They hide the reality of more complicated lives and the lives of trans people who are not rich or white or neatly fitting into gendered norms. They present as simple the choices that can be difficult, and as quick and clear those transitions that can be long and complex. They feed a prurient interest in the bodies of trans people, offering the private details of their genitals, surgeries, and medications for public consumption in a way that those of cisgender people never would be. They obscure the very real dangers and obstacles experienced

by trans people on a daily basis. And at times, trans people fear that media attention like this is liable to provoke a backlash.[1]

For many trans people, the events I have described in this book form part of a
complex and painful history in which access to medical treatments required that
they hide important parts of themselves, that they subject themselves to invasive
scrutiny and conform to a medical establishment's definition of what gender
should be like. In the decades since Harry Benjamin's death, this dynamic has
been increasingly challenged. With the rise of a transgender rights movement,
trans people have rejected the conceptualization of trans phenomena as pathological and have refused the medical categories that were used by Benjamin and
his peers. During the 1990s, the term "transgender" began to gain popularity,
becoming a broad category meant to include many varieties of lived experience,
encompassing not only those who had previously been called transvestites and
transsexuals but also a whole new range of ways in which people experience
gender. Some trans people seek medical intervention; others do not. Some
reject the gender binary altogether.[2]

Trans communities have developed a rich body of literature, art, and scholarship. The academic field of trans studies has emerged to explore the experience
of transgender from humanistic and social science perspectives. In previous
decades and still today, trans people have been portrayed in movies as the punch
line to jokes, as the "big reveal" to a crime mystery, and very often as victims.
They have been depicted as if being trans is the defining feature of their character. In recent years, trans writers, filmmakers, and performing artists have begun
to give us a far wider range of ways to understand the experience of trans lives.[3]

In earlier decades sexual and gender minorities did not always find common
cause, but in the 1990s a new political sensibility emerged, leading to the inclu-
sion of transgender people in formerly gay, lesbian, and bisexual organizations;
the use of the term "LGBT+ community" represented a new phase in sexual
and gender identity politics.

To the contemporary transgender community, Harry Benjamin might seem
a somewhat off-putting, old-fashioned figure, surrounded by HGs: "His Girls."
Historian Susan Stryker writes in the *GLBTQ Encyclopedia* that Benjamin was
"justly regarded as the world's most prominent expert on the subject" after
the publication of his book and remembered as "a compassionate if somewhat
paternalistic advocate for his transsexual patients." She adds, though, that most
transgender activists regard the standards of care that bore his name to be "offen-
sively patronizing and pathologizing."[4] What would Benjamin make of today's

rich, confident culture of genderqueer, nonbinary, and gender nonconforming people? Charles Ihlenfeld feels Benjamin would have been very delighted to see his views vindicated.[5] I too suspect that Benjamin would have felt quite at home.

———

Most of the historians who have been interested in Benjamin's work have viewed him through the lens of the contributions he made late in life to transgender medicine. Benjamin's role as a leading proponent of the Steinach operation is usually seen as a rather dubious though colorful episode of his early years. Other historians have been interested in Benjamin's connection to Eugen Steinach, Gertrude Atherton, and rejuvenation, and for them, his later fame as the "Father of Transsexualism" forms a curious coda. My initial intention in writing this book was to focus on Benjamin's glandular rejuvenation work, but I came to realize that the real story lay in exploring the meaningful link between his early fascination with glandular science and the transgender medicine for which he is better known. When one looks more closely at the evolution of Benjamin's medical practice, it is clear that it is a story of continuity rather than disjunction. For Benjamin, the techniques he used in treating his aging patients evolved as science and commerce made new treatments available. And the reasoning he applied in offering treatments to his patients, whether aging or transgender, drew from the same conviction that much suffering had a biological basis and could be helped through the use of hormones along with other therapies.

Writing this book in my role as a historian has been a journey of understanding how the subject that has engaged my interest for years—the history of the science of hormones—forms one part of the complex genealogy of today's discussions of transgender. It has also been a journey of educating myself, a cisgender person, about trans studies and trans lives. Transgender writer and activist Jennifer Finney Boylan says, "If you've met one transgender person, you've met . . . one transgender person."[6] As I have reflected on the transgender people I've known—in work, school, church, and neighborhood—this simple truth resonates. I have known trans people as individuals who care passionately about the environment or who create intricate computer code; as persons of quiet and sure faith and those in the process of figuring it out; as conscientious, imaginative, generous, prickly, dependable, sensible, and wry. And I have come to know that, as trans writer CN Lester puts it, "being trans" is never the most interesting thing about them.[7]

Ethel Spector Person published her book *The Sexual Century* in 1999, making the story of Benjamin its culminating chapter. In it, she revealed the story of his visit with Freud and Freud's suggestion that Benjamin was a latent homosexual. This was a secret that Benjamin had asked her to keep until after his death, just as Freud had asked Benjamin to keep his own story of having undergone the Steinach operation a secret until after his death. Person concluded that Benjamin had been a lifelong medical maverick and that his late-in-life ideas were a logical result of his lifetime of experiences. She felt his commitment to nonconformity had emerged from his early social ostracism and had been stimulated by his encounter with the ideas of Auguste Forel. She argued that this attitude consolidated over the years in his aversion to the conventionality of other doctors who were content with their standard practices and standard fees and in his persistent faith in scientific progress. Moreover, she acknowledged his rejection of any absolute positions, saying that despite a notable loyalty in his convictions, he was "always ready to abandon the entrenched position and move on."[8] Person concluded that the delineation of transsexualism was the result of many strands being brought together: the ideas of sexual liberation, research into hormones, new surgical techniques, the "creative imagination" of Christine Jorgensen, and "the perceptivity, open mindedness and scientific background of Harry Benjamin."[9]

When sexologist and historian Erwin Haeberle interviewed Benjamin on his one hundredth birthday, Benjamin remarked, "As a born Berliner I would, of course, be very happy if I could still see the return of sexology to Berlin. When I remember that this city was once the world center of this science, then it is very sad to see how this proud heritage is now practically forgotten."[10] In the early 1980s, a new generation of scholars and gay activists in Germany began to recover their lost history. A search was begun for the papers and publications of Magnus Hirschfeld, and in time, materials were recovered from private collections, including items that Li Shiu Tong had carried with him to Vancouver. After Li's death in 1993, Hirschfeld's final diaries, artifacts, and death mask were rescued from a dumpster by a neighbor and eventually acquired by Ralf Dose, one of the foremost Hirschfeld scholars. In 1982, as the fiftieth anniversary of the destruction of Hirschfeld's archives approached, a historical society was formed which ultimately led to the creation of the Research Center for the Cultural History of Sexuality in 2012 at Humboldt University in Berlin.[11]

For many years, when Eugen Steinach's name was remembered it was usually for its association with a discredited therapy. More recently, however, historians have recovered his significance as one of the leading physiologists of his day.[12] Paul Kammerer's case was reexamined in Arthur Koestler's popular 1971 book *The Case of the Midwife Toad*, in which Koestler argued that Kammerer's specimen may have been deliberately sabotaged. In more recent studies, scholars have argued that his laboratory results were quite likely to have been genuine.[13] The leading role that the Vivarium had held in theoretical biology was forgotten for decades and the illustrious names of its Jewish scientists obliterated in history books. In the 1990s, historians began to recover this lost history. In 2014, the Austrian Academy of Science held a two-day symposium in celebration of the donation of the Vivarium to the Austrian Imperial Academy of Science by its three founders. This resulted in a volume of essays acknowledging the important legacy and global influence of the institute's scientists.[14] The Vivarium's lasting contribution has been in providing an alternative approach to biological inheritance. The institute had fostered the formation of techniques to precisely measure the effects of the environment on heredity. A century ago, when evolutionary biology was overwhelmingly focused on the gene, this approach was overlooked. Today, it has come to the fore in studies of epigenetic inheritance, evolutionary developmental biology, and niche construction theory.

In the course of our lives, we all undergo transformations over which we often have little control, and perhaps this is part of the fascination that the popular accounts of rejuvenation or gender transition have held. The story that I have told of the history of hormone use in medicine began in 1891 when George Redmayne Murray injected a thyroid extract into his myxedematous patient, "Mrs. S." The 101 years spanned by Benjamin's life saw what had begun as a marvelous pink liquid squeezed through Murray's handkerchief become a multibillion-dollar global industry. Insulin, cortisone, adrenaline, "the Pill," hormone replacement therapy, testosterone, growth hormone, and their synthetic counterparts: commercial hormone products course through our world in medicine, sports, and agriculture, much as the hormones themselves course through our bodies. Endocrinology has become even more powerful as researchers use the tools of molecular biology to clone hormones and their receptors and to study the underlying causes of endocrine disease. Physicians can also use drugs to block hormone production or action (for example, in tamoxifen therapy for breast cancer, which blocks the production of estrogen). Now, as then, the right hormone product in the right situation can mean the difference between life and death, between sickness and health. But now, as then, the hormones also hint at the possibility of transformation. Benjamin saw this potential in 1915 and embraced it in his work with reactivation in the 1920s and 1930s and again with transgender individuals beginning in 1949.

Science is our human attempt to make sense of the natural world. But what questions we choose to ask, how we understand what we observe, and how we decide to use the knowledge that results are all shaped by particular human minds born of particular times, places, and cultures. Hormone molecules speed through the vessels of the body, binding to other molecules, triggering cascades of chemical events. But the layers of meaning we attribute to the phenomena are all our own. The ways in which Benjamin and his contemporaries under-stood these chemical events were all filtered through a screen of their cultural understanding of gender, sexuality, and age. Benjamin's interpretation of trans-sexuality was a product of its time and the collaborative creation of specific minds with specific agendas.

Rejuvenation therapy, like hope, springs eternal. Human growth hormone, which in 1985 was marketed as a tool to help growth-stunted children, has spread to being used as a performance-enhancing agent by bodybuilders and athletes and increasingly, as an anti-aging drug with over $1 billion in sales in the United States alone. Perhaps the question posed in *Black Oxen* by Atherton's character Prince Hohenhauer resonates still: If our medical science gives us the power to shape our bodies, ourselves, and our destinies, what are we going to do with this power? What good will we create in the world?

As a society, we continue to wrestle with the question that Benjamin posed: Does it sometimes make more sense to change society through education than to change the individual? While transgender people have made important strides in gaining civil rights and social acceptance in some parts of the world, even now, their hard-won rights are being threatened in many jurisdictions. Stigma, discrimination, and violence continue to create a chronic stress for many transgender people.

In 2006, the Harry Benjamin International Gender Dysphoria Association changed its name to the World Professional Association for Transgender Health in order to dissociate itself from a pathological view of gender nonconformity.

In 2010, the association issued a statement urging that gender nonconformity not be considered a disease but a matter of diversity. The seventh version of the Standards of Care marked a shift from the earlier six versions (often referred to as the Harry Benjamin Standards of Care), which had often been perceived as barriers to care. A broader spectrum of identities was available, not just the gender binary, and the guidelines for care were more flexible. It accepted that the journey taken by each individual might be very different and that hormones and surgery were just two among many options available to help people achieve a comfort with themselves and their identity.

The dreams, goals, and lived experiences of transgender people are as many and varied as there are transgender people. Perhaps the most valuable prize for individuals is simply the freedom to get on with their lives and, as Reed Erickson hoped, to bring full expression of their selves, talents, and passions to the world. If there is a message that we can take from Benjamin's story, then it might be the fundamental importance of learning to see each other as human beings, even when—perhaps especially when—we find it a challenge to imagine or understand each other's lives.

Aleshia Brevard was interviewed by historian Susan Stryker in 1997.[15] She gave a lively overview of her life and later wrote an autobiography. "The journey is a serious one," she said. "We joke. We sometimes cavort outlandishly. Each transsexual follows his or her own ritualistic path, but finally we all try to desensitize the pain. Ultimately, ours is a journey born of anguish. We make that journey in order to live as we are . . . without having to hide from anyone."[16] It was not that she didn't remember the chill of fear she had felt walking down the street or the bottles thrown out of car windows. But she also fondly remembered Harry Benjamin as a real gentleman who did so much to smooth the way for her and make things as easy as possible. Without his help and that of other key supporters, she felt she would likely have ended up dead. At the same time, she wondered whether she might have been just as happy to live as a woman without having undergone surgery. In the 1960s, she had believed surgery was what she wanted, but in retrospect, she wondered whether it had been not so much her own wish as it had been that of the man with whom she was then deeply in love and whom she would marry. She recalled a time when her friend Stormy's boyfriend literally made her and Stormy hide in a closet while the moving men were bringing their belongings into their new home because he was worried that their appearance might raise doubts about his own sexuality. "We accepted without question that we were . . . an embarrassment."[17]

"I mean that's my whole purpose . . . in talking with you," she told Stryker. "I want to make as much noise as we can so that we can keep any child from ever feeling that again."[18]

Brevard went back to Middle Tennessee State University and completed her bachelor of arts degree. She worked as an actress, including creating the character Tex on the daytime soap opera *One Life to Live*, and taught theater at East Tennessee State University, all while having a tumultuous romantic life often dominated by husbands and boyfriends. Late in life, she came to the happy realization that she didn't need a man to be content. Age brought other revelations as well. "I awoke one morning in my mid-fifties to discover that, overnight, men had stopped turning around in the street to watch me sashay past." With it came a new sense of oneness that she had never experienced before: "As we mature, the genders physically tend to become more akin. Waists are less defined, features tend to blur, and a once-firm chin comes to rest on the chest. Now, as a senior citizen, I sometimes even hear myself, vocally, sounding exactly like my father."[19] These moments make her laugh. Her greatest joys come in the freedom to be herself, without fear that gender might suddenly become an issue in a trip to the market without makeup on or during a casual chat with a passerby at twilight as she waters her roses. "Being accepted, respected, and appreciated was all I ever wanted."[20]

Jennifer Finney Boylan, approaching sixty, suffered a traumatic hearing loss thanks to a lifetime of playing in rock and roll bands and a more recent bout with an insistent smoke detector as she seared a steak in her apartment. Suddenly, fitted with hearing aids and learning to read lips, she dusted off the memory of a friend of her grandmother's whose predicament had once inspired jokes rather than compassion from her: "It wasn't that I didn't understand that she suffered, back when she was old and deaf and I was young and not. It's that whatever she suffered from was something I didn't need to be concerned with. It didn't occur to me that imagining the humanity of people other than myself was my responsibility. And yet the root cause of so much grief is our failure to do just that."[21]

Jan Morris wrote a highly respected trilogy on the history of the British Empire, the first volume as a man, the second in transition, and the third as Jan. She traveled the world from Trieste and Venice to Hong Kong, writing dozens of acclaimed books that featured her fluid prose, keen insight, and deeply personal perspective. In her 1974 book, *Conundrum*, her only work until then to take an autobiographical slant, she too examined her choices and asked what might have been. "Would my conflict have been so bitter if I had been born now, when the gender line is so much less rigid?" she asked. "If society had allowed me to live in the gender I preferred would I have bothered to change sex? Is mine only a transient phenomenon, between the dogmatism of the last century, when men were men and women were ladies, and the eclecticism of the next, when citizens will be free to live in the gender role they prefer? Will people read of our pilgrimage to Casablanca, a hundred years hence, as we might read of the search for the philosopher's stone, or Simeon Stylites on his pillar?"[22]

Her love of Elizabeth Tuckniss remained a constant. When they first met, they enjoyed each other's company so much that Morris rode the bus with Tuckniss when she went to work, just so they could be together a little longer. They survived the death of one of their five children and faced the scrutiny of a critical, sometimes hostile public. They spent months apart and each had their own lovers, but they always sustained a "passionate amity" between them. With Morris's transition in 1972, they were required to divorce but quietly continued to live together in the Welsh village of Llanystumdwy in a stone farmhouse lined with a thousand books. Morris referred to Tuckniss as her "sister-in-law," the only term she could come up with to describe their relationship.

"So there we were," explained Tuckniss. "It did not make any difference to me. We still had our family. We just carried on."[23]

In 2008, when laws changed in the UK allowing civil partnerships for same-sex couples, and fifty-eight years after they had first wed as man and wife, they quietly remarried in a simple private ceremony. Perhaps because she had made her transition half a lifetime before, Morris became exasperated by the continuing questions about transgender matters, saying, "I've never believed it to be quite as important as everyone made it out to be." In *Conundrum*, she wrote, "To me gender is not physical at all, but is altogether insubstantial. It is soul, perhaps, it is talent, it is taste, it is environment, it is how one feels, it is light and shade, it is inner music, it is a spring in one's step or an exchange of glances, it is more truly life and love than any combination of genitals, ovaries and hormones."

Morris was the second-last surviving member of the Everest team. In time, Tuckniss developed dementia. Although what Morris called "extreme old age" proved not to be so fun, especially when she had to give up her beloved travels, she continued to write her elegant, kind, and gently crusty prose until her final days, leaving one volume of essays with her publisher to be issued after her death.[24]

Morris always said wryly that no matter what she accomplished, she expected that her obituary would read "Sex-Change Author Dies." Her story was much with me as I worked on this book. Her dramatic descent of Everest had been the scene with which my earlier drafts had begun. Morris died on 20 November 2020 at the age of ninety-four, as I was completing my final revisions. I smiled with her in spirit as I combed through the reports of her death and found that, in fact, her gender transition rarely featured first in the headlines, especially in better publications. The stories instead gave space to the richness of her life and to her accomplishments in writing and the art of living. Years before, she had a headstone carved. When the time comes, it is to be placed on an island where her ashes will lie beside Tuckniss's. It says in Welsh and English, "Here are two friends, at the end of one life." Theirs is a story of two people who managed to hold on through it all. And it is not so much about what changed but what remained steadfast and true in the face of all the changes.[25]

Acknowledgments

I am grateful to the archivists and institutions who have made my research possible: Liana Hong Zhou and Shawn Wilson at the Kinsey Institute at Indiana University; Arlene Shaner at the New York Academy of Medicine; Amber Dushman at the American Medical Association; Imbritt Wiese and Yong-Mi Rauch at the Haeberle-Hirschfeld Archives of Sexology, Humboldt-Universität zu Berlin; the Bancroft Library, University of California, Berkeley; the Archives and Special Collections of Columbia University Medical Center; the Staatsbibliothek zu Berlin; the Universitätsarchiv Tübingen; the University Archives of the University of Chicago; and Paddy Bradley and Darren Luke of cornishmemory.com for sharing wonderful pictures of Redruth in the opening days of the Great War.

I am especially grateful to Dr. Charles Ihlenfeld and Dr. Christine Wheeler, who graciously shared their memories of their mentor and friend with me. Their special insights served as a guiding light for this entire work.

The Toronto Public Library provided much-needed quiet and space through its excellent Jack Rabinovitch Reading Room Writers' Suite. Marina Endicott, as writer-in-residence at the library, provided sage advice and encouragement at a key moment. Ken McGoogan and classmates at the University of Toronto summer school course on creative nonfiction helped to launch this project. Thanks go to Marc-André DuBord, Eric Boodman, and Gregory Ross for research assistance and to Elisabeth Kissel for transcription services.

Colleagues in two writing groups offered thoughtful critique and gentle nurture of this book through its long gestation: Ursula Devine, Kimberly de Witte, Marianne Fedunkiw, Michelle Harvey, Charles Hayter, Susan Heinrich, Sherri Klassen, Mohammed Mia, and Carla Murphy. Guidance came from James

Bennett, Erwin Haeberle, Bert Hansen, Chris McIntosh, Michael Pettit, and Judy Wearing. Valuable feedback and moral support were appreciated from early readers: Elsa Armstrong, Dana Bortolin, Emma Castelhano, Sheila Cressman, Martha Drake, Luciana Gentili, Colette Harper, Terri Pickering, Leslie Robbins, and Krista Wylie. Susan Olding, my marvelous mentor and coach, offered the perfect blend of encouragement and criticism. I am especially grateful to the peer reviewers for the University of North Carolina Press for their generosity in providing constructive, expert, and incredibly detailed critiques. In the course of its long journey, my project has had the benefit of advice from several editors and reviewers; their contributions have all helped to make this a better book.

Special thanks go to agents extraordinaire Tisse Takagi and Peter Tallack, who shepherded my book through ups and downs. Its successful completion owes much to their intellectual engagement, astute advice, and unfailing support. My warm thanks go to my editor Lucas Church for his careful handling of this project, Julie Bush for her superb copyediting, Lindsay Starr and the design team for the striking cover, and Thomas Bedenbaugh and Valerie Burton for seeing it through to publication.

Finally, this book would not have been possible without the love and support of my family, especially my late mother, Anita Li, my husband, Ernie Hamm, and our children, Clara and David. Thank you for helping me free up the time and intellectual space for this work, for your keen interest and expert advice, for your many challenging questions, and for your steadfast belief that I could—and should—get it done.

Notes

Abbreviations

GAP   Gertrude Franklin Horn Atherton Papers, The Bancroft Library, University of California, Berkeley

HB   Harry Benjamin (in correspondence notes)

HBC Harry Benjamin Collection, Kinsey Institute for Research in Sex, Gender, and Reproduction, Indiana University, Bloomington

HHA Haeberle-Hirschfeld Archives of Sexology, Humboldt University, Berlin

SBC   Eugen Steinach–Harry Benjamin Correspondence, New York Academy of Medicine, New York

UC   Morris Fishbein Papers, Special Collections Research Center, University of Chicago, Chicago

Preface

1. Schaefer and Wheeler, "Harry Benjamin's First Ten Cases"; Meyerowitz, *How Sex Changed*, 47–48, 171.

2. Benjamin, *Transsexual Phenomenon.*

3. The most complete biographical source on Benjamin is the final chapter of Person, *Sexual Century*. See also Matte, "Putting Patients First." Benjamin's career is treated extensively and put into context in Meyerowitz, *How Sex Changed*; and Stryker, *Transgender History*. Specific dimensions of Benjamin's work are examined in Sengoopta, "Tales from the Vienna Labs"; Velocci, "Standards of Care"; Ihlenfeld, "Harry Benjamin and Psychiatrists"; Matte, "Historicizing Liberal American Trans-normativities"; Ekins, "Science, Politics and Clinical Intervention"; Hill, "Dear Doctor Benjamin"; and Reay, "Transsexual Phenomenon."

Chapter 1

1. Harry Benjamin, "The Winter of Our Discontent," typescript, c. 1942, box 23, folders 38, 39, 40, 41, HBC; Kaplan, "Endocrine Interpretation of the Dental Apparatus." See discussion by Kaplan, who reported findings "gathered from the observations and studies pursued by Dr. Joseph Fraenkel and his followers, who are students of constitutional medicine, particularly as applied to therapeutics," 219.

2. Haeberle, "Transatlantic Commuter"; Benjamin, "Winter of Our Discontent," chap. 3, p. 2.

3. "German Soprano with Company at Lyceum," *Pittsburgh Press*, 8 February 1916; passenger manifest, SS *Bergensfjord* sailing from Bergen, Norway, to New York, date unknown, August–9 September 1916. *Passenger and Crew Lists of Vessels Arriving at New York, New York, 1897–1957*. Microfilm Publication T715, 8892 rolls. NAI: 300346. Records of the Immigration and Naturalization Service; National Archives at Washington, DC, online database, Ancestry.com. The Motion Picture Studios Directory of 1919 notes she had a career on stage and screen and that she "rows, swims, dances." *Motion Picture Studios Directory, 1919 and 1921*, 122, online database, Ancestry.com.

4. Benjamin, "Winter of Our Discontent," chap. 3, p. 3.

5. Murray, "Note on the Treatment of Myxoedema."

6. Benjamin, "Winter of Our Discontent," chap. 1, pp. 8–9.

7. Geroulanos and Meyers, *Human Body in the Age of Catastrophe*, 4.

8. Key scholarship in the history of endocrinology includes Sengoopta, *Most Secret Quintessence of Life*; Logan, *Hormones, Heredity, and Race*; Oudshoorn, *Beyond the Natural Body*; Nordlund, *Hormones of Life*; Watkins, *Estrogen Elixir*; Medeiros, *Heightened Expectations*; and Medvei, *History of Endocrinology*.

9. Walsh, "Glands on the Market"; Walsh and Li, "Remembering Insulin."

10. Benjamin, "Winter of Our Discontent," chap. 3, pp. 8–9.

11. Dana, "Correspondence."

12. Kaplan, "Endocrine Interpretation of the Dental Apparatus." Fraenkel lectured on internal secretions but did not publish. Details of what he might have said during these Wednesday meetings are suggested in publications of his followers.

13. Tracy, "George Draper and American Constitutional Medicine."

14. Feder, *Gustav Mahler*; Hilmes, *Malevolent Muse*.

15. Benjamin, "Winter of Our Discontent," chap. 3, pp. 4–7; Dana, "Correspondence."

Chapter 2

1. Harry Julius Benjamin, birth certificate, 12 January 1885, in *Germany, Lutheran Baptisms, Marriages, and Burials, 1518–1921*, online database, Ancestry.com, 2017.

2. Richie, *Faust's Metropolis*, 145; Emmerson, *1913*, 62; Schnurr, "Berlin's Turn of the Century Growing Pains."

3. Julius Benjamin, Taufe (Baptism), 31 July 1847, in *Germany, Lutheran Baptisms, Marriages, and Burials, 1518–1921*, online database, Ancestry.com, 2017.

4. Richie, *Faust's Metropolis*, 243. In 1871, the Jewish population in Berlin was just under 50,000 in a population of 826,000; by 1910, it was 170,000 in a population of over 2 million.

5. Bertha's father is described as *Schlosser* (locksmith) in the birth certificate for Bertha in 1852 and as *Handelsmann* (businessman) in the birth certificate for her sister Johanne, born in 1858. Bertha Caroline Friederike Hoffmann, birth 6 February 1852, baptism 15 February 1852; Johanne Hermine Wilhelmine, birth 31 August 1858, baptism 17 October 1858, in *Germany, Lutheran Baptisms, Marriages, and Burials, 1518–1921*, online database, Ancestry.com, 2017.

6. Walter Julius Benjamin, birth certificate, 30 December 1888; Julius Benjamin, death certificate, 27 November 1913, in *Germany, Lutheran Baptisms, Marriages, and Burials, 1518–1921*, online database, Ancestry.com, 2017; Edith Seelig, born 29 August 1890, petition for citizenship, United States of America, 5 February 1932, New York, US, State and Federal Naturalization Records, 1794–1943, online database, Ancestry.com, 2013.

7. Benjamin, "Winter of Our Discontent," chap. 3, pp. 4–7.

8. Person, *Sexual Century*, 352. Julius was baptized in the Lutheran Church at birth, but in the documents at the time of Harry's birth, Julius's religion was listed as Jewish. At death, he was listed as *Evangelisher* (Protestant, Lutheran).

9. Richie, *Faust's Metropolis*, 242.

10. Ihlenfeld, "Memorial for Harry Benjamin"; Urban, "Buffalo Bill in Florence"; "Wild West in Berlin!"

11. Woessmann, Becker, and Hornung, "Being the Educational World Leader Helped Prussia."

12. Königliches Wilhelms-Gymnasium in Berlin, *Jahresbericht über das Schuljahr Ostern . . . bis Ostern*. See 1886–87, 1887–88.

13. Person, *Sexual Century*, 351; Königliches Wilhelms-Gymnasium in Berlin, *Jahresbericht über das Schuljahr Ostern . . . bis Ostern*, 1895–96, 1899–1900. In an interview with Harry Benjamin in the 1970s, Person reported that about 10 percent of the students were from the wealthiest Jewish families. The Königliches Wilhelms-Gymnasium yearbook for 1895–96 indicates there were about 400 Lutheran and 270 to 280 Jewish students. About 95 percent were local. By 1899–1900, the student population was about half Lutheran and half Jewish, with tiny numbers of Catholics and Dissenters.

14. Ethel Spector Person, "Manuscript Interview Notes, Harry Benjamin Reference Materials and Drafts, 1948–1986," box 33, folder 6, Ethel Spector Person Papers, Archives and Special Collections, Columbia University Health Sciences Library, New York; "Jahres-Bericht über das Dorotheenstädtische Realgymnasium zu Berlin."

15. Person, "Manuscript Interview Notes."

16. Notebook "Postillonlied," undated, box 2, series IIB Diaries, item 5, HBC.

17. Person, *Sexual Century*, 352; Haeberle, "Transatlantic Commuter."

18. Person, *Sexual Century*.

19. Diary "Tagebuch," 1904–6, 6 June 1904, box 2, series IIB Diaries, item 7, HBC.

20. Diary "Tagebuch," 1904–6, 6 June 1904.

21. Diary "Tagebuch," 1904–6, 9 April 1906.

22. Diary "Tagebuch," 1904–6, 12 July 1904.

23. Diary "Tagebuch," 1904–6, 19 July 1904.

24. Cushing, *Life of Sir William Osler*, 215–16.

25. "Jahres-Bericht über das Dorotheenstädtische Realgymnasium zu Berlin."

26. Richie, *Faust's Metropolis*, 206, 232.

27. Benjamin, "Winter of Our Discontent," chap. 1, p. 6.

28. Zabecki, *Germany at War*, 494–95; Benjamin, "Winter of Our Discontent," chap. 1, p. 6.

29. Mazón, *Gender and the Modern Research University*, 80–81.

30. Warner, *Therapeutic Perspective*.

31. Benjamin, "Winter of Our Discontent," chap. 1, p. 7a–b. The dialogue is taken from Benjamin's account written in 1941.

32. Stud. med. aus Berlin, 1909–11, Dr. med. Tübingen (Rigorosum: 12.5.1911, Diplom: 6.4.1912), Bestellsignatur; 258/1102. Vermerk über seine Promotion zum Thema "Anwendung des Antiforminverfahrens für den Tuberkelbazillennachweis," Note: "gut," UAT 125/93, Universitätsarchiv Tübingen; Benjamin, "Anwendung des Antiforminverfahrens."

33. Benjamin, "Winter of Our Discontent," chap. 1, pp. 8–9.

34. Richie, *Faust's Metropolis*, 206.

35. Benjamin, "Winter of Our Discontent," chap. 1, pp. 10–11.

Chapter 3

1. "Has Dr. Friedmann Really Found a Tuberculosis Cure?," *New York Times*, 23 February 1913.

2. "Dr. Friedmann Is Here," *New York Times*, 26 February 1913; "Dr Friedmann Is Here to Try Experiments," *Evening Republican* (Columbus, IN), 26 February 1913.

3. "Call Out the Police to Aid Friedmann," *New York Times*, 20 March 1913; "Dr. Friedmann Mobbed," *Asbury Park Press* (Asbury, NJ), 21 March 1913; "In Desperation Many Kneel at Friedmann Feet," *Evening Review* (East Liverpool, OH), 21 March 1913; "Friedmann Wants Place to Treat Poor," *New York Times*, 21 March 1913; "Warn Dr. Friedmann to Observe the Law," *New York Times*, 4 March 1913; "Dr. Friedmann Postpones Clinic," *New York Tribune*, 2 March 1913; "Sick Seek in Vain for Dr. Friedmann," *New York Times*, 2 March 1913; "Dr. Friedmann Is Here with Reputed Tubercular Cure," *Santa Ana (CA) Register*, 27 February 1913; "Friedmann Ordered to Leave Waldorf," *Brooklyn Daily Eagle*, 5 March 1913; "Sees Danger for Friedmann Cases," *New York Times*, 23 March 1913; "Friedmann Patient Dies in Bellevue," *New York Times*, 25 March 1913; "Forbids Friedmann to Treat in Clinics," *New York Times*, 5 March 1913; *Dr. Friedmann's New Treatment for Tuberculosis. Message from the President of the United States. Transmitting in Response to Senate Resolution of 2 January 1913, a Memorandum of the Secretary of State Submitting a Report by the Consul General at Berlin relative to the Friedmann Cure for Tuberculosis*, 17 January 1913 (Washington: Government Printing Office, 1913); "Translations of Dr. Friedrich Friedmann's Statements," *New York Times*, 11 February 1913.

4. Harry Benjamin, "The Winter of Our Discontent," typescript, c. 1942, box 23, folders 38, 39, 40, 41, chap. 2, pp. 1–2, HBC.

5. Benjamin, "Winter of Our Discontent," chap. 2, p. 3.

6. "Refuses Offer of a Million," *Pittsburgh Press*, 26 February 1913.

7. Benjamin, "Winter of Our Discontent," chap. 2, pp. 4–5.

8. "Two Report Cures by Dr. Friedmann," *New York Times*, 21 April 1913.

9. "Friedmann Asserts Patients Are Better," *New York Times*, 19 March 1913.

10. "Friedmann Calls on Col. Roosevelt," *New York Times*, 23 April 1913; "Roosevelt Sees Him," *Evening Chronicle* (Charlotte, NC), 26 April 1913.

11. "Friedmann Sells for $1,925,000," *New York Times*, 27 April 1913.

12. In June, Benjamin brought suit against Friedmann for an accounting of the profits from the sale of the remedy and for the treatment of private patients, but it seems this came to nothing. "Friedmann Aid to Sue," *New York Times*, 6 June 1913; "Dr. Friedmann Sued by Former Associate," *Pittsburgh Daily Post*, 6 June 1913.

13. Benjamin, "Winter of Our Discontent," chap. 2, p. 9.

14. Werner, "Der 'Wunderheiler' Friedmann"; Werner, *Der Heiler*; Hüntelmann, "Das Friedrich Franz Friedmannsche Tuberkulosemittel Schildkröten." Friedmann's serum was one in a long succession of failed attempts to treat the white plague. Petra Werner posits that Friedmann was a sincere believer in the efficacy of his serum until late in life, though his motives remain controversial. On the other hand, immune therapy was a respectable idea for the science of its time, and the fact that we do not now believe the serum to have been effective is not in itself a reason for damning its inventor; there were scores of remedies in circulation in those days and there remained no scientific consensus about its efficacy. Friedmann's remedy was used by fewer and fewer physicians after World War I, though he continued to offer it in his own clinic. Later, during the Weimar Republic, the critiques of his science and of his shady business associations began to be streaked with anti-Semitism. Hüntelmann describes the serum as a "precarious substance."

15. Diary, 1913, box 2, series IIB Diaries, item 9, HBC; Benjamin, "Winter of Our Discontent," chap. 2, p. 12; Tom Dewe Mathews, "Nowhere Man," *The Guardian*, 16 January 2000.

16. "Dr. Friedmann Assailed," *Pioneer* (Bemidji, MN), 11 August 1913; "Charge Dr. Friedmann with Unprofessional Conduct," *Courier-Journal* (Louisville, KY), 12 August 1913.

17. Benjamin, "Winter of Our Discontent," chap. 2, pp. 12–13.

18. McDowell, Green, and Zuckerman, *Hospital for Joint Diseases*.

19. Person, *Sexual Century*, 345; Benjamin, "Winter of Our Discontent," chap. 2, p. 14.

20. Benjamin, "Winter of Our Discontent," chap. 1, pp. 1–3. Benjamin's account is echoed by that of pianist Selmar Jansen. "Tech Piano Professor on Captured Steamer," *Pittsburg Daily Post*, 26 August 1914.

21. "In a Cornish Village," *Middlesex Chronicle*, 15 August 1914.

22. "Two Transatlantic Liners Bring Home Refugees, Tourists Reach Home," *Courier-Journal*, 24 August 1914; T. K. Breakell, "RFC Pilot's Autobiography," Wirksworth Parish Records, 1 April 2017, www.wirksworth.org.uk/TKB-BIO.htm; Benjamin, "Winter of Our Discontent," chap. 1, p. 2.

23. London, *Cornwall in the First World War*, 8–10. A wonderful set of images of this event are available in the Paddy Bradley Collection on the Cornish Memory website, www.cornishmemory.com.

24. German foreigners had to get a permit if they traveled more than five miles from their registered address. They were also forbidden from possessing weapons, signal devices, carrier pigeons, motor cars, or ciphers. "Bekanntmachung fuer Auslaender Deutscher Nation," box 3 Correspondence, folder Bertha Benjamin, HBC.

25. HB to Bertha Benjar, 16 August 1914, box 3 Correspondence, folder Bertha Benjamin, HBC.

26. Memorandum, box 3 Correspondence, folder Bertha Benjamin, HBC; Notebook "1914," box 2, series IIB Diaries, item 10, HBC; Benjamin, "Winter of Our Discontent," chap. 1, pp. 3–4.

27. Passenger manifest, SS *Dominion*, 16–28 September 1914, Liverpool to Philadelphia *Pennsylvania, US, Arriving Passenger and Crew Lists, 1798–1962* [database on-line], Ancestry.com, 2006; Benjamin, "Winter of Our Discontent," chap. 1, p. 5.

28. Bonner, *Becoming a Physician*; Bonner, "German Doctors in America"; Kirschbaum, "Whatever Happened to German America?"; Kirschbaum, *Eradication of German Culture in the United States*.

29. Benjamin, "Winter of Our Discontent," chap. 3, p. 2.

Chapter 4

1. Harry Benjamin, "The Winter of Our Discontent," typescript, c. 1942, box 23, folders 38, 39, 40, 41, chap. 6, 2–5, HBC.

2. Benjamin, "Winter of Our Discontent," chap. 6, pp. 2–5.

3. The diary's lock was removed for me by the archivist at the Kinsey Institute. The transcription of the German Fraktur into modern script was by Elisabeth Kissel; the translation is my own. Diary "Tagebuch," 1906–9, 14 August 1906, box 2, series IIB Diaries, item 8, HBC.

4. Diary "Tagebuch," 1906–9, 14 August 1906.

5. Diary "Tagebuch," 1906–9, 23 August 1906.

6. Diary "Tagebuch," 1906–9, 17 August 1906.

7. Benjamin, "Winter of Our Discontent," chap. 6, pp. 1–2.

8. Benjamin, "Winter of Our Discontent," chap. 6, pp. 1–2.

9. Logan, *Hormones, Heredity, and Race*. Logan provides an insightful examination of hormone science in interwar Vienna.

10. Thorne, "Dr. Steinach and Rejuvenation."

11. Coen, "Living Precisely in Fin-de-Siècle Vienna"; Müller, *Vivarium*.

12. Benjamin, "Winter of Our Discontent," chap. 6.

13. Benjamin, "Reminiscences."

14. Borell, "Setting the Standards for a New Science"; Borell, "Brown-Séquard's Organotherapy"; Borell, "Organotherapy and the Emergence of Reproductive Endocrinology"; Krementsov, "Hormones and the Bolsheviks."

15. Logan, *Hormones, Heredity, and Race*, 28.

16. Sengoopta, "Tales from the Vienna Labs"; Sengoopta, *Most Secret Quintessence of Life*.

17. Postcard, Paul Kammerer to HB, 11 August 1921, box 5 Correspondence, folder Kammerer, HBC.

18. Benjamin, "Winter of Our Discontent," chap. 6.

19. Benjamin, "Winter of Our Discontent," chap. 6.

Chapter 5

1. Berghahn, review of *Gay Berlin*; Dose, *Magnus Hirschfeld*.

2. Ihlenfeld, "Memorial for Harry Benjamin."

3. Harry Benjamin, "The Winter of Our Discontent," typescript, c. 1942, box 23, folders 38, 39, 40, 41, chap. 4, pp. 12–13.

4. Benjamin, "Reminiscences."

5. Benjamin, "Reminiscences."

6. Dose, *Magnus Hirschfeld*, 45. Dose says that Hirschfeld unwisely made claims about the unconscious homosexuality of Moltke without having personally examined him. He was forced to revise his opinion during a second trial, and his reputation never fully recovered.

7. Benjamin, "Reminiscences."

8. Ethel Spector Person, "Manuscript Interview Notes, Harry Benjamin Reference Materials and Drafts, 1948–1986," box 33, folder 6, Ethel Spector Person Papers, Archives and Special Collections, Columbia University Health Sciences Library, New York. Person wrote a note saying Benjamin "hoped to make her bisex."

9. Diary "Tagebuch," 1906–9, 10 February 1907, box 2, series IIB Diaries, item 8, HBC.

10. Diary "Tagebuch," 1906–9, 10 February 1907, 15 January 1909.

11. Person, "Manuscript Interview Notes."

12. Diary "Tagebuch," 1906–9, 30 January 1909, box 2, series IIB Diaries, item 8, HBC. In an interview given when Benjamin was in his nineties, Ethel Person jotted the following in her yellow pad: "Last exam → Dr.→ Asked for hand in marriage / she was shocked / broke into tears, rushed out of room." Person, "Manuscript Interview Notes."

13. Sengoopta, "Glandular Politics," 450. Sengoopta argues that the idea that homosexuality was a disease was not overthrown, as in a paradigm shift, but rather, only slowly displaced by the notion that it was a developmental error.

14. Sengoopta, "Glandular Politics," 453.

15. Timm and Taylor, "Historicizing Transgender Terminology."

16. Sengoopta, "Glandular Politics."

17. Sengoopta, "Glandular Politics."

18. Sengoopta, "Glandular Politics."

19. Dose, *Magnus Hirschfeld*; Marhoefer, *Sex and the Weimar Republic*.

20. Isherwood, *Christopher and His Kind*, 15.

21. Isherwood, *Christopher and His Kind*, 14–19.

22. Timm, "'I Am So Grateful to All You Men of Medicine'"; Bauer, *Hirschfeld Archives*. While an oasis for many victims of violence, Bauer argues that the institute also reflected the sexual and racial oppressions of a colonial Germany.

23. Benjamin, "Reminiscences."

24. "Sex Problems to Be Discussed by Scientists," *Lima (OH) Gazette*, 6 August 1921; "Love Is Complex Reflex Action, Says Physician," *Omaha Daily Bee*, 28 October 1921; Dose, "World League for Sexual Reform."

Chapter 6

1. "Gland Operation to Retard Senility," *New York Times*, 20 November 1921.

2. HB to Eugen Steinach, 17 November 1921, SBC.

3. Harry Benjamin, "The Winter of Our Discontent," typescript, c. 1942, box 23, folders 38, 39, 40, 41, chap. 3, pp. 11–12, HBC.

4. "Dr. Steinach Coming to Make Old Young," *New York Times*, 9 February 1922.

5. HB to Eugen Steinach, 12 February 1922, SBC; "Youth of Woman Renewed as Well as Man's through the Steinach Operation," *St. Louis Post-Dispatch*, 14 February 1922.

6. Atherton, *Adventures of a Novelist*, 554–59; Leider, *California's Daughter*. The best source on Atherton's life is Leider's excellent biography, on which much of this section depends.

7. Leider, *California's Daughter*, 47.

8. Churchwell, *Careless People*.

9. Atherton, *Adventures of a Novelist*, 537–39; Atherton, "Alpine School of Fiction."

10. Bill from Parsons, Closson & McIlvaine to Gertrude Atherton, 20 February 1922, box 13, GAP.

11. "Sleet Ties Traffic, Causes Two Deaths," *New York Times*, 13 February 1922; Ambrose, *Knickerbocker Snowstorm*.

12. Atherton, *Adventures of a Novelist*, 556.

13. Cassedy, *Connected*.

14. Churchwell, *Careless People*, 100–101; "'Broadcasting Boom' of 1922," United States Early Radio History website, 16 January 2023, http://earlyradiohistory.us/sec018.htm.

15. Glands, Glandex Company, 1920, 0293–12; Rejuvenation, 1903–1989; CN Exhilarator of Life Company, 1921–1948, American Medical Association Historical Health Fraud and Alternative Medicine Collection, Chicago.

16. "City's 1921 Death Rate Lowest on Record," *New York Times*, 1 January 1922.

17. Smith, "Half Century of Public Health," 5.

18. Atherton, *Adventures of a Novelist*, 558.

19. Atherton, *Adventures of a Novelist*; HB to Eugen Steinach, 16 February 1922, SBC.

20. Atherton, *Adventures of a Novelist*, 553–59.

21. HB to Eugen Steinach, 31 May 1922, SBC.

22. Leider, *California's Daughter*. Letter to Charlotte Hallowell quoted in Leider, 293.

23. Dardis, *Firebrand*, xii.

24. Atherton, *Black Oxen*.

25. Dawson, introduction to *Black Oxen*.

26. Atherton, *Black Oxen*, 132–33, 178–88.

27. Atherton, *Adventures of a Novelist*, 560, quoting William Butler Yeats, *The Countess Cathleen* (1892).

28. Atherton, *Adventures of a Novelist*, 559–60.

29. Gilmore, *Horace Liveright*, 98.

30. Van Vechten, "Lady Who Defies Time."

31. Atherton, *Black Oxen*, Melanie V. Dawson, note on the text, 37–38; Horace Liveright to Gertrude Atherton, 18 October 1923, box 6, GAP.

32. Leider, *California's Daughter*, 294; HB to Gertrude Atherton, 30 July 1923, box 1, GAP.

33. *Black Oxen* (film).

34. Atherton, *Black Oxen*, Melanie V. Dawson, note on the text, 37–38.

35. Grand Theatre *Black Oxen* advertisement, *Jacksonville Daily Journal*, 30 March 1924.

36. "Is Mrs. Atherton Rejuvenated Like Heroine of Book?," *Brooklyn Daily Eagle*, 18 March 1924.

37. "Women Here Made Younger, Like Heroine in 'Black Oxen,' by Rejuvenation Treatment," *New York Herald Tribune*, 16 March 1924; "Is Mrs. Atherton Rejuvenated Like Heroine of Book?," *Brooklyn Daily Eagle*, 18 March 1924.

38. "Women Here Made Younger, Like Heroine in 'Black Oxen,' by Rejuvenation Treatment," *New York Herald Tribune*, 16 March 1924.

39. Harry Benjamin, "The Steinach Method as Applied to Women," 753.

40. Benjamin, "Control of Old Age," 345.

41. Pettit, "Becoming Glandular."

42. SL to Gertrude Atherton, 29 December 1935, box 6, GAP.

43. Atherton, *Adventures of a Novelist*, 560.

44. Pettit, "Becoming Glandular." Pettit explores this intriguing question in his excellent article by using letters that Atherton received from ordinary people as a means of investigating the creation of this new identity.

45. H. E. Krehbiel, "Marie Jeritza Acclaimed in Korngold Opera," *New York Tribune*, 20 November 1921; Oscar Thompson, "Korngold Opera at Metropolitan Yields Triumph for Mme. Jeritza," *Musical America*, 26 November 1921.

46. HB to Eugen Steinach, 7 December 1921, SBC.

47. Maria Jeritza is identified as a friend and client of Benjamin by the Archive for Sexology, www .sexarchive.info/GESUND/ARCHIV/COLLBEN.HTM.

48. Farrar was actually only six years older than Jeritza, who was thirty-four at her debut at the Met. Robert Baxter, "Geraldine Farrar, compact disc liner notes," Ward Marston, 2003, www.marstonrecords .com/products/farrar; "Hail Farrar Queen as She Sings Adieu," *New York Times*, 23 April 1922.

49. Translation by Lisa Lockhart, lyrics "Glück, das mir verblieb" (Marietta's lied), from Act I of the German opera *Die Tote Stadt* by Erich Korngold, 18 January 1999, www.aria-database.com.

Chapter 7

1. Harry Benjamin, "The Winter of Our Discontent," typescript, c. 1942, box 23, folders 38, 39, 40, 41, chap. 9, p. 8, HBC.

2. Pettit, "Becoming Glandular."

3. Leider, *California's Daughter*, 305.

4. Nordlund, "Endocrinology and Expectations in 1930s America."

5. Horace Liveright to Gertrude Atherton, 21 May 1923, 5 September 1923, 29 September 1923, box 6, GAP.

6. Krementsov, *Revolutionary Experiments*; McLaren, *Reproduction by Design*.

7. Sayers, "Incredible Elopement of Lord Peter Wimsey," 44–45.

8. Sayers, *Unpleasantness at the Bellona Club*, 121.

9. HB to Gertrude Atherton, 4 September 1924, box 1, GAP; "Slayer's Gland Systems Blamed for Diseased Minds," *Chicago Sunday Tribune*, 10 August 1924; "Gland Theory Is Far Fetched, Woodyatt Says," *Chicago Daily Tribune*, 16 August 1924.

10. Ethel Spector Person, "Manuscript Interview Notes, Harry Benjamin Reference Materials and Drafts, 1948–1986," box 33, folder 6, Ethel Spector Person Papers, Archives and Special Collections, Columbia University Health Sciences Library, New York.

11. Greta Gülzow to HB, 13 September 1922, box 3 Correspondence, folder Greta Benjamin, HBC; Person, "Manuscript Interview Notes."

12. Greta Gülzow to HB, 13 September 1922.

13. Greta Gülzow to HB, 13 September 1922; Person, "Manuscript Interview Notes."

14. Greta Gülzow to HB, 11 December 1922.

15. "Rejuvenator," *Shamokin (PA) News-Dispatch*, 27 July 1927. I have no indication she was a film star, so this was likely invented by the paper.

16. Person, "Manuscript Interview Notes."

17. Clipping, "Eye on Gotham," undated, box 21, HBC; Buckley, "Transsexual Operation."

18. Person, "Manuscript Interview Notes."

19. Benjamin, "Reminiscences."

20. Person, *Sexual Century*; Person, "Manuscript Interview Notes."

21. Charles Ihlenfeld, interviews by author, 13 November 2017, 20 November 2017, 1 July 2018, via video conference.

22. Meyerowitz, *How Sex Changed*.

23. Aleshia Brevard Crenshaw, interview by Susan Stryker, 2 August 1997, Gay and Lesbian Historical Society, www.glbthistory.org.

24. HB to Alfred Kinsey, 17 July 1951, HBC, *LGBT Thought and Culture* database, accessed 20 June 2018.

25. "Giving Youth to American Women Now Regular Industry in Vienna," *New York World*, 5 August 1923; Harriman, "Profile—Elizabeth Arden."

26. HB to Eugen Steinach, 10 June 1929, 17 September 1929, SBC; United States Patent Office, 1,715,027, Greta Benjamin of New York, 28 May 1929, Metallic Face Mask and Process of Making Same, filed 16 January 1928, Serial No. 246,934.

27. Lisser, "First Forty Years," 9.

28. Bliss, *Discovery of Insulin*.

29. HB diary entry, 26 May 1923, Notebook "1923 Europe," box 2, series IIB Diaries, item 12, HBC.

30. *New York Medical Week*, 13 October 1923; contract between UFA and Harry Benjamin, 20 June 1923; advertisement for *Steinach-Film*, 1923, both in Archive for Sexology, www.sexarchive.info /GESUND/ARCHIV/COLLSTE.HTM; Haeberle, "Transatlantic Commuter."

31. Logan, *Hormones, Heredity, and Race*, 59–61, 182.

32. Benjamin, "Winter of Our Discontent," chap. 6, p. 6.

33. Gliboff, "'Protoplasm . . . Is Soft Wax in Our Hands.'"

34. HB form letter, 2 September 1922, box 5 Correspondence, folder Kammerer, HBC.

35. Kammerer to Benjamin, 11 July 1923 and 31 August 1923, quoted in and translation by Logan, *Hormones, Heredity, and Race*, 184.

36. Benjamin, introduction to *Rejuvenation and the Prolongation of Human Efficiency*.

37. Haeckel published his best-selling manifesto for monism, *The Riddle of the Universe*, in 1899 and founded the German Monist League in 1906.

38. Logan, *Hormones, Heredity, and Race*, 89–116; Kammerer, *Rejuvenation and the Prolongation of Human Efficiency*.

39. "Biologist to Tell How Species Alter," *New York Times*, 28 November 1923.

40. Gertrude Atherton to HB, 15 October 1926, box 14, GAP.

41. Order blank for Sanitablets and Polycrines, the Harrower Laboratory, c. 1925, in possession of author.

42. Parkes, "Prospect and Retrospect in the Physiology of Reproduction."

43. Parkes, "Prospect and Retrospect in the Physiology of Reproduction."

44. Medvei, *A History of Endocrinology*, 396–401.

45. Arthur J. Cramp to Miss Davy, memorandum, 28 July 1928, American Medical Association Historical Health Fraud and Alternative Medicine Collection, Chicago.

46. Rogers, *Alternate Path*; Thomas, "Dr. Morris Fishbein Dead at 87."

47. Fishbein, *Medical Follies*, 165, 168–69.

48. Rosenberg, "Martin Arrowsmith"; "Sinclair Lewis at Work"; De Kruif, "An Intimate Glimpse of a Great American Novel in the Making."

49. Fishbein, *New Medical Follies*, 105.

50. Fishbein, *New Medical Follies*, 104; HB to Morris Fishbein, 13 July 1927, box 101, folder 4, UC.

51. Benjamin, "New Clinical Aspects of the Steinach Operation."

52. H. Marks, *The Progress of Experiment*.

53. Benjamin, "New Clinical Aspects of the Steinach Operation"; Harry Benjamin, "Steinach and the Journal of the American Medical Association," enclosure in HB to Olin West, 16 April 1929, box 101, folder 4, UC; Benjamin, "The Control of Old Age," 336; Benjamin quotes Goethe's *Faust* as translated by Bayard Taylor.

54. Morris Fishbein to Horace Liveright, telegram 29 January 1929, box 4, folder 9; Liveright to Fishbein, 10 May 1929, box 4, folder 9, UC.

55. Morris Fishbein to Horace Liveright, 7 May 1929, box 4 folder 9; Fishbein to Liveright, 1 February 1929, box 4, folder 9; Fishbein to R. R. Simmons, 23 April 1929, box 101, folder 4, UC.

56. Horace Liveright to Morris Fishbein, 8 March 1929, box 4, folder 9, UC.

57. Arthur Garfield Hays to Morris Fishbein, 22 September 1930, box 101, folder 4, UC.

58. HB to editor, *Journal of the Iowa State Medical Society*, 26 March 1929, box 101, folder 4, UC. The editor chose not to print Benjamin's letter, replying that "the subject matter of this discussion is one which, at best, is limited to the realm of speculation." He then duly forwarded the correspondence to Fishbein, who replied that he "greatly admired" his response to Benjamin, saying, "The gentleman is a publicity hound." R. R. Simmons to HB, 19 April 1929; Morris Fishbein to R. R. Simmons, 23 April 1929, box 101, folder 4, UC.

59. Stokes, "Max Thorek and Testicular Transplantation."

60. Max Thorek to HB, 16 August 1929, box 101, folder 4; Morris Fishbein to Arthur Garfield Hays, 26 September 1930, box 101, folder 4, UC.

61. Price, *Carl Richard Moore*.

62. Benjamin would hold the post of Consulting Endocrinologist at City College from 1930 to 1941. Curriculum vitae, box 23, folder 18, HBC.

63. Harrow, *Glands in Health and Disease.*

64. Griminger, "Casimir Funk."

65. Benjamin Harrow to HB, 12 July [1928], box 5 Correspondence, folder Harrow, HBC.

66. McCormick would be the fourth of Walska's six husbands, who would include a Russian baron, a carpet tycoon, and the British inventor of the death ray.

67. "Ganna Walska to Open Beauty Shop in Paris: Voronoff Will Give Monkey Gland Treatment," *New York Times*, 13 April 1927; "Ganna, Voronoff to Sell Beauty, Youth in Shop," *New York Daily News*, 22 July 1927; "Dr. V. D. Lespinasse. Chicago Gland Surgeon in 1922 Operated on Harold McCormick," *New York Times*, 16 December 1946; "Secret Operation on H. F. M'Cormick. Family Refuses to Say Whether His Stay in Hospital Is for Gland Transplanting," *New York Times*, 18 June 1922.

68. Harrow, *Casimir Funk*, 108.

69. Harrow, *Casimir Funk*, 136.

70. "Thirteenth International Physiological Congress at Boston"; Rall, "The XIIIth International Physiological Congress in Boston in 1929."

71. Casimir Funk to HB, dated Wednesday [23 August 1929], on letterhead of the XIIIth International Physiological Congress, Harvard Medical School, Boston, 19–23 August 1929, box 4 Correspondence, folder Funk, HBC.

72. "Tells of Gains Made in Fight on Old Age. Drs. Funk and Voronoff at Boston Congress Report Recent Discoveries," *New York Times*, 29 August 1929.

73. Ihlenfeld, "Memorial for Harry Benjamin."

74. Casimir Funk to Mr. McHugh, 9 November 1930, box 4 Correspondence, folder Funk, HBC.

75. HB to Casimir Funk, 30 October 1930, box 4 Correspondence, folder Funk, HBC.

76. HB to Casimir Funk, 5 April 1930, box 4 Correspondence, folder Funk, HBC.

77. HB to Casimir Funk, 13 May 1929, box 4 Correspondence, folder Funk, HBC.

78. "Says Lord Lee Sold Holbein for $250,000," *New York Times*, 5 December 1928; "J. S. Bache Acquires a $600,000 Raphael," *New York Times*, 12 March 1929.

79. Harrow, *Casimir Funk*, 91.

80. HB to Casimir Funk, draft of letter unsent, undated, box 4 Correspondence, folder Funk, HBC.

81. Harrow, *Casimir Funk*, v.

82. HB to Magnus Hirschfeld, 24 March 1932, 4 May 1932, Briefwechsel Hirschfeld-Benjamin, HHA.

83. Person, "Manuscript Interview Notes."

84. Person, *Sexual Century*, 359.

85. HB to Magnus Hirschfeld, 20 April 1934, Briefwechsel Hirschfeld-Benjamin, HHA.

86. BR [initials used to hide identity of patient] to Gertrude Atherton, 20 November 1946, box 3 Correspondence, folder Atherton, HBC.

87. Ihlenfeld, "Memorial for Harry Benjamin," 7.

Chapter 8

1. Haeberle, "Transatlantic Commuter"; Benjamin, "Reminiscences."

2. Isherwood, *Mr. Norris Changes Trains*; Isherwood, *Goodbye to Berlin.*

3. Isherwood, *Christopher and His Kind*, 15–16. I thank the anonymous reviewer for the press for the helpful rewording of these sentences.

4. Isherwood, *Christopher and His Kind*, 16, 27.

5. Hansson et al., "'He Gave Us the Cornerstone of Sexual Medicine'"; the Nobel Prize Nomination Archive, accessed 17 January 2023, www.nobelprize.org/nomination/archive/.

6. Gertrude Atherton to HB, 9 October [1933?], box 14, GAP.

7. Atherton says, "It costs $3.50 a bottle here, and as I take four a day you may imagine how far that would go." I assume this means she is taking four pills a day rather than four bottles. Thank you to Julie Bush for her attention to this detail. Gertrude Atherton to HB, 2 January 1934, 2 January 1937, box 14, GAP.

8. Li, "Marketing Menopause"; Li, *J. B. Collip*; Oudshoorn, *Beyond the Natural Body*.

9. Dose, *Magnus Hirschfeld*, 31.

10. HB to Magnus Hirschfeld, 28 January 1928, Briefwechsel Hirschfeld-Benjamin, HHA.

11. Benjamin, "Male Hormone."

12. Medvei, *History of Endocrinology*, 405.

13. Meyerowitz, *How Sex Changed*. Meyerowitz suggests he probably meant that it would be impossible for surgeons to give her a functioning penis or make it possible for her to reproduce, 29.

14. Meyerowitz, *How Sex Changed*, 30.

15. Meyerowitz, *How Sex Changed*, 19–20.

16. Elbe (Einar Wegener) received surgeries to remove her testicles and penis, to transplant human ovaries, and to create a vagina.

17. Amin, "Glands, Eugenics, and Rejuvenation in Man into Woman."

18. Amin, "Glands, Eugenics, and Rejuvenation in Man into Woman." The Lili Elbe Digital Archive is an excellent resource documenting Elbe's life and providing the several texts and context for *Man into Woman*. Caughie et al., Lili Elbe Digital Archive.

19. Haeberle, "Transatlantic Commuter"; Haeberle, "Movement of Inverts."

20. Stryker, *Transgender History*, 57.

21. Benjamin, "Reminiscences"; Dose, "World League for Sexual Reform"; Dose, *Magnus Hirschfeld*, 51.

22. HB to Magnus Hirschfeld, 28 January 1928, Briefwechsel Hirschfeld-Benjamin, HHA.

23. Dose, "World League for Sexual Reform"; HB to Magnus Hirschfeld, 10 June 1930, 20 September 1933, Briefwechsel Hirschfeld-Benjamin, HHA.

24. Dardis, *Firebrand*.

25. "Endocrine Glands," 76, 81.

26. Pettit, "Becoming Glandular."

27. McLaren, *Reproduction by Design*, 81–108.

28. Logan, *Hormones, Heredity, and Race*, 34–35.

29. Diana Long Hall, quoted in Oudshoorn, *Beyond the Natural Body*, 39.

30. Sengoopta, *Most Secret Quintessence of Life*; Oudshoorn, *Beyond the Natural Body*.

31. Dose, *Magnus Hirschfeld*, 31.

32. Benjamin, "Reminiscences," 4.

33. Dose, *Magnus Hirschfeld*, 59. Viereck would later become notorious as a Nazi sympathizer. Alarmed at some of the reports coming from Germany in 1933, Benjamin remarked to Hirschfeld that he feared Viereck might start a propaganda campaign in favor of the Hitler government and that if he were to do so, he was likely to lose the great majority of his friends. Viereck served five years in jail

as a Nazi propagandist from 1942 to 1947. However, there is some evidence Benjamin continued to have some contact with Viereck in later years, as he wrote to Alfred Kinsey in 1949 reminding him of his promise to send a picture of himself, saying, "Whenever I see it in Viereck's place I am somewhat jealous." HB to Magnus Hirschfeld, 20 September 1933, Briefwechsel Hirschfeld-Benjamin, HHA; HB to Alfred Kinsey, 11 April 1949, *LGBT Thought and Culture* database, HBC; Timm, "'I Am So Grateful to All You Men of Medicine.'"

34. Benjamin, "Reminiscences"; Dose, *Magnus Hirschfeld*, 27.

35. Dose, *Magnus Hirschfeld*, 60.

36. HB to Magnus Hirschfeld, 20 February 1931, Briefwechsel Hirschfeld-Benjamin, HHA. His diabetes had been diagnosed in Berlin. Ludwig Levy-Lenz noted Hirschfeld lived simply but was denied his favorite dishes because of his diabetes. He had difficulty controlling his diet as he knew he should, often eating several pieces of cake if he were not watched. Dose, *Magnus Hirschfeld*, 27.

37. Magnus Hirschfeld to HB, 26 September 1931, 16 March 1932, 11 April 1932; HB to Hirschfeld, 24 March 1932, 4 May 1932, Briefwechsel Hirschfeld-Benjamin, HHA.

38. Dose, *Magnus Hirschfeld*, 78–81. Laurie Marhoefer has written a dual biography of Hirschfeld and Li and their journey, showing how complex issues of racism and colonialism played out in the creation of Hirschfeld's ideas and activism. Marhoefer, *Racism and the Making of Gay Rights*.

39. Gretchen Benjamin to Max Thorek, 17 September 1930, box 101, folder 4, UC. Thorek forwarded Gretchen's letter to Fishbein, along with a copy of the letter he had written to Harry.

40. HB to Magnus Hirschfeld, 11 July 1934, Briefwechsel Hirschfeld-Benjamin, HHA.

41. Person, *Sexual Century*.

42. Arthur Garfield Hays to Morris Fishbein, 12 March 1934; Hays to Fishbein, 29 August 1930; Fishbein to Hays, 5 September 1930, box 101, folder 4, UC.

43. Olin West to Morris Fishbein, undated, attached to Arthur Garfield Hays to Morris Fishbein, 29 August 1930, box 101, folder 4, UC.

44. Arthur Garfield Hays to Morris Fishbein, 24 September 1935, box 101, folder 4, UC.

45. "Guide to the Morris Fishbein Papers 1912–1976," University of Chicago Library, 2007, www .lib.uchicago.edu/e/scrc/findingaids/view.php?eadid=ICU.SPCL.FISHBEIN.

46. Benjamin, "Prostitution Re-assessed"; Ellis, "Prostitution Re-assessed"; Benjamin and Ellis, "Objective Examination of Prostitution"; Ihlenfeld, "Memorial for Harry Benjamin," 10. Also see recording of Ellis's remarks in the documentary film *Harry Benjamin, M.D. 1885–1986*, at www .sexsmartfilms.com/premium/film/763/HARRY+BENJAMIN%2C+M.

47. Benjamin, "Humane Necessity," 79; Gumpert, "False Mercy," 80.

48. Davis, "'Not Marriage at All, but Simple Harlotry.'"

49. Benjamin's own version was that Lindsey, happily married and never divorced, became enraged when the bishop called him "that divorced man." Benjamin, "Reminiscences," 9; "Divorce Termed Dishonor by Bishop Manning in Paris," *Baltimore Sun*, 1 August 1927; "Judge Lindsey to Hear Manning Sermon Today; Says He May 'Rise Up' and Retort to Bishop," *New York Times*, 7 December 1930; "Lindsey Is Freed, Rebuked by Court," *New York Times*, 18 December 1930.

50. Evans, "Rejuvenation."

51. HLW [initials used to hide identity of patient] to Gertrude Atherton, 12 December 1935, 22 December 1935, box 12, GAP; Gertrude Atherton to HB, 25 December 1935, box 14, GAP.

52. HB to Norman Haire, 14 November 1936, 16 December 1936; Haire to HB, 16 December 1936, box 4 Correspondence, folder Haire, HBC.

53. Platt, "Lazarus Beside Me."

54. HB diary entry, 15 April 1937, Notebook "1937 Europe," box 2, series IIB Diaries, item 18, HBC.

55. Platt, "Lazarus Beside Me." This account is drawn entirely from Platt's own telling of the events. Over the years, Platt looked back wistfully upon her meeting with Yeats and came to see it as one of the high points of her life. She wrote an account of it in 1946 and toyed with sharing the story with Yeats's biographers but never did. After Platt's death in 1976, her executor was left with a jumble of papers, the manuscript left in a plastic bag at the back of a dusty drawer, alongside faded letters and diaries. In 2015, this executor took the lot to the home of her cousin and her cousin's husband, the poet Peter Scupham. "Do you think there is anything of interest or should I just throw it all away?" she asked. Over a cup of coffee, Scupham reached into the pile and pulled out Platt's story of her encounter with Yeats. He realized immediately that it should be published. Sarah Hughes, "WB Yeats, the Art Teacher and a Night at the Sexologist's," *The Guardian*, 8 August 2015.

56. Benjamin, "Reminiscences," 7–8.

57. Pettit, "Becoming Glandular"; Medeiros, *Heightened Expectations*; Watkins, *Estrogen Elixir*; McLaren, *Reproduction by Design*; Krementsov, "Hormones and the Bolsheviks."

58. Nordlund, "Endocrinology and Expectations in 1930s America."

59. HB to Magnus Hirschfeld, 22 August 1932, Briefwechsel Hirschfeld-Benjamin, HHA.

60. Harry Benjamin, "The Winter of Our Discontent," typescript, c. 1942, box 23, folders 38, 39, 40, 41, chap. 4, p. 11, HBC; Kevles, *In the Name of Eugenics*.

61. Meyerowitz, *How Sex Changed*, 29–40.

62. Henry, *Sex Variants*, 487–98; Schaefer and Wheeler, "Harry Benjamin's First Ten Cases"; Ihlenfeld, "Memorial for Harry Benjamin"; Meyerowitz, *How Sex Changed*, 46n105. Meyerowitz convincingly argues that "Rudolph von H.," whose case history appears in Henry, *Sex Variants*, is the pseudonym for Spengler.

63. Bakker et al., *Others of My Kind*, 13–40; Timm, "'I Am So Grateful to All You Men of Medicine'"; Talmey, "Transvestism"; Henry, *Sex Variants*, 495. Spengler is "Case I" in Talmey's article. Schaefer and Wheeler say Benjamin started treating Spengler for arthritis in 1938. Spengler's birthdate is 18 April 1873, so he would have been fifty-two in 1925 or 1926. Otto Spengler, draft registration card, US, World War I Draft Registration Cards, 1917–1918, online database, Ancestry.com. Progynon became available after 1928.

64. Otto Spengler to Gertrude Atherton, 10 September 1938, box 3 Correspondence, folder Atherton, HBC; Timm, "'I Am So Grateful to All You Men of Medicine.'"

65. Otto Spengler to Gertrude Atherton, 10 September 1938; Gertrude Atherton to HB, handwritten note on the bottom of letter received from Spengler, 10 September 1938; HB to Atherton, 27 September 1938, box 3 Correspondence, folder Atherton, HBC; HB to Atherton, 5 October 1938, box 1, GAP.

66. Buckley, "Transsexual Operation."

67. Müller, *Vivarium*.

68. HB to Gertrude Atherton, 21 March 1938, box 3 Correspondence, folder Atherton, HBC.

69. Benjamin, "Reminiscences."

70. HB to Magnus Hirschfeld, 27 April 1931, Briefwechsel Hirschfeld-Benjamin, HHA.

71. Benjamin, "Winter of Our Discontent," chap. 3, p. 10.

72. Haeberle, "Transatlantic Commuter."

73. Haeberle, "Transatlantic Commuter."

Chapter 9

1. HB to Eugen Steinach, 4 August 1938, SBC.

2. Charles Ihlenfeld, interviews by author, 13 November 2017, 20 November 2017, 1 July 2018, via video conference.

3. Notebook "1938," section labeled "Trip by car 1935 to California," box 2, series IIB Diaries, item 19, HBC.

4. Christine Wheeler, interview by author, 11 September 2013, New York.

5. "J. Harlow," entry in miscellaneous unbound pages, box 2, series IIB Diaries, item 4, HBC.

6. Magnus Hirschfeld to HB, 3 June 1934; HB to Hirschfeld, 11 July 1934, Briefwechsel Hirschfeld-Benjamin, HHA.

7. Person, *Sexual Century*, 361.

8. Leider, *California's Daughter*.

9. Benjamin and Masters, *Prostitution and Morality*, 8.

10. Don Lucas, interview by Susan Stryker, 13 June 1997, Gay and Lesbian Historical Society, www.glbthistory.org.

11. Harry Benjamin, "The Winter of Our Discontent," typescript, c. 1942, box 23, folders 38, 39, 40, 41, chap. 3, p. 10, HBC.

12. Benjamin, "The Winter of Our Discontent," chap. 3, p. 10.

13. HB to Magnus Hirschfeld, 22 January 1931, Briefwechsel Hirschfeld-Benjamin, HHA.

14. Sengoopta, "Tales from the Vienna Labs"; HB to Paul Smith, 23 January 1941, SBC.

15. HB to Gertrude Atherton, 3 January 1943; HB to Atherton, 13 January 1943, box 1, GAP.

16. Benjamin, "Winter of Our Discontent," chap. 8, p. 1, chap. 9, p. 11.

17. Benjamin, "Winter of Our Discontent," chap. 2, p. 10.

18. Benjamin, "Winter of Our Discontent," chap. 9, p. 2.

19. "Guide to the Morris Fishbein Papers 1912–1976," University of Chicago Library, 2007, www .lib.uchicago.edu/e/scrc/findingaids/view.php?eadid=ICU.SPCL.FISHBEIN.

20. Benjamin, "Winter of Our Discontent," chap. 4, p. 15.

21. Gertrude Atherton to HB, 30 July 1941, box 14, GAP.

22. Maugham, *Razor's Edge*, 243.

23. W. S. Maugham to HB, 29 November [1941], box 23, folder 41, HBC.

24. W. S. Maugham to HB, 16 January [1942], box 23, folder 41, HBC.

25. Julie Medlock to HB, 13 January 1942, box 23, folder 41, HBC.

26. Greta and Harry Benjamin to Eugen Steinach, telegram, 12 May 1944, SBC; HB to Gertrude Atherton, 27 December 1945, box 3 Correspondence, folder Atherton, HBC.

27. Benjamin, "Eugen Steinach, 1861–1944."

28. Editorial note to abstract, Harry Benjamin, "Endocrine Gerontotherapy: The Use of Sex Hormone Combinations in Female Patients," *Journal of Gerontology* 4 (1949): 22, abstracted in *Obstetrical and Gynecological Survey* 5, no. 3 (1950): 394.

29. Gertrude Atherton to HB, 14 March 1948, box 3, folder Gertrude Atherton, HBC.

30. Leider, *California's Daughter*, 306–7.

31. HB to Gertrude Atherton, 14 October 1947, box 1, GAP.

32. HB to Gertrude Atherton, 26 December 1947, box 1, GAP.

33. HB to Gertrude Atherton, 21 January 1948, 6 February 1948, box 1, GAP.

34. HB to Gertrude Atherton, 13 January 1943, box 1, GAP; HB to Norman Haire, 17 August 1938, box 4 Correspondence, folder Haire, HBC.

35. "History," 450 Sutter Building website, accessed 22 April 2013, www.450sutter.com/.

36. Kinsey, Pomeroy, and Martin, *Sexual Behavior in the Human Male*; Kinsey et al., *Sexual Behavior in the Human Female*.

37. Ihlenfeld, "Memorial for Harry Benjamin"; Meyerowitz, *How Sex Changed*, 47–48.

38. Ihlenfeld, "Memorial for Harry Benjamin," 14; Ethel Spector Person, "Manuscript Interview Notes, Harry Benjamin Reference Materials and Drafts, 1948–1986," box 33, folder 6, Ethel Spector Person Papers, Archives and Special Collections, Columbia University Health Sciences Library, New York. He said he had no misgivings or sense of revulsion and felt perfectly justified in this approach.

39. Meyerowitz, *How Sex Changed*, 47. HB to VB [initials used to hide patient identity], 31 May 1949, and HB to Edmund G. Brown, 22 November 1949, both in box 3, series IIC, folder VB, HBC, quoted in Meyerowitz, 47n107.

40. Meyerowitz, *How Sex Changed*, 46–48, 120–21; Schaefer and Wheeler, "Harry Benjamin's First Ten Cases"; Stryker, *Transgender History*, 62; Haeberle, "Transatlantic Commuter."

41. Schaefer and Wheeler, "Harry Benjamin's First Ten Cases"; Person, "Manuscript Interview Notes."

42. Oudshoorn, *Beyond the Natural Body*; Rasmussen, "Steroids in Arms"; H. Marks, "Cortisone, 1949"; Sengoopta, *The Most Secret Quintessence of Life*; Krementsov, "Hormones and the Bolsheviks"; Nordlund, *Hormones of Life*; Liebenau, *Medical Science and Medical Industry*; Swann, *Academic Scientists and the Pharmaceutical Industry*.

43. Skidmore, *True Sex*; Reay, *Trans America*; Bakker et al., *Others of My Kind*.

44. Stryker, *Transgender History*, 61–62.

45. Schaefer and Wheeler, "Harry Benjamin's First Ten Cases," 80. I've used the pseudonyms given by Schaefer and Wheeler here.

46. Schaefer and Wheeler, "Harry Benjamin's First Ten Cases," 83.

47. Meyerowitz, *How Sex Changed*, 185–86.

48. Meyerowitz, *How Sex Changed*, 154.

49. Meyerowitz, *How Sex Changed*, 92, 181–82.

50. De Kruif, *Male Hormone*, 226.

51. De Kruif, *Male Hormone*, 117.

52. Beach, *Hormones and Behavior*.

53. Meyerowitz, *How Sex Changed*, 55.

54. Doctor, *Becoming a Woman*, 67–69; Meyerowitz, *How Sex Changed*, 56. Richard Doctor, author of a biography of Jorgensen, suggests Jorgensen made up this story to protect the identity of the physician. Meyerowitz, looking at Jorgensen's correspondence from around this date, agrees that she obtained estradiol from Angelo.

55. Ihlenfeld, "Memorial for Harry Benjamin."

56. Ihlenfeld, "Memorial for Harry Benjamin."

57. Person, "Manuscript Interview Notes."

58. Ihlenfeld, "Memorial for Harry Benjamin," 26–27.

Chapter 10

1. Jorgensen, *Christine Jorgensen*; Meyerowitz, *How Sex Changed*, 49–98.

2. Quoted in Meyerowitz, *How Sex Changed*, 59.

3. Jorgensen received first an orchiectomy (surgical removal of testicles) and a year later a penectomy (surgical removal of penis).

4. Meyerowitz, *How Sex Changed*, 120.

5. Murray, Schraufnagel, and Hopewell, "Treatment of Tuberculosis."

6. HB to Robert Wood, 14 February 1955, box 4 Correspondence, folder Haire, HBC.

7. "Dr. Paul Niehans, Swiss Surgeon, 89," *New York Times*, 4 September 1971; Gobind Behari Lal, "Control of Aging Organs Reported in Swiss Tests," *Seattle Post-Intelligencer*, 2 December 1956.

8. "It was not the most sensible thing I've done from a mountaineering point of view," Westmacott later said. "Obituary, Mike Westmacott," *The Telegraph* (London), 24 June 2012.

9. Westmacott initially never mentioned saving Morris's life. Even Westmacott's wife, Sally, did not learn of this until she read it in Morris's book years later. "Obituary, Mike Westmacott"; James Morris, *Coronation Everest*, 134.

10. James Morris, *Coronation Everest*, 116–43; Conefrey, *Everest 1953*; "Journalist Recalls the Battle to Break Everest Story," *BBC News*, 29 May 2013; David Holden, "James and Jan," *New York Times*, 17 March 1974.

11. Ethel Spector Person, "Manuscript Interview Notes, Harry Benjamin Reference Materials and Drafts, 1948–1986," box 33, folder 6, Ethel Spector Person Papers, Archives and Special Collections, Columbia University Health Sciences Library, New York.

12. HB to Alfred Kinsey, 16 April 1953, *LGBT Thought and Culture* database, HBC.

13. Ihlenfeld, "Memorial for Harry Benjamin," 25.

14. Benjamin, introduction to *Christine Jorgensen*, viii; Hill, "Dear Doctor Benjamin."

15. Meyerowitz, *How Sex Changed*, 63–69.

16. Meyerowitz, *How Sex Changed*, 62–81.

17. Meyerowitz, *How Sex Changed*, 74–76.

18. Meyerowitz, *How Sex Changed*, 114–15.

19. Meyerowitz, *How Sex Changed*, 114–15; Dreger, "'Ambiguous Sex'—or Ambivalent Medicine?"

20. Schaefer and Wheeler, "Harry Benjamin's First Ten Cases," 74; Person, *Sexual Century*; Matte, "Historicizing Liberal American Transnormativities"; Matte, "Putting Patients First"; Meyerowitz, *How Sex Changed*; Stryker, *Transgender History*. Person's chapter on Benjamin is the most significant source on Benjamin's life and career. Meyerowitz, Stryker, and Matte have developed the argument that Benjamin's readiness to provide treatment for transgender people was due to the influence of Steinach and Hirschfeld in combination with his decades of hormone therapy in gerontology. They also develop the argument that Benjamin's collaboration with his patients was critical in shaping his ideas about transsexuality.

21. Meyerowitz, *How Sex Changed*, 59.

22. For an excellent discussion of the origins of the term "transsexualism" and the complexities of translation, see Timm and Taylor, "Historicizing Transgender Terminology"; Meyerowitz, *How Sex Changed*, 43–44.

23. Benjamin, "Transvestism and Transsexualism," 13.

24. Benjamin, "Transvestism and Transsexualism," 14.

25. Elmer Belt to HB, 22 February 1960, HBC, quoted in Velocci, "Standards of Care."

26. Velocci, "Standards of Care."

27. Meyerowitz, *How Sex Changed*, 141–43.

28. Meyerowitz, *How Sex Changed*, 133.

29. Ronquillo, "Former UCLA Football Player Ira Pauly Reminisces on Game"; Anderson, "From the Archives"; Ira B. Pauly, interview by Maija Anderson, 18 February 2015, Oregon Health and Science University.

30. Anderson, "From the Archives"; Pauly interview by Anderson.

31. Ihlenfeld, "Memorial for Harry Benjamin," 17.

32. Benjamin, "Newer Aspects of the Transsexual Phenomenon," 138; Meyerowitz, *How Sex Changed*, 164.

33. Meyerowitz, *How Sex Changed*, 164.

34. Meyerowitz, *How Sex Changed*, 164.

35. Anderson, "From the Archives."

36. Meyerowitz, *How Sex Changed*, 163–64; Reay, "Transsexual Phenomenon"; HB to HF [initials used to hide patient identity], 1 September 1955, box 4, series IIC, folder HF, HBC, as quoted in Meyerowitz, 164.

37. Jan Morris, "Conundrum," 61–65.

38. "Reed Erickson and the Erickson Educational Foundation," Transgender Archives, University of Victoria, accessed 20 May 2016, www.uvic.ca/transgenderarchives/collections/reed-erickson /index.php; Lewis, "Trans History in a Moment of Danger."

39. Meyerowitz, *How Sex Changed*, 209–10; Devor and Matte, "Building a Better World for Transpeople."

40. Meyerowitz, *How Sex Changed*; Devor and Matte, "Building a Better World for Transpeople."

41. Ihlenfeld, "Memorial for Harry Benjamin."

42. Meyerowitz, *How Sex Changed*, 214–16.

43. Ihlenfeld, "Memorial for Harry Benjamin," 22.

44. Ihlenfeld, "Memorial for Harry Benjamin."

45. Brevard, *Woman I Was Not Born to Be*; Aleshia Brevard Crenshaw, interview by Susan Stryker, 2 August 1997, Gay and Lesbian Historical Society, www.glbthistory.org.

46. Brevard, *Woman I Was Not Born to Be*, 127.

47. Brevard, *Woman I Was Not Born to Be*, 59–60.

48. Brevard, *Woman I Was Not Born to Be*, 7.

49. Brevard, *Woman I Was Not Born to Be*, 12.

50. Crenshaw interview by Stryker; Meyerowitz, *How Sex Changed*, 232.

51. Brevard, *Woman I Was Not Born to Be*, 28–30.

52. Benjamin, "Reminiscences."

53. Benjamin and Masters, *Prostitution and Morality*, 6.

54. Benjamin and Masters, *Prostitution and Morality*, 166–68.

55. Benjamin and Masters, *Prostitution and Morality*, 8.

56. Benjamin and Masters, *Prostitution and Morality*, 472–74.

57. Ihlenfeld, "Memorial for Harry Benjamin," 27.

58. Benjamin and Masters, *Prostitution and Morality*, 6.

Chapter 11

1. Meyerowitz, *How Sex Changed*, 230; Stryker, *Transgender History*, 98; Elliot Blackstone, interview by Susan Stryker, 6 November 1996, Gay and Lesbian Historical Society, www.glbthistory.org.

2. Benjamin, *Transsexual Phenomenon*, 47.

3. Benjamin, *Transsexual Phenomenon*, 91.

4. HB to Peter Benjamin, 6 December 1966, box 3 Correspondence, folder Peter Benjamin, HBC.

5. Stryker, *Transgender History*, 96.

6. Meyerowitz, *How Sex Changed*, 215.

7. Meyerowitz, *How Sex Changed*, 222.

8. Ihlenfeld, "Memorial for Harry Benjamin."

9. Meyerowitz, *How Sex Changed*, 218–26.

10. Ihlenfeld, "Memorial for Harry Benjamin."

11. Meyerowitz, *How Sex Changed*, 226.

12. Ihlenfeld, "Memorial for Harry Benjamin"; Blackstone interview by Stryker; Stryker, *Transgender History*, 98.

13. Suzan Cooke, interview by Susan Stryker and Joanne Meyerowitz, 10 January 1998, Gay and Lesbian Historical Society, www.glbthistory.org; Stryker, *Transgender History*, 79–113.

14. Meyerowitz, *How Sex Changed*, 153–55, 171.

15. Hacking, "Looping Effects of Human Kinds."

16. Skidmore, *True Sex*.

17. Bakker et al., *Others of My Kind*.

18. Li, "Marketing Menopause"; Watkins, *Estrogen Elixir*; Houck, *Hot and Bothered*; L. Marks, *Sexual Chemistry*.

19. Medeiros, *Heightened Expectations*; Tomes, *Remaking the American Patient*.

20. Devor, "Reed Erickson and the Erickson Educational Foundation."

21. Meyerowitz, *How Sex Changed*, 214–16.

22. Devor and Matte, "Building a Better World for Transpeople."

23. Devor and Matte, "Building a Better World for Transpeople."

24. HB to Wardell Pomeroy, 23 July 1968, *LGBT Thought and Culture* database, HBC.

25. Ihlenfeld, "Memorial for Harry Benjamin."

26. Charles Ihlenfeld, interviews by author, 13 November 2017, 20 November 2017, 1 July 2018, via video conference.

27. Ihlenfeld, "Memorial for Harry Benjamin"; Ihlenfeld interviews by author.

28. Person, *Sexual Century*.

29. Person, *Sexual Century*.

30. Christine Wheeler, interview by author, 11 September 2013, New York; Ihlenfeld, "Memorial for Harry Benjamin."

31. Ihlenfeld, "Memorial for Harry Benjamin," 7.

32. Ihlenfeld, "Memorial for Harry Benjamin."

33. Ihlenfeld, "Memorial for Harry Benjamin"; Ihlenfeld interviews by author.

34. HB to Hans Burchard, 17 September 1971, box 3 Correspondence, folder Burchard, HBC.

35. Person, *Sexual Century*, 361.

36. Person, *Sexual Century*, 359n6.

37. Ihlenfeld, "Memorial for Harry Benjamin."

38. *The Rocky Horror Picture Show*, "Sweet Transvestite."

39. Ihlenfeld, "Memorial for Harry Benjamin"; Meyerowitz, *How Sex Changed*, 277.

40. Jan Morris, *Conundrum*, 58.

41. Morris, *Conundrum*, 61–65.

42. Morris, *Conundrum*, 123.

43. Morris, *Conundrum*, 124.

44. Morris, *Conundrum*, 96–97.

45. Bakker et al., *Others of My Kind*. This excellent collection of essays focuses on trans people as the agents of change, rather than on the scientists and doctors who studied them. It gathers the histories and images created by trans individuals to create communities and help shape transgender identity.

46. Buckley, "Transsexual Operation," 113.

47. Buckley, "Transsexual Operation," 111, 113–14.

48. HB to Greta Benjamin, 4 March 1972, box 3 Correspondence, folder Greta Benjamin, HBC.

49. Benjamin, *Transsexual Phenomenon*, dedication page.

50. HB to Greta Benjamin, 26 September 1965, box 3 Correspondence, folder Greta Benjamin, HBC.

51. HB to Greta Benjamin, 18 May 1972, box 3 Correspondence, folder Greta Benjamin, HBC.

52. Charles Ihlenfeld, "I Remember Harry," notes, Series II, folder 8, Charles L. Ihlenfeld Collection, Kinsey Institute for Research in Sex, Gender, and Reproduction, Indiana University, Bloomington.

53. Buckley, "Transsexuality Expert, 90, Recalls 'Maverick' Career."

54. Ihlenfeld, "I Remember Harry."

55. Person, *Sexual Century*, 348; Ethel Spector Person, "Manuscript Interview Notes, Harry Benjamin Reference Materials and Drafts, 1948–1986," box 33, folder 6, Ethel Spector Person Papers, Archives and Special Collections, Columbia University Health Sciences Library, New York.

56. Goethe, *Faust*, part 2, act 5.

57. "Dr. Alvarez," *Tuscan Daily Citizen*, 23 April 1971.

58. Walter C. Alvarez to HB, 7 May 1974, box 3 Correspondence, folder Alvarez, HBC.

Chapter 12

1. Ihlenfeld, "Memorial for Harry Benjamin," 23.

2. Ihlenfeld, "Memorial for Harry Benjamin," 23.

3. Ihlenfeld, "Memorial for Harry Benjamin," 5.

4. Ihlenfeld, "Memorial for Harry Benjamin," 8.

5. HB to Anthony A. Bliss, undated, box 6 Correspondence, folder Metropolitan Opera, HBC.

6. HB to Walter Benjar, 8 April 1978, box 3 Correspondence, folder Walter Benjar, HBC.

7. HB to Walter Benjar, 13 August 1979 and 3 September 1979, box 3 Correspondence, folder Walter Benjar, HBC.

8. Leider, *California's Daughter*, 294, 306–7.

9. Ihlenfeld, "Memorial for Harry Benjamin"; Christine Wheeler, interview by author, 11 September 2013, New York.

10. Ihlenfeld, "Memorial for Harry Benjamin," 16.

11. Ihlenfeld, "Memorial for Harry Benjamin," 5.

12. Ihlenfeld, "Memorial for Harry Benjamin."

13. Ihlenfeld, "Memorial for Harry Benjamin," 29.

14. Haeberle, "Transatlantic Commuter."

15. Ihlenfeld, "Memorial for Harry Benjamin."

16. Stryker, *Transgender History*, 139.

17. Stryker, *Transgender History*, 140; Ihlenfeld, "Memorial for Harry Benjamin."

18. Wheeler interview by author.

19. Ihlenfeld, "Harry Benjamin and Psychiatrists."

20. Richards and Ames, *Second Serve*; Richards and Ames, *No Way Renée*.

21. Green and Fleming, "Transsexual Surgery Follow-Up"; Pfäfflin, "Regrets after Sex Reassignment Surgery."

22. Haeberle, "Transatlantic Commuter."

23. Haeberle, "Transatlantic Commuter."

24. Ihlenfeld, "Memorial for Harry Benjamin," 5, 30.

25. Ihlenfeld, "Memorial for Harry Benjamin," 9.

26. Ihlenfeld, "Memorial for Harry Benjamin." A documentary, *Harry Benjamin, M.D. 1885–1986*, including excerpts from this memorial can be found online at www.sexsmartfilms.com/premium /film/763/HARRY+BENJAMIN%2C+M.D.

27. Charles Ihlenfeld, "I Remember Harry," notes, Series II, folder 8, Charles L. Ihlenfeld Collection, Kinsey Institute for Research in Sex, Gender, and Reproduction, Indiana University, Bloomington.

Epilogue

1. Lester, *Trans like Me*.

2. Stryker, *Transgender History*.

3. *Disclosure* documentary.

4. Susan Stryker, "Dr. Harry Benjamin (1885–1986)," *GLBTQ Encyclopedia*, 2003, www.glbtq.com.

5. Charles Ihlenfeld, interviews by author, 13 November 2017, 20 November 2017, 1 July 2018, via video conference.

6. Jennifer Finney Boylan, "The Modern Trans Memoir Comes of Age," *New York Times*, 13 June 2017.

7. Lester, *Trans like Me*, 11.

8. Person, *Sexual Century*, 360–61.

9. Person, *Sexual Century*, 366.

10. Haeberle, "Transatlantic Commuter."

11. Bauer, *Hirschfeld Archives*, 4; Dose, *Magnus Hirschfeld*, 79–95.

12. Sengoopta, *Most Secret Quintessence of Life*; Logan, *Hormones, Heredity, and Race*.

13. Gliboff, "'Protoplasm . . . Is Soft Wax in Our Hands.'"

14. Müller, *Vivarium*.

15. Aleshia Brevard Crenshaw, interview by Susan Stryker, 2 August 1997, Gay and Lesbian Historical Society, www.glbthistory.org.

16. Brevard, *Woman I Was Not Born to Be*, 62.

17. Crenshaw interview by Stryker.

18. Crenshaw interview by Stryker.

19. Brevard, *Woman I Was Not Born to Be*, 241–44.

20. Brevard, *Woman I Was Not Born to Be*, 244.

21. Jennifer Finney Boylan, "Bring Moral Imagination Back in Style," *New York Times*, 22 July 2016.

22. Jan Morris, *Conundrum*, 189.

23. Tom Peterkin, "Sex-Change Author Jan Morris Remarries Wife She Wed as a Man," *The Telegraph*, 3 June 2008.

24. Jan Morris, *Allegorizings*.

25. Garner, "Jan Morris, A Distinctive Guide Who Took Readers around the World"; Lea, "Jan Morris, Historian, Travel Writer and Trans Pioneer, Dies Aged 94."

Bibliography

Ambrose, Kevin. *The Knickerbocker Snowstorm*. Charleston, SC: Arcadia, 2013.

Amin, Kadji. "Glands, Eugenics, and Rejuvenation in Man into Woman: A Biopolitical Genealogy of Transsexuality." *Transgender Studies Quarterly* 5, no. 4 (2018): 589–605.

Anderson, Maija. "From the Archives: Dr. Ira Pauly, Pioneer in Transgender Health Care." *OHSU School of Medicine* (blog), 20 January 2016.

Atherton, Gertrude. *Adventures of a Novelist*. New York: Liveright, 1932.

———. "The Alpine School of Fiction." *Bookman* (New York) 55 (1922): 26–33.

———. *Black Oxen*. Edited by Melanie V. Dawson. Peterborough, ON: Broadview Editions, 2012. First published 1923 by Boni and Liveright (New York).

Bakker, Alex, Rainer Herrn, Michael Thomas Taylor, and Annette F. Timm. *Others of My Kind: Transatlantic Transgender Histories*. Calgary, AB: University of Calgary Press, 2020.

Bauer, Heike. *The Hirschfeld Archives: Violence, Death, and Modern Queer Culture*. Philadelphia: Temple University Press, 2017.

Beach, Frank A. *Hormones and Behavior: A Survey of Interrelationships between Endocrine Secretions and Patterns of Overt Response*. New York: P. B. Hoeber, 1948.

Benjamin, Harry. "Anwendung des Antiforminverfahrens für den Tuberkelbazillennachweis." Dr. med. Diss. Eberhard-Karls-Universität, Tübingen, 1911.

———. "The Control of Old Age; with Special Reference to Gonadal Therapy." *American Medicine* 22 (June 1927): 337–54.

———. "Eugen Steinach, 1861–1944: A Life of Research." *Scientific Monthly* 61 (December 1945): 427–42.

———. "For the Sake of Morality." *Medical Journal and Record*, 15 April 1931.

———. "A Humane Necessity." *The Nation*, 28 January 1950, 79–80.

———. Introduction to *Christine Jorgensen: A Personal Autobiography*, by Christine Jorgensen, vii–viii. New York: Paul S. Eriksson, 1967.

———. Introduction to *Rejuvenation and the Prolongation of Human Efficiency. Experiences with the Steinach-Operation on Man and Animals*, by Paul Kammerer, 17–20. New York: Boni and Liveright, 1923.

———. "The Male Hormone: A Summary of Laboratory and Clinical Experiences." Presented at the Sacramento County Medical Society, Sacramento, CA, 21 November 1933.

———. "New Clinical Aspects of the Steinach Operation." *Medical Journal and Record*, 21 November 1925.

———. "Newer Aspects of the Transsexual Phenomenon." *Journal of Sex Research* 5, no. 2 (May 1969): 138.

———. "Prostitution Re-assessed." *International Journal of Sexology* 4 (1951): 154–60.

———. "Reminiscences." *Journal of Sex Research* 6, no. 1 (February 1970): 3–9.

———. "The Steinach Method as Applied to Women: Preliminary Report." *New York Medical Journal and Medical Record* 18 (1923): 750–3.

———. *The Transsexual Phenomenon*. New York: Julian Press, 1966.

———. "Transvestism and Transsexualism." *International Journal of Sexology* 7, no. 1 (1953): 12–14.

Benjamin, Harry, and Albert Ellis. "An Objective Examination of Prostitution." *International Journal of Sexology* 8, no. 2 (1954): 100–105.

Benjamin, Harry, and R. E. L. Masters. *Prostitution and Morality: A Definitive Report on the Prostitute in Contemporary Society and an Analysis of the Causes and Effects of the Suppression of Prostitution*. New York: Julian Press, 1964.

Berghahn, V. R. Review of *Gay Berlin*, by Robert Beachy. *New York Times*, 31 October 2014, Sunday Book Review.

Berman, Louis. *The Glands Regulating Personality: A Study of the Glands of Internal Secretion in Relation to the Types of Human Nature*. New York: Macmillan, 1921.

Black Oxen. Directed by Frank Lloyd. First National Pictures, 1923.

Bliss, Michael. *The Discovery of Insulin*. Toronto: McClelland and Stewart, 1982.

Bonner, Thomas Neville. *Becoming a Physician: Medical Education in Britain, France, Germany, and the United States, 1750–1945*. Baltimore, MD: Johns Hopkins University Press, 1995.

———. "German Doctors in America—1887–1914: Their Views and Impressions of American Life and Medicine." *Journal of the History of Medicine and Allied Sciences* 14, no. 1 (1959): 1–17.

Borell, Merriley. "Brown-Séquard's Organotherapy and Its Appearance in America at the End of the Nineteenth Century." *Bulletin of the History of Medicine* 50 (1976): 309–20.

———. "Organotherapy and the Emergence of Reproductive Endocrinology." *Journal of the History of Biology* 18, no. 1 (1985): 1–30.

———. "Setting the Standards for a New Science: Edward Schäfer and Endocrinology." *Medical History* 22 (1978): 282–90.

Brevard, Aleshia. *The Woman I Was Not Born to Be: A Transsexual Journey*. Philadelphia: Temple University Press, 2001.

Buckley, Tom. "Transsexuality Expert, 90, Recalls 'Maverick' Career." *New York Times*, 11 January 1975.

———. "The Transsexual Operation." *Esquire*, 1 April 1967.

Cassedy, Steven. *Connected: How Trains, Genes, Pineapples, Piano Keys, and a Few Disasters Transformed Americans at the Dawn of the Twentieth Century*. Stanford: Stanford University Press, 2014.

Caughie, Pamela L., Emily Datskou, Sabine Meyer, Rebecca J. Parker, and Nikolaus Wasmoen, eds. Lili Elbe Digital Archive. 5 October 1922. www.lilielbe.org.

Churchwell, Sarah. *Careless People: Murder, Mayhem, and the Invention of "The Great Gatsby."* London: Virago, 2013.

Coen, Deborah R. "Living Precisely in Fin-de-Siècle Vienna." *Journal of the History of Biology* 39, no. 3 (2006): 493–523.

Conefrey, Mick. *Everest 1953: The Epic Story of the First Ascent.* Seattle: Mountaineers Books, 2014.

Cushing, Harvey. *The Life of Sir William Osler.* Oxford: Clarendon Press, 1925.

Dana, Charles L. "Correspondence: The Late Dr. Joseph Fraenkel." *Medical Record* 97, no. 23 (June 1920): 966.

Dardis, Tom. *Firebrand: The Life of Horace Liveright, the Man Who Changed American Publishing.* New York: Random House, 1995.

Davis, Rebecca L. "'Not Marriage at All, but Simple Harlotry': The Companionate Marriage Controversy." *Journal of American History* 94, no. 4 (March 2008): 1137–63.

Dawson, Melanie V. Introduction to *Black Oxen*, by Gertrude Atherton, 9–32. New York: Broadview Editions, 2012.

De Kruif, Paul. "An Intimate Glimpse of a Great American Novel in the Making." *Designer and the Woman's Magazine*, June 1924.

———. *The Male Hormone.* New York: Garden City Publishing, 1945.

Devor, Aaron. "Reed Erickson and the Erickson Educational Foundation." *Aaron H. Devor* (blog), 20 May 2016. https://onlineacademiccommunity.uvic.ca/ahdevor/publications/erickson/.

Devor, Aaron, and Nicolas Matte. "Building a Better World for Transpeople: Reed Erickson and the Erickson Educational Foundation." *International Journal of Transgenderism* 10, no. 1 (2007): 47–68.

Disclosure. Directed by Sam Feder. Documentary. Netflix, 2020.

Doctor, Richard F. *Becoming a Woman: A Biography of Christine Jorgensen.* New York: Haworth Press, 2008.

Dose, Ralf. *Magnus Hirschfeld: The Origins of the Gay Liberation Movement.* Translated by Edward H. Willis. New York: Monthly Review Press, 2014.

———. "The World League for Sexual Reform: Some Possible Approaches." *Journal of the History of Sexuality* 12, no. 1 (January 2003): 1–15.

Doyle, Arthur Conan. "The Adventure of the Creeping Man." *Strand Magazine*, March 1923.

Dreger, Alice Domurat. "'Ambiguous Sex'—or Ambivalent Medicine? Ethical Problems in the Treatment of Intersexuality." *Hastings Center Report* 28, no. 3 (June 1998): 24–35.

Ekins, Richard. "Science, Politics and Clinical Intervention: Harry Benjamin, Transsexualism and the Problem of Heteronormativity." *Sexualities*, no. 3 (2005): 306–28.

Ellis, Albert. "Prostitution Re-assessed." *International Journal of Sexology* 5 (1951): 41–42.

Emmerson, Charles. *1913: In Search of the World before the Great War.* New York: Public Affairs, 2013.

"The Endocrine Glands." *Fortune*, November 1933.

Epstein, Randi Hutter. *Aroused: The History of Hormones and How They Control Just About Everything.* New York: W. W. Norton, 2018.

Evans, Wainwright. "Rejuvenation." *Esquire*, December 1935.

Feder, Stuart. *Gustav Mahler: A Life in Crisis.* New Haven, CT: Yale University Press, 2004.

Fishbein, Morris. *The Medical Follies; An Analysis of the Foibles of Some Healing Cults: Including Osteopathy, Homeopathy, Chiropractic, and the Electronic Reactions of Abrams, with Essays on the Antivivisectionists, Health Legislation, Physical Culture, Birth Control, and Rejuvenation.* New York: Boni and Liveright, 1925.

———. *The New Medical Follies: An Encyclopedia of Cultism and Quackery in These United States, with Essays on the Cult of Beauty, the Craze for Reduction, Rejuvenation, Eclecticism, Bread and Dietary Fads, Physical Therapy, and a Forecast as to the Physician of the Future.* New York: Boni and Liveright, 1927.

Garner, Dwight. "Jan Morris, a Distinctive Guide Who Took Readers around the World." *New York Times*, 21 November 2020.

Geroulanos, Stefanos, and Todd Meyers. *The Human Body in the Age of Catastrophe: Brittleness, Integration, Science, and the Great War*. Chicago: University of Chicago Press, 2018.

Gilmore, Walker. *Horace Liveright, Publisher of the Twenties*. New York: David Lewis, 1970.

Gliboff, Sandor. "'Protoplasm . . . Is Soft Wax in Our Hands': Paul Kammerer and the Art of Biological Transformation." *Endeavour* 29, no. 4 (December 2005): 162–67.

Goethe, Johann Wolfgang. *Faust: A Tragedy*. Translated by Walter Arndt. New York: Norton Critical Editions, 1998.

Green, Richard, and Davis Fleming. "Transsexual Surgery Follow-Up: Status in the 1990s." *Annual Review of Sex Research* 1, no. 1 (1990): 163–74.

Griminger, Paul. "Casimir Funk: A Biographical Sketch (1884–1967)." *Journal of Nutrition* 102, no. 9 (September 1972): 1105–13.

Gumpert, Martin. "A False Mercy." *The Nation*, 28 January 1950, 80.

Hacking, Ian. "The Looping Effects of Human Kinds." In *Causal Cognition*, edited by Dan Sperber, David Premack, and Ann Premack, 351–94. Oxford: Clarendon Press, 1995.

Haeberle, Erwin J. "A Movement of Inverts: An Early Plan for a Homosexual Organization in the United States." *Journal of Homosexuality* 10, nos. 1–2 (2008): 127–33.

———. "The Transatlantic Commuter: An Interview with Harry Benjamin (b. January 12, 1885) on the Occasion of His 100th Birthday." *Sexualmedizin* 14, no. 1 (1985): 44–47. English translation. Archive for Sexology. 20 April 2012. www.sexarchive.info/GESUND/ARCHIV/TRANS_B5.HTM.

Hansson, Nils, Matthis Krischel, Per Södersten, Friedrich H. Moll, and Heiner Fangerau. "'He Gave Us the Cornerstone of Sexual Medicine': A Nobel Plan but No Nobel Prize for Eugen Steinach." *Urologia Internationalis* 104 (2020): 501–9.

Harriman, Margaret Case. "Profile—Elizabeth Arden: Glamour, Inc." *New Yorker*, 6 April 1935.

Harrow, Benjamin. *Casimir Funk, Pioneer in Vitamins and Hormones*. New York: Dodd, Mead, 1955.

———. *Glands in Health and Disease*. New York: E. P. Dutton, 1922.

Henry, George W. *Sex Variants: A Study of Homosexual Patterns*. New York: P. B. Hoeber, 1948.

Hill, Darryl B. "Dear Doctor Benjamin: Letters from Transsexual Youth (1963–1976)." *International Journal of Transgenderism* 10, nos. 3–4 (n.d.): 149–70.

Hilmes, Oliver. *Malevolent Muse: The Life of Alma Mahler*. Boston: Northeastern University Press, 2015.

Houck, Judith A. *Hot and Bothered: Women, Medicine, and Menopause in Modern America*. Cambridge, MA: Harvard University Press, 2008.

Hüntelmann, Axel C. "Das Friedrich Franz Friedmannsche Tuberkulosemittel. Schildkröten, Tuberkelbazillen, Heil- und Schutzstoffe und andere prekäre Stoffe." In *Precarious Matters / Prekäre Stoffe: The History of Dangerous and Endangered Substances in the 19th and 20th Centuries*, edited by Viola Balz, Alexander v. Schwerin, and Heiko Stoff, 153–67. Berlin: Max-Planck-Institut für Wissenschaftsgeschichte, 2008.

Ihlenfeld, Charles. "Harry Benjamin and Psychiatrists." *Journal of Gay and Lesbian Psychotherapy* 8, no. 1/2 (2004): 147–52.

———. "Memorial for Harry Benjamin." *Archives of Sexual Behavior* 17, no. 1 (1988): 2–31.

Isherwood, Christopher. *Christopher and His Kind*. London: Vintage, 1976.

———. *Goodbye to Berlin*. New York: New Directions, 1939.

———. *Mr. Norris Changes Trains*. New York: New Directions, 1935.

"Jahres-Bericht über das Dorotheenstädtische Realgymnasium zu Berlin: Für das Schuljahr . . . Schulprogramme—Digital Collections," 1883–1924. http://digital.ub.uni-duesseldorf.de/ulbdsp /periodical/titleinfo/4408772?query=dorotheenstadt.

Jorgensen, Christine. *Christine Jorgensen: A Personal Autobiography*. New York: Paul S. Eriksson, 1967.

Kammerer, Paul. *The Inheritance of Acquired Characteristics*. New York: Boni and Liveright, 1924.

———. *Rejuvenation and the Prolongation of Human Efficiency: Experiences with the Steinach-Operation on Man and Animals*. New York: Boni and Liveright, 1923.

Kaplan, D. M. "An Endocrine Interpretation of the Dental Apparatus." *Endocrinology* 1 (April 1917): 208–21.

Kevles, Daniel. *In the Name of Eugenics: Genetics and the Uses of Human Heredity*. Cambridge, MA: Harvard University Press, 1995.

Kinsey, Alfred C., Wardell B. Pomeroy, and Clyde E. Martin. *Sexual Behavior in the Human Male*. Philadelphia: W. B. Saunders, 1948.

Kinsey, Alfred C., Wardell B. Pomeroy, Clyde E. Martin, and Paul H. Gebhard. *Sexual Behavior in the Human Female*. Philadelphia: W. B. Saunders, 1953.

Kirschbaum, Erik. *The Eradication of German Culture in the United States, 1917–1918*. Stuttgart: Hans-Dieter Heinz Akademischer Verlag, 1986.

———. "Whatever Happened to German America?" *New York Times*, 23 September 2015. www .nytimes.com/2015/09/23/opinion/whatever-happened-to-german-america.html.

Königliches Wilhelms-Gymnasium in Berlin. *Jahresbericht über das Schuljahr Ostern . . . bis Ostern*. Berlin, 1865, 1886–87, 1887–88. http://digital.ub.uni-duesseldorf.de/ulbdsp/periodical/titleinfo /3995666?query=wilhelms%20gymnasium%20oberlin.

Krementsov, Nikolai. "Hormones and the Bolsheviks: From Organotherapy to Experimental Endo-crinology, 1918–1929." *ISIS* 99 (2008): 486–518.

———. *Revolutionary Experiments: The Quest for Immortality in Bolshevik Science and Fiction*. Oxford: Oxford University Press, 2013.

Lea, Richard. "Jan Morris, Historian, Travel Writer and Trans Pioneer, Dies Aged 94." *The Guardian*, 20 November 2020.

Leider, Emily. *California's Daughter: Gertrude Atherton and Her Times*. Stanford: Stanford University Press, 1991.

Lester, CN. *Trans Like Me: Conversations for All of Us*. New York: Seal Press, 2018.

Lewis, Abram J. "Trans History in a Moment of Danger: Organizing within and beyond 'Visibility' in the 1970s." In *Trap Door: Trans Cultural Production and the Politics of Visibility*, edited by Reina Gossett, Eric A. Stanley, and Johanna Burton, 57–89. Cambridge, MA: MIT Press, 2017.

Li, Alison. *J. B. Collip and the Development of Medical Research in Canada*. Montreal: McGill-Queens University Press, 2003.

———. "Marketing Menopause: Science and the Public Relations of Premarin." In *Women, Health and Nation: Canada and the United States since 1945*, edited by Gina Feldberg, Molly Ladd-Taylor, Alison Li, and Kathryn McPherson, 101–22. Montreal: McGill-Queens University Press, 2003.

———. "Wondrous Transformations: Endocrinology After Insulin." In *Essays in Honour of Michael Bliss*, edited by E. A. Heaman, Alison Li, and Shelley McKellar, 351–77. Toronto: University of Toronto Press, 2008.

Liebenau, Jonathan. *Medical Science and Medical Industry: The Formation of the American Pharmaceutical Industry*. London: Macmillan, 1987.

Lisser, Hans. "The First Forty Years (1917–1957)." *Endocrinology* 80 (January 1967): 5–28.

Logan, Cheryl A. *Hormones, Heredity, and Race: Spectacular Failure in Interwar Vienna*. New Brunswick, NJ: Rutgers University Press, 2013.

London, Pete. *Cornwall in the First World War*. London: Truran, 2013.

Marhoefer, Laurie. *Racism and the Making of Gay Rights: A Sexologist, His Student, and the Empire of
Queer Love*. Toronto: University of Toronto Press, 2022.

———. *Sex and the Weimar Republic: German Homosexual Emancipation and the Rise of the Nazis*.
Toronto: University of Toronto Press, 2015.

Marks, Harry. "Cortisone, 1949: A Year in the Political Life of a Drug." *Bulletin of the History of
Medicine* 66 (1992): 419–39.

———. *The Progress of Experiment: Science and Therapeutic Reform in the United States, 1900–1990*.
Cambridge: Cambridge University Press, 1997.

Marks, Lara V. *Sexual Chemistry: A History of the Contraceptive Pill*. New Haven, CT: Yale University
Press, 2001.

Matte, Nicholas. "Historicizing Liberal American Transnormativities: Medicine, Media, Activism,
1960–1990." PhD diss., University of Toronto, 2014.

———. "Putting Patients First: Harry Benjamin and the Development of Transgender Medicine in
the Twentieth Century." MA thesis, University of Victoria, 2001.

Maugham, W. Somerset. *The Razor's Edge*. 1st International Edition. New York: Vintage International,
2003. First published in 1944 by Doubleday, Doran & Company (New York). Page references are to
the 2003 edition.

Mazón, Patricia M. *Gender and the Modern Research University: The Admission of Women to German
Higher Education, 1865–1914*. Stanford: Stanford University Press, 2003.

McDowell, Baynon, William S. Green, and Joseph D. Zuckerman. *Hospital for Joint Diseases, 1905–
2005: One Hundred Years of Excellence*, 17 May 2018. https://documents.pub/document/hospital
-for-joint-diseases-1905-2005-new-york-hospital-for-joint-diseases.html?page=1.

McLaren, Angus. *Reproduction by Design: Sex, Robots, Trees, and Test-Tube Babies in Interwar Britain*.
Chicago: University of Chicago Press, 2012.

Medeiros, Aimee. *Heightened Expectations: The Rise of the Human Growth Hormone Industry in America*. Tuscaloosa: University of Alabama Press, 2016.

Medvei, Victor Cornelius. *A History of Endocrinology*. Lancaster, UK: MTP Press, 1982.

Meyerowitz, Joanne. *How Sex Changed: A History of Transsexuality in the United States*. Cambridge,
MA: Harvard University Press, 2002.

Morris, James. *Coronation Everest*. London: Faber and Faber, 1958.

Morris, Jan. *Allegorizings*. New York: Liveright, 2021.

———. *Conundrum*. New York: Harcourt Brace Jovanovich, 1974.

Müller, Gerd B., ed. *Vivarium: Experimental, Quantitative, and Theoretical Biology at Vienna's
Biologische Versuchanstalt*. The Vienna Series in Theoretical Biology. Cambridge, MA: MIT Press,
2017.

Murray, George R. "Note on the Treatment of Myxoedema by Hypodermic Injections of an Extract
of the Thyroid Gland of a Sheep." *British Medical Association Journal*, 10 October 1891, 796–97.

Murray, John F., Dean E. Schraufnagel, and Philip C. Hopewell. "Treatment of Tuberculosis: A Historical Perspective." *Annals of the American Thoracic Society* 12, no. 12 (December 2015): 1750–59.

Nordlund, Christer. "Endocrinology and Expectations in 1930s America: Louis Berman's Ideas on New Creations in Human Beings." *British Journal for the History of Science* 40, no. 1 (2007): 83–104.

———. *Hormones of Life: Endocrinology, the Pharmaceutical Industry, and the Dream of a Remedy for Sterility, 1930 to 1970.* Sagamore Beach, MA: Science History Publications, 2011.

Oudshoorn, Nelly. *Beyond the Natural Body: An Archeology of Sex Hormones.* London: Routledge, 1994.

Parkes, A. S. "Prospect and Retrospect in the Physiology of Reproduction." *British Medical Journal* 2 (1962): 71–75.

Person, Ethel Spector. *The Sexual Century.* New Haven, CT: Yale University Press, 1999.

Pettit, Michael. "Becoming Glandular: Endocrinology, Mass Culture, and Experimental Lives in the Interwar Age." *American Historical Review* 118, no. 4 (2013): 1052–76.

Pfäfflin, Friedemann. "Regrets after Sex Reassignment Surgery." *Journal of Psychology and Human Sexuality* 5, no. 4 (1993): 69–85.

Platt, Avies. "A Lazarus beside Me." *London Review of Books* 37, no. 16 (27 August 2015): 29–32.

Price, Dorothy. *Carl Richard Moore, 1892–1955.* Washington, DC: National Academy of Sciences, 1974.

Rall, Jack A. "The XIIIth International Physiological Congress in Boston in 1929: American Physiology Comes of Age." *Advances in Physiology Education* 40 (2016): 5–16.

Rasmussen, Nicolas. "Steroids in Arms: Science, Government, Industry, and the Hormones of the Adrenal Cortex in the United States, 1930–1950." *Medical History* 46 (2002): 299–324.

Reay, Barry. *Trans America: A Counter-History.* Cambridge, UK: Polity, 2020.

———. "The Transsexual Phenomenon: A Counter-History." *Journal of Social History* 47, no. 4 (Summer 2014): 1042–70.

Richards, Renée, and John Ames. *No Way Renée: The Second Half of My Notorious Life.* New York: Simon and Schuster, 2007.

———. *Second Serve: The Renée Richards Story.* New York: Stein and Day, 1983.

Richie, Alexandra. *Faust's Metropolis: A History of Berlin.* New York: Carroll and Graf, 1998.

Rogers, Naomi. *An Alternative Path: The Making and Remaking of Hahnemann Medical College and Hospital in Philadelphia.* New Brunswick, NJ: Rutgers University Press, 1998.

Ronquillo, Emilio. "Former UCLA Football Player Ira Pauly Reminisces on Game." *Daily Bruin,* 26 August 2013. http://dailybruin.com/2013/08/26/former-ucla-football-player-ira-pauly-reminisces-on-game/.

Rosenberg, Charles E. "Martin Arrowsmith: The Scientist as Hero." *American Quarterly* 15, no. 4 (1963): 447–58.

Sayers, Dorothy L. "The Incredible Elopement of Lord Peter Wimsey." In *Hangman's Holiday,* 33–67. London: Hodder and Stoughton, 2016.

———. *The Unpleasantness at the Bellona Club.* New York: Avon, 1963.

Schaefer, Leah Cahan, and Connie Christine Wheeler. "Harry Benjamin's First Ten Cases (1938–1953): A Clinical Historical Note." *Archives of Sexual Behavior* 24, no. 1 (1995): 73–93.

Schnurr, Eva-Maria. "Berlin's Turn of the Century Growing Pains." *Spiegel Online,* 22 November 2012. www.spiegel.de/international/germany/the-late-19th-century-saw-the-birth-of-modern-berlin-a-866321.html.

Schoen, Mark, dir. *Harry Benjamin, M.D. 1885–1986.* SexSmartFilms, 2007, 13 min. www.sexsmartfilms.com/premium/film/763/HARRY+BENJAMIN%2C+M.

Sengoopta, Chandak. "Glandular Politics: Experimental Biology, Clinical Medicine, and Homosexual Emancipation in Fin-de-Siècle Central Europe." *ISIS* 89 (1998): 445–73.

———. *The Most Secret Quintessence of Life: Sex, Glands, and Hormones, 1850–1950*. Chicago: University of Chicago Press, 2006.

———. "Tales from the Vienna Labs: The Eugen Steinach–Harry Benjamin Correspondence." *Favourite Edition: Newsletter of the Friends of the Rare Book Room, New York Academy of Medicine*, Spring 2000.

"Sinclair Lewis at Work." *Designer and the Woman's Magazine*, June 1924.

Sharman, Jim, dir. *The Rocky Horror Picture Show*. Los Angeles: 20th Century Fox, 1975. 100 minutes.

Skidmore, Emily. *True Sex: The Lives of Trans Men at the Turn of the 20th Century*. New York: New York University Press, 2017.

Smith, Stephen. "A Half Century of Public Health." *American Journal of Public Health* 12, no. 1 (1 January 1922): 3–6.

Stokes, Monica. "A Note from the Library: Max Thorek and Testicular Transplantation." *International Museum of Surgical Science* (blog), 18 May 2017. https://imss.org/2017/05/18/a-note-from-the-library-max-thorek-and-testicular-transplantation/.

Stryker, Susan. *Transgender History: The Roots of Today's Revolution*. 2nd ed. New York: Seal, 2008.

Swann, John P. *Academic Scientists and the Pharmaceutical Industry: Cooperative Research in Twentieth Century America*. Baltimore, MD: Johns Hopkins University Press, 1988.

Talmey, B. S. "Transvestism." *New York Medical Journal* 99 (1914): 362–68.

"The Thirteenth International Physiological Congress at Boston." *British Medical Journal* 2 (1929): 595–97.

Thomas, Robert McG., Jr. "Dr. Morris Fishbein Dead at 87; Former Editor of A.M.A. Journal." *New York Times*, 28 September 1976.

Thorne, Van Buren, MD. "Dr. Steinach and Rejuvenation." *New York Times*, 26 June 1921.

Timm, Annette F. "'I Am So Grateful to All You Men of Medicine': Trans Circles of Knowledge and Intimacy." In *Others of My Kind: Transatlantic Transgender Histories*, by Alex Bakker, Rainer Herrn, Michael Thomas Taylor, and Annette F. Timm, 71–131. Calgary: University of Calgary Press, 2020.

Timm, Annette F., and Michael Thomas Taylor. "Historicizing Transgender Terminology." In *Others of My Kind: Transatlantic Transgender Histories*, by Alex Bakker, Rainer Herrn, Michael Thomas Taylor, and Annette F. Timm, 251–65. Calgary: University of Calgary Press, 2020.

Tomes, Nancy. *Remaking the American Patient: How Madison Avenue and Modern Medicine Turned Patients into Consumers*. Chapel Hill: University of North Carolina Press, 2016.

Tracy, Sarah. "George Draper and American Constitutional Medicine, 1916–1946." *Bulletin of the History of Medicine* 66 (1992): 53–89.

Urban, William. "Buffalo Bill in Florence." *Illinois Quarterly* 40, no. 3 (1978): 5–21. http://department.monm.edu/history/urban/wyatt_earp/Buffalo_Bill_in_Florence.htm.

Van Vechten, Carl. "A Lady Who Defies Time." *The Nation*, 14 February 1923.

Velocci, Beans. "Standards of Care: Uncertainty and Risk in Harry Benjamin's Transsexual Classifications." *Transgender Studies Quarterly* 8, no. 4 (2021): 462–80.

Walsh, Patrick M. "Glands on the Market: Doctors, Drug Companies, and the Making of American Endocrinology, 1889–1919." PhD diss., University of Wisconsin-Madison, 2023.

Walsh, Patrick M., and Alison Li. "Remembering Insulin et al." *History of Pharmacy and Pharmaceuticals* 64, no. 1 (January 2022): 104–13.

Warner, John Harley. *The Therapeutic Perspective: Medical Practice, Knowledge, and Identity in America, 1820–1885*. Princeton, NJ: Princeton University Press, 1997.

Watkins, Elizabeth Siegel. *The Estrogen Elixir: A History of Hormone Replacement Therapy in America.* Baltimore, MD: Johns Hopkins University Press, 2007.

Werner, Petra. *Der Heiler: Tuberkuloseforscher Friedrich Franz Friedmann.* Munich: Koehler & Amelang, 2002.

———. "Der 'Wunderheiler' Friedmann." *Gegenworte (Berlin-Brandenburgische Akademie der Wissenschaften)* 2 (1998): 59–63.

"Wild West in Berlin!" *Norddeutsche Allgemeine Zeitung,* 24 July 1890. http://codyarchive.org/texts/wfc.nsp11424.html#en.

Woessmann, Ludger, Sascha O. Becker, and Erik Hornung. "Being the Educational World Leader Helped Prussia Catch Up in the Industrial Revolution." *VoxEU.Org* (blog), 9 May 2010. http://voxeu.org/article/education-helped-prussia-catch-industrial-revolution.

Zabecki, David T., ed. *Germany at War: 400 Years of Military History.* 4 vols. Santa Barbara, CA: ABC-CLIO, 2014.

Index

53–55, 112; homosexuality, 48, 114–15; *Prostitution and Morality*, 176; sexual liberty, commitment to, 114, 121, 176–77; sex work, 121–22, 136, 176–77; Society for the Scientific Study of Sex, 169
—transsexualism: collaboration with transgender colleagues, 146–48, 156–57, 159, 164; compassion and respect in treating, xi, 143, 161, 164–65, 167, 195; defining of, 159–64, 183; early experience with transgender individuals, xi, 47, 112, 114; Erikson Educational Foundation, 168–70, 186; evolving views of, 145–48, 159–64, 181; first transgender patients, 130–32, 141–45, 146–47; hormones in, use of, 131, 143–44, 145, 147, 156, 161, 163–64, 166, 174, 185; gender dysphoria, as term, 160; gerontology work, continuity with, xi, 132; Harry Benjamin Foundation, 170; Harry Benjamin International Gender Dysphoria Association, 187, 199; "His Girls," 175; inquiring into causes of, 148, 175, 178–79, 200; as pioneering expert, xii, 158–59, 164, 178–80, 195; practical and legal support, 144, 146, 157, 172, 174–75, 182; on psychiatry and psychotherapy in, 146, 161, 165–66, 180; rationale in treating, 143–44, 146, 167–68, 179, 201; research on, 170, 174, 186, 187, 198–99, 201; Sexual Orientation Scale, 159–60, 179, 199; sex work and, 176; standards of care, 163; as term, 160; university-based gender-reassignment clinics, 180, 200; worries in treating, 162–63, 165
—travels: arrival in New York, 22–24, 75, 76; attending congresses, 54–55, 115, 168; to Berlin, 44, 53–55, 86, 109, 133; eagerness to travel, 20; outbreak of World War I, 27–30; as transatlantic commuter, 109, 133; in United States, 134–35; to Vienna, 32–43, 86–87, 109, 132
—views: on Austria and Vienna, 37, 43, 73, 133; on biological causation, 148, 160, 200; on the British, 29; on easing suffering, 192; on eugenics, 129; on euthanasia, 122;

on Germany, 133, 136; on moderation, 138–39; on monism, 36, 92; on New York, 23, 154; on psychiatry and psychoanalysis, 87, 200–201; on San Francisco, 136, 141; on scientific medicine, 97–98, 134
—written works: *Prostitution and Morality*, 176–77; *The Transsexual Phenomenon*, 151, 178–80; *The Winter of Our Discontent* (unpublished), 137–39
Benjamin, Julius, 10, 11, 12, 13, 17, 20, 21, 26, 31, 45, 107, 136, 193
Benjamin, Max Louis, 136
Benjamin-Benjar, Walter, 10, 11, 13, 26, 28, 120, 136, 193, 197
Benjamin Seelig, Edith, 2–3, 10, 13, 26, 28, 136, 140, 193, 197
Best, Charles, 89–90
Berlin, xi; anti-Semitism in, 11, 12–13, 47, 140, 220n14; culture of, 2, 9–10, 11–12, 14, 15, 17, 45–46, 90, 109–10, 193; homosexuality, transvestism in, xi, 44–45, 46–47, 50, 109–10, 112–13; interwar inflation in, 84–85; Jews in, 10–11; policing in, 45, 46–47; post–World War II, 140; scientific and industrial developments in, 9–10, 16–17, 20–21; sex-change surgery in, 112–13; sexology in, 44, 46, 52–53, 54–55, 109–10, 112–13, 115, 133, 208
Berman, Louis, 82, 129
Black Oxen (film), x, 67–68, 70
Blackstone, Elliot, 178, 182
Bowman, Karl, 144, 146
Boylan, Jennifer Finney, 207, 212
Brevard, Aleshia, 88, 172–75, 211–12
Brinkley, John, 82
Brown, Edmund G., 144
Brown-Séquard, Charles-Édouard, 40
Buckley, Tom, 192, 193–94
Burou, Georges, 191
Butenandt, Adolf, 95, 112

Carlson, Carroll, 162
Caruso, Enrico, 14, 73, 189
Casablanca, 171, 191, 213
Cauldwell, David, 160